Intraoperative MRI-Guided Neurosurgery

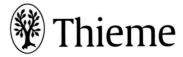

Intraoperative MRI-Guided Neurosurgery

Walter A. Hall, MD, MBA
The Robert B. and Molly G. King Professor of Neurosurgery
Department of Neurosurgery
SUNY Upstate Medical University
Syracuse, New York

Christopher Nimsky, MD, PhD
Professor and Chairman
Department of Neurosurgery
University of Marburg
Marburg, Germany

Charles L. Truwit, MD
Chairman
Department of Radiology
Hennepin County Medical Center
Professor and Margaret and H. O. Peterson Chair in Neuroradiology
University of Minnesota School of Medicine
Minneapolis, Minnesota

Thieme
New York • Stuttgart

Thieme Medical Publishers, Inc.
333 Seventh Ave.
New York, NY 10001

Executive Editor: Kay D. Conerly
Editorial Assistant: Lauren Henry
Editorial Director: Michael Wachinger
Production Editor: Kenneth L. Chumbley, Publication Services
International Production Director: Andreas Schabert
Vice President, International Marketing and Sales: Cornelia Schulze
Chief Financial Officer: James W. Mitos
President: Brian D. Scanlan
Compositor: Thomson Digital
Printer: Replika

Library of Congress Cataloging-in-Publication Data

Intraoperative MR-guided neurosurgery / [edited by] Walter A. Hall, Christopher Nimsky, Charles L. Truwit.
     p. ; cm.
  Includes bibliographical references.
  Summary: "Intraoperative MR-Guided Neurosurgery contains detailed coverage of this state-of-the-art technology from the pioneers who developed it. World-renowned neurosurgeons and neuroradiologists combine their collective wisdom and experience to demonstrate how MR-guided neuronavigation can be used to view real-time images of a patient's brain during surgery to help remove tumors with greater precision. The authors provide step-by-step descriptions of how to perform procedures, including advice based on their clinical results. Readers will learn about the advantages and drawbacks of the various MR imaging systems, clinical indications for MR-guidance, anesthesia considerations, safety concerns related to working in a magnetic environment, and much more"–Provided by publisher.
  ISBN 978-1-60406-305-9 (hardback : alk. paper) 1. Computer-assisted neurosurgery. 2. Magnetic resonance imaging. I. Hall, Walter A., 1957- II. Nimsky, Christopher. III. Truwit, Charles L.
  [DNLM: 1. Neurosurgical Procedures–methods. 2. Brain Neoplasms–surgery. 3. Magnetic Resonance Imaging–methods. 4. Neuronavigation–methods. WL 368 I616 2011]
  RD593.5.I58 2011
  617.4'807548—dc22
                    2010017471

Important note: Medical knowledge is ever-changing. As new research and clinical experience broaden our knowledge, changes in treatment and drug therapy may be required. The authors and editors of the material herein have consulted sources believed to be reliable in their efforts to provide information that is complete and in accord with the standards accepted at the time of publication. However, in view of the possibility of human error by the authors, editors, or publisher of the work herein or changes in medical knowledge, neither the authors, editors, nor publisher, nor any other party who has been involved in the preparation of this work, warrants that the information contained herein is in every respect accurate or complete, and they are not responsible for any errors or omissions or for the results obtained from use of such information. Readers are encouraged to confirm the information contained herein with other sources. For example, readers are advised to check the product information sheet included in the package of each drug they plan to administer to be certain that the information contained in this publication is accurate and that changes have not been made in the recommended dose or in the contraindications for administration. This recommendation is of particular importance in connection with new or infrequently used drugs.

Some of the product names, patents, and registered designs referred to in this book are in fact registered trademarks or proprietary names even though specific reference to this fact is not always made in the text. Therefore, the appearance of a name without designation as proprietary is not to be construed as a representation by the publisher that it is in the public domain.

Printed in India

5 4 3 2 1

ISBN 978-1-60406-305-9

Corporate Acknowledgments

The editors and publisher thank the following companies for their kind support of this book:

GE Healthcare
Waukesha, Wisconsin, USA

Philips Healthcare
Andover, Massachusetts, USA

IMRIS Inc.
Winnipeg, Manitoba, Canada

Acknowledgments

This book is dedicated first and foremost to the patients that we have had the privilege of helping with intraoperative MRI (ioMRI)-guided neurosurgery. We have seen several thousand patients with a wide array of neurosurgical disorders, primarily brain tumors. We believe that ioMRI has made a quantum difference in the management of these patients both by minimizing the effects of intraoperative brain shift and by revealing to neurosurgeons the extent of residual tumor that remains despite the belief that a "gross total" resection had been achieved.

The book is also dedicated to the investigators: past, present, and future. Of these, none deserves more thanks than Ferenc Jolesz, MD, PhD at the Brigham and Women's Hospital in Boston, who was the first to conceive of performing surgery under real-time MRI-guidance. Other investigators that deserve recognition are the radiologists, surgeons, physicists, and engineers that have helped to solve the multitude of problems, both foreseen and unforeseen, that were encountered and had to be overcome in order to establish the field to where it stands today, as demonstrated in this book.

Lastly, we want to acknowledge the MRI equipment manufacturers that were willing to commit resources to solve seemingly insoluble manufacturing difficulties and to deal with the regulatory agencies that have enabled patients to benefit from these technologies. To the MRI equipment vendors, we are grateful for your commitment to invention and to excellence.

Walter A. Hall, MD, MBA
Chip Truwit, MD
Christopher Nimsky, MD, PhD

Contents

Foreword ix
    L. Dade Lunsford

Foreword x
    William G. Bradley Jr.

Preface xi

Contributors xiii

I   Background 1

  Chapter 1   Low-Field Suite Design 3
                  Michael Schulder

  Chapter 2   Mid-Field Suite Design 12
                  Nicolas Foroglou and Peter M. Black

  Chapter 3   High-Field Suite Design 18
                  Charles L. Truwit, Yogesh Kumar, and Walter A. Hall

  Chapter 4   Optimal Pulse Sequences 29
                  Gurpreet Singh Sandhu, Jonathan S. Lewin, and Sherif Gamal Nour

  Chapter 5   Anesthesia Considerations 48
                  Reza Gorji

  Chapter 6   Safety Considerations 56
                  Alastair J. Martin

II   Minimally Invasive Cranial Applications 65

  Chapter 7   Low-Field Brain Biopsy 67
                  John Koivukangas and Sanna Yrjänä

  Chapter 8   High-Field Brain Biopsy 73
                  Walter A. Hall and Charles L. Truwit

  Chapter 9   MRI-Guided Catheter Placement 80
                  Gregory T. Sherr and Cornelius H. Lam

  Chapter 10 Implantation of Deep Brain Stimulator Electrodes Using Interventional MRI 88
                  Philip A. Starr, Alastair J. Martin, and Paul S. Larson

III   Intracranial Tumor Resection **97**

Chapter 11 Utilization of Low-Field Intraoperative MRI in Glioma Surgery–An Overview 99
Volker Seifert and Christian Senft

Chapter 12 Intraoperative MRI Scanning in High-Grade Gliomas 108
Hubertus Maximillian Mehdorn, Arya Nabavi, Felix Schwartz, and Lutz Dörner

Chapter 13 Pituitary Tumor Resection–iMRI in Transsphenoidal Surgery 119
Rudolf Fahlbusch and Vincenzo Paternó

Chapter 14 Functional Magnetic Resonance Imaging-Guided Brain Tumor Resections 130
Peter D. Kim, Charles L. Truwit, and Walter A. Hall

Chapter 15 Diffusion Tensor Imaging-Guided Resection 139
Christopher Nimsky

IV   Nonneoplastic Surgical Indications **151**

Chapter 16 Intraoperative Magnetic Resonance Imaging for Epilepsy Surgery 153
Michael Buchfelder, Christopher Nimsky, and Daniel Weigel

Chapter 17 Awake Craniotomy and Intraoperative MRI for the Resection of Gliomas 162
Arya Nabavi, Simone Goebel, Lutz Dörner, Nils Warneke,
Stephan Ulmer, and Hubertus Maximillian Mehdorn

Chapter 18 Intraoperative Magnetic Resonance Imaging and Cerebrovascular Surgery 170
Taro Kaibara, Robert F. Spetzler, and Garnette R. Sutherland

Chapter 19 Skull Base Surgery and Intraoperative Magnetic Resonance Imaging 178
Taro Kaibara and Robert F. Spetzler

Chapter 20 Treatment of Spinal Disorders 186
Carlo M. DeLuna

V   Design, Equipment, and Logistics **197**

Chapter 21 Promising Advances in Intraoperative MRI-Guided Neurosurgery 199
Ferenc A. Jolesz and Alexandra J. Golby

Chapter 22 Equipment Integration: Neuronavigation 212
Christopher Nimsky and Oliver Ganslandt

Chapter 23 Neurosurgical Robots: A Review 222
Shelly Lwu and Garnette R. Sutherland

Chapter 24 MRI-Guided Focused Ultrasound Surgery in the Brain 233
Rivka R. Colen and Ferenc A. Jolesz

Chapter 25 Cost and Benefit Analysis of Intraoperative MRI-Guided Neurosurgery 241
William C. Broaddus, Zhijian Chen, G. T. Gillies, John Kucharczyk,
and Wayne L. Monsky

Index **249**

Contents

Foreword

It is a pleasure to be asked to write the foreword for this pioneering and innovative guide to the use of the intraoperative MRI in the field of neurosurgery. In 1980, the evolution in CT imaging raised the issue of combining high-resolution imaging with surgical technologies in the operating room itself. By 1982, we placed the first dedicated CT scanner in the operating room at the University of Pittsburgh Medical Center at a time when only two other CT scanners existed in the entire city. Intraoperative imaging was not taken seriously by most colleagues or industry itself, despite the enormous benefit from this innovative union of surgery and imaging tools. In over twenty years, the field dramatically expanded. With the advent of MRI, the multiplanar imaging revolution was underway. It was logical that all brain and spinal surgery would ultimately become image-guided because the incorporation of imaging provides preoperative mapping and critical precision, thereby facilitating minimally invasive surgical techniques.

The editors have assembled an outstanding group of chapter authors who describe their use of advanced MRI within the context of the surgical environment. In the last decade, the outcomes of patients worldwide have benefited from the emergence of MRI guidance. In this volume, the reader will be able to glean answers to many questions, including some of those that have perplexed me over the last thirty years.

1. Will better resection of gliomas result in better long-term outcomes?

2. How do we balance the goal of the operation, e.g., tumor removal, with the goal of making the imaging technology work efficiently?

3. Which MRI system (low-field versus high-field) is better, more efficient, and less intrusive?

4. Can we expand the role of intraoperative imaging to functional and vascular disorders?

5. How do we effectively incorporate multimodality imaging, CT, MRI, angiography, PET, functional MRI scan, and MEG within the portfolio of data that we use to enhance outcomes in patients undergoing brain or spinal surgery?

6. What emerging surgical techniques such as focused ultrasound will incorporate MRI data into the surgical procedure itself?

Doctors Hall, Nimsky, and Truwit have provided a timely and important contribution to our understanding of the role of advanced imaging in the context of surgical procedures. The reader will find this a valuable addition to the knowledge base of a fully mature technology now available at many centers of excellence.

L. Dade Lunsford, MD, FACS
Lars Leksell Professor and Distinguished Professor
University of Pittsburgh
Pittsburgh, Pennsylvania

Foreword

Intraoperative MRI-Guided Neurosurgery has been written and edited by intraoperative MRI (iMRI) pioneers Walter Hall and Christopher Nimsky (both neurosurgeons) and neuroradiologist Chip Truwit. This is the first comprehensive book on neurosurgical iMRI that covers the gamut of current (and some future) applications of iMRI in neurosurgery. Experience using all MRI manufacturers includes that from the editors using Philips (Drs. Hall and Truwit) and Siemens (Dr. Nimsky) and that from General Electric by the Brigham group headed by Ferenc Jolesz, who originally conceived of iMRI in 1990 and developed the first "double donut" iMRI unit in 1995. That over one thousand neurosurgical procedures were performed by neurosurgeon Peter Black and colleagues at the Brigham before the double donut system was decommissioned attests to the clinical utility of iMRI in the neurosurgical setting.

In addition to experience from the three major MRI vendors, the authors cover the gamut of field strengths from the .12T PoleStar to the 3T whole body systems. The three major configurations of iMRI are all discussed, including moving the patient to the magnet (e.g., University of Erlangen), moving the magnet to the patient (e.g., IMRIS), and keeping the patient on the MRI couch and either sliding the couch in and out of the magnet for imaging or imaging directly during the procedure (double donut and University of Minnesota using robotics). A cost-benefit analysis of iMRI is discussed, which includes systems dedicated to iMRI and those that are shared with additional revenue-producing diagnostic and interventional radiology procedures.

This unique book comes at a critical time during the evolution of neurosurgical iMRI; almost every neurosurgeon I know would like to have one. On a personal note, I had to fight the hospital administration tooth and nail to get iMRI at my former institution twelve years ago and was only vindicated when we (and others) showed that 80 percent of the time when a neurosurgeon thought he had a gross total resection, the tumor could still be seen by MRI–with obvious survival implications for low-grade gliomas. In contrast, over the last year at University of California–San Diego, nine of the ten candidates I interviewed for chief of neurosurgery cited iMRI as the most important equipment component of their recruitment package. While this book is of obvious value to any neurosurgeon (including those involved in skull base and spinal surgery), it will also be quite useful to neuroradiologists who will be needed to support such ventures, ENT surgeons, orthopedic surgeons, and medical informatics experts who will be involved in integrating the pre- and intraoperative fMRI, DTI, and MR perfusion and diffusion studies into the iMRI sytem at the time of surgery.

In summary, I would say that this book should be required reading for anyone considering getting into neurosurgical iMRI or for anyone putting in a new neurosurgical suite in their hospital.

William G. Bradley Jr., MD, PhD, FACR
Professor and Chair
Department of Radiology
University of California–San Diego
San Diego, California

Preface

With the advent of computed tomography (CT) and, subsequently, magnetic resonance imaging (MRI), neurosurgeons have become increasingly dependent on image guidance to perform safe and cost effective surgery. Initially, this took the form of stereotactic neurosurgery, including brain biopsies, depth electrode placement, and, eventually, more advanced, functional neurosurgeries. This type of image-guidance, although still in vogue in some circles, evolved to frameless stereotactic image-guided surgery. Again, CT and MRI formed the backbone of these technical advances. As neurosurgery and neuroimaging continued to evolve and become technologically more sophisticated, it was only natural that the two specialty areas would become increasingly more interrelated in their daily performance. Thus, it was natural that the next meaningful merger of these two fields would be the development of intraoperative MRI-guided neurosurgery. Unlike any of the prior computer-generated, imaging-guidance techniques, intraoperative MRI-guidance is performed in near-real time, allowing the neurosurgeon to make adjustments in the surgical approach after the brain has shifted due to the egress of cerebrospinal fluid, or as a brain tumor is progressively resected.

This work chronicles the development of intraoperative MRI-guided neurosurgery since its inception when various magnets of different field strengths and configurations were being tested for their advantages and disadvantages as aids to surgery. The first section of the book discusses the benefits of different strength MRI systems and some general principles that are pertinent to operating in an MRI environment, such as those related to anesthesia and safety issues. The various clinical indications for MRI guidance are discussed in the second section of the text, where the authors describe either the clinical results obtained at their sites or the technical aspects of safely performing surgery in a magnetic environment. In the last section of the book, the reader is introduced to other forms of technology that have been combined with intraoperative MRI guidance; these include focused ultrasound and robotics and some of the anticipated, promising directions in the field.

Even though the field was initially slow to develop prior to the new millennium, there has been a steadily progressive growth in the number of system installations, particularly in recent years. These systems have not been limited to academic health centers but have also been sited in the community setting where the hospital administration has recognized the benefit of avoiding return trips to the operating room and the obvious benefit of shortening the patient's length of stay. Industry has likewise recognized the universal interest in this technology, and several vendors now offer a variety of solutions to meet virtually every individual institutional need. Although initially used by neurosurgeons, the technology is now being embraced by surgeons and interventionalists from other medical specialties such as otolaryngology and orthopedic surgery. This volume is appropriate for radiologists and surgeons at all levels of their career, whether they are in training or have numerous years of operative experience because of the novelty of operating in an entirely new clinical environment.

As we have watched the development of this technology from two continents, we have selected those contributors who pioneered this field and have witnessed and overcome the challenges inherent and unique to a new surgical technology. From the beginning of the concept of performing surgery using MRI visualization of the operative field, to the optimal design of the operating room in which to utilize these systems, we have attempted to be inclusive in our coverage. For those contemplating whether to begin a program for intraoperative MRI-guided neurosurgery, we hope this text will serve as a useful guide for their transition from the conventional operating theatre into an operative arena where the success and goals of planned invasive procedures have been achieved prior to the patient's emergence from anesthesia.

Walter A. Hall, MD, MBA
Charles L. Truwit, MD
Christopher Nimsky, MD, PhD

Contributors

Peter M. Black, MD, PhD
Franc D. Ingraham Professor of Neurosurgery
Harvard Medical School
Boston, Massachusetts

William C. Broaddus, MD, PhD
F. Norton Hord Jr. Professor
Department of Neurosurgery
Medical College of Virginia Hospitals
Virginia Commonwealth University
Richmond, Virginia

Michael Buchfelder, MD, PhD
Professor and Chairman
Department of Neurosurgery
University of Erlangen–Nürnberg
Erlangen, Germany

Zhijian Chen, MD, PhD
Assistant Professor
Department of Neurosurgery
Medical College of Virginia Hospitals
Virginia Commonwealth University
Richmond, Virginia

Rivka R. Colen, MD
Fellow in Radiology
Brigham and Women's Hospital
Harvard Medical School
Boston, Massachusetts

Carlo M. DeLuna, MD
Associate Professor
Department of Neurosurgery
Milton S. Hershey Medical Center
Chief
Section of Neurosurgery
Wilkes-Barre General Hospital
Penn State University
Hershey, Pennsylvania

Lutz Dörner, MD
Department of Neurosurgery
University of Kiel–Schleswig-Holstein
Kiel, Germany

Rudolf Fahlbusch, MD, PhD
Director
Center of Endocrine Neurosurgery
Center of Intraoperative MRI
International Neuroscience Institute
Hannover, Germany

Nicolas Foroglou, MD, PhD
Assistant Professor
Department of Neurosurgery
AHEPA University Hospital
Aristotle University of Thessaloniki
Thessaloniki, Greece

Oliver Ganslandt, MD, PhD
Professor and Vice Chairman
Department of Neurosurgery
University Erlangen–Nuremberg
Erlangen, Germany

G. T. Gillies, PhD
Research Professor
Department of Biomedical Engineering
University of Virginia
Charlottesville, Virginia

Simone Goebel, PhD
Clinical and Experimental Neuropsychologist
Department of Neurosurgery
University of Kiel–Schleswig-Holstein
Kiel, Germany

Alexandra J. Golby, MD
Assistant Professor of Surgery
Assistant Professor of Radiology
Harvard Medical School
Associate Surgeon
Director of Image-guided Neurosurgery
Department of Neurosurgery
Brigham and Women's Hospital
Harvard Medical School
Boston, Massachusetts

Reza Gorji, MD
Associate Professor of Anesthesia
SUNY Upstate Medical University
Syracuse, New York

Walter A. Hall, MD, MBA
The Robert B. and Molly G. King Professor of Neurosurgery
Department of Neurosurgery
SUNY Upstate Medical University
Syracuse, New York

Ferenc A. Jolesz, MD
B. Leonard Holman Professor of Radiology
Director, Division of MRI and Image Guided
    Therapy Program
Department of Radiology
Brigham and Women's Hospital
Harvard Medical School
Boston, Massachusetts

Taro Kaibara, MD, FACS, FRCS(C)
Department of Neurosurgery
Barrow Neurological Institute
Phoenix, Arizona

Peter D. Kim, MD, PhD
Chief Resident
Department of Neurosurgery
SUNY Upstate Medical University
Syracuse, New York

John Koivukangas, MD, PhD
Professor and Head
Department of Neurosurgery
Oulu University Hospital
University of Oulu
Oulu, Finland

John Kucharczyk, PhD
Professor
Department of Radiology
University of Minnesota School of Medicine
Minneapolis, Minnesota

Yogesh Kumar, MD
Fellow
Department of Neuroradiology
University of Minnesota School of Medicine
Minneapolis, Minnesota

Cornelius H. Lam, MD
Associate Professor
Department of Neurosurgery
University of Minnesota School of Medicine
Minneapolis, Minnesota

Paul S. Larson, MD
Associate Professor
Department of Neurological Surgery
University of California–San Francisco
Chief of Neurosurgery
San Francisco VA Medical Center
San Francisco, California

Jonathan S. Lewin, MD, FACR
Martin W. Donner Professor and Chairman
Department of Radiology and Radiological Science
Professor of Oncology, Neurosurgery, and Biomedical
    Engineering
Johns Hopkins School of Medicine
Radiologist-in-Chief
The Johns Hopkins Hospital
Baltimore, Maryland

Shelly Lwu, MD, MSc
Resident
Department of Clinical Neurosciences
University of Calgary
Calgary, Canada

Alastair J. Martin, PhD
Professor
Department of Radiology and Biomedical Imaging
University of California–San Francisco
San Francisco, California

Hubertus Maximillian Mehdorn, MD, PhD
Professor and Chairman
Department of Neurosurgery
University of Kiel–Schleswig-Holstein
Kiel, Germany

Wayne L. Monsky, MD, PhD
Assistant Professor
Department of Radiology
University of California–Davis Medical Center
Sacramento, California

Arya Nabavi, MD, PhD, MaHM
Vice-Chairman
Department of Neurosurgery
University of Kiel–Schleswig-Holstein
Kiel, Germany

Christopher Nimsky, MD, PhD
Professor and Chairman
Department of Neurosurgery
University of Marburg
Marburg, Germany

Sherif Gamal Nour, MD, FRCR
Associate Professor
Department of Radiology
Division of Abdominal Imaging
Director
MR-Guided Intervention
Interventional Radiology and Image-Guided Medicine
Emory University Hospitals and School of Medicine
Atlanta, Georgia

Vincenzo Paternó, MD
Associate Neurosurgeon
Department of Neurosurgery
International Neuroscience Institute
Hannover, Germany

Gurpreet Singh Sandhu, MD, MBBS, MMST
Research Fellow
Department of Radiology
University Hospitals
Case Western Reserve University
Cleveland, Ohio

Michael Schulder, MD
Professor and Vice Chairman
Department of Neurosurgery
Hofstra University School of Medicine
Manhasset, New York

Felix Schwartz, MD
Resident
Department of Neurosurgery
University of Kiel–Schleswig-Holstein
Kiel, Germany

Volker Seifert, MD, PhD
Professor and Chairman
Department of Neurosurgery
Director
Center of Clinical Neurosciences
Johann Wolfgang Goethe University
Frankfurt am Main, Germany

Christian Senft, MD
Assistant Professor
Department of Neurosurgery
Johann Wolfgang Goethe University
Frankfurt am Main, Germany

Gregory T. Sherr, MD
Chief Neurosurgical Resident
Department of Neurosurgery
University of Minnesota School of Medicine
Minneapolis, Minnesota

Robert F. Spetzler, MD
Director
Barrow Neurological Institute
J. N. Harber Chairman
Division of Neurological Surgery
Barrow Neurological Institute
Phoenix, Arizona

Philip A. Starr, MD, PhD
Professor
Department of Neurological Surgery
University of California–San Francisco
San Francisco, California

Garnette R. Sutherland, MD, FRCS
Professor of Neurosurgery
Department of Clinical Neurosciences
University of Calgary
Calgary, Canada

Charles L. Truwit, MD
Chairman
Department of Radiology
Hennepin County Medical Center
Professor and Margaret and H. O. Peterson Chair in
    Neuroradiology
University of Minnesota School of Medicine
Minneapolis, Minnesota

Stephan Ulmer, MD
Assistant Professor
Department of Neuroradiology
University of Spita–Basel
Basel, Switzerland

Nils Warneke, MD
Resident
Department of Neurosurgery
University of Kiel–Schleswig-Holstein
Kiel, Germany

Daniel Weigel, MD
Senior Neurosurgeon
Department of Neurosurgery
University of Erlangen–Nuremberg
Erlangen, Germany

Sanna Yrjänä, PhD
Hospital Physicist
Department of Neurosurgery
Oulu University Hospital
Oulu, Finland

I

Background

1

Low-Field Suite Design

Michael Schulder

Magnetic resonance imaging (MRI), known originally as nuclear magnetic resonance imaging (NMRI), was first proposed some 40 years ago.[1,2] Practical human anatomic imaging was reported in the early 1980s and became widely applied several years later.[3] Twenty years after the discovery that living tissues had different MR signals that might yield useful images, work was under way to bring MRI into the operating room (OR). The clinicians involved in these projects tended to be neurosurgeons, who were used to diagnostic MRI (dMRI) and understood the great benefit that would result from the ability to image patients during surgery. In 1995 the first intraoperative MRI (iMRI) unit was ready for use at the Brigham and Women's Hospital in Boston. This pioneering device was constructed from the ground up in collaboration with General Electric Medical Systems (Waukesha, WI), in a specially designed suite near the Radiology Department.[4] Built around a 0.5 tesla (0.5 T) superconducting magnet, the room was shielded for magnetic and radiofrequency interference. All objects in the room had to be MRI-compatible, requiring the new design and manufacture of many items normally taken for granted in the OR (including scalpels). Several other centers around the world installed this iMRI. Although this device is no longer marketed, Mittal and colleagues[5] defined many of the advantages and challenges that come with iMRI. What has remained unique about this system is that the surgical, stereotactic, and imaging spaces were identical.

Other iMRI systems were described soon after. Some groups devised their iMRI around an existing magnet of various field strength, such as the 0.2 T Siemens Magnetom[6] (SiemensAG, Erlangen, Germany) or the 1.5 T Philips dMRI (Philips Healthcare, Andover, MA).[7] The OR/imaging suites were either modified rooms in Radiology (as done by Hall et al at the University of Minnesota[7]) or were newly built rooms created to accommodate iMRI in the OR environment (as in Erlangen[6]), where arrangements were made to move patients from the surgical area into the MRI when it was time to image. This latter strategy obviated much of the difficulty involved regarding the need for MRI-compatible instruments.

Yet another approach by Sutherland et al incorporated a high-field (1.5 T) MRI in a regular if modified OR.[8] Their magnet is stored in a shielded alcove next to the OR, and moves as needed on a ceiling track for imaging. The OR must be sturdy enough to accommodate the weight of the magnet, and also ensure that environmental vibrations do not affect the image acquisitions. A newer development is the concept of an intraoperative imaging suite, in which 1.5 T[9] or more recently 3 T[10,11] imagers are situated in a separate room. Patients are moved from the OR itself to the nearby room for imaging. When such movement no longer constitutes true "intraoperative imaging" is a matter of debate.

For all of the justifiable interest in high-field iMRI, there is still a good deal of activity centered around low-field-strength units. This chapter will discuss the design and practical use of low-field iMRI.

◆ Low-Field iMRI–The PoleStar System

Early iMRI innovations all asked the surgeon to alter his or her routine in some way, as described above. The PoleStar system was conceived to bring iMRI into a regular OR with as few modifications as possible, so that surgery could be done as per routine, but with the addition of imaging. The first-generation device, the PoleStar N-10, used a 0.12 T magnet.[12] The two poles were separated by 25 cm and were mounted on a small, mobile gantry. The magnet was "parked" under the OR table and raised for imaging. Other authors also described their experience with the PoleStar N-10.[13–15] Inevitably, and as with other iMRI designs, the limitations of this device loomed larger after the initial excitement wore off. The images themselves were limited by variable quality and a relatively small field of view (FOV). The next generation device, the PoleStar N20, was meant to address these concerns. Field strength was increased to 0.15 T,

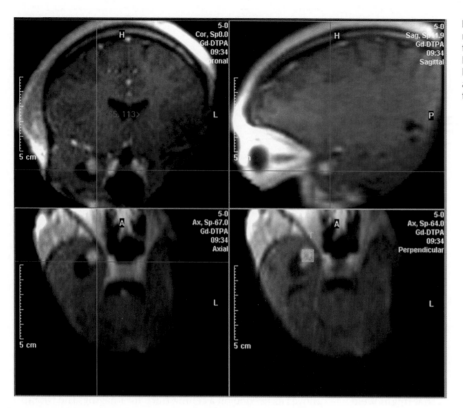

Fig. 1.1 Contrast-enhanced magnetic resonance image of a patient with a right temporal ganglioglioma, acquired with PoleStar N20 (Medtronic Navigation Inc., Louisville, CO). This was a coronal scan with axial (lower left), sagittal (upper right), and target-centered reformatting.

which allowed for the gap between the poles to be widened to 27 cm – a seemingly small difference, but one that greatly increased flexibility in patient positioning for surgery. In addition, the FOV was significantly expanded, giving the images a look more familiar to neurosurgeons (**Fig. 1.1**). Increasing magnet strength did require the device to be larger, and the N20 weighs in at 670 kg, 220 more than its predecessor. It is also sits 10 cm higher than the N10, so that it has a larger footprint. Still, the PoleStar N20 can be parked under the head of the OR table without hindering access to the surgical field (**Fig. 1.2**).

As noted, the PoleStar system was designed to work in a regular OR. When not in use, the magnet is stored in a cage that is recessed into one of the OR walls (**Fig. 1.3**). This stainless steel cage contains the magnetic field, and when the PoleStar is stored the room can be used for any and all surgical applications, including various computerized devices, without concern for interference or device damage. The initial configurations of the cage were slightly larger than the MRI device itself, with doors just over 4 feet high. This makes removing and replacing the magnet a bit laborious for most surgeons and OR staff. More recent installations have included full-height cages that allow most people to enter without bending to manipulate the MRI and its cables. Retrofitting an OR with a larger cage is logistically difficult, and expensive. These are the sort of ergonomic considerations to incorporate at the beginning of an iMRI installation. Still, "workarounds"

are possible. A pneumatic-assist mechanism can be placed in a half-height cage; this device can push or pull the magnet out of or into the cage, thus bypassing one of the annoyances of PoleStar iMRI use.

◆ iMRI and Integrated Navigation

Intraoperative imaging provides useful information regarding the presence of any residual lesion, catheter placement, etc. However, without the ability to navigate based on this updated information, the new images are half a help, at best. Indeed, various authors have emphasized that compensating for brain shift is one of the main benefits of intraoperative imaging of any kind.[16–19] "Conventional" surgical navigation is achieved by registering a preoperative image to physical space (i.e., the patient's head for the purposes of this discussion). It is possible to use iMRI to update the registration and maintain the accuracy of surgical navigation during surgery.[20] The PoleStar, however, provides another, simpler solution. Rather than relying on registration, the system includes infrared-emitting cameras that track a "passive" navigation wand on which are mounted reflective spheres. A reference frame, likewise with infrared reflecting spheres, is attached to the proprietary, MRI-compatible headholder. Once an image is acquired, the wand is tracked automatically (**Fig. 1.4**). This navigation will remain accurate as long as the spatial relationship between the surgical

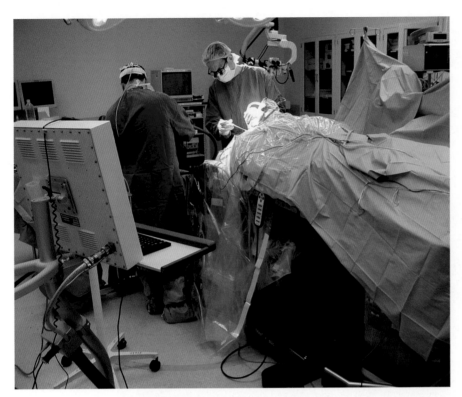

field and the reference frame remains unchanged. If there should be some unexpected movement that invalidates this tracking, imaging can be repeated and accurate navigation restored. This is a significant advantage over reliance on preoperative imaging and registration alone. The navigational accuracy of the PoleStar N20 system has been shown, using a pegboard-water phantom, to be under 2 mm on average, hence in line with traditional surgical navigation systems.[21]

Any iMRI technology, of any field strength, must include integrated surgical navigation of some kind to take full advantage of the imaging capability.

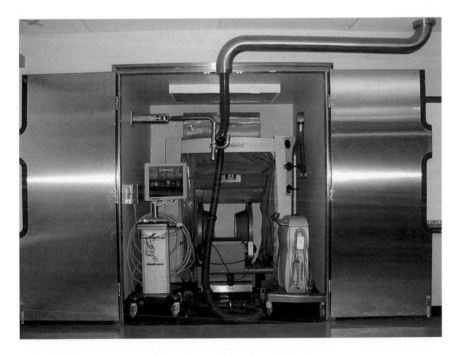

Fig. 1.3 Full-height magnet storage cage for PoleStar N20 (Medtronic Navigation, Inc., Louisville, CO).

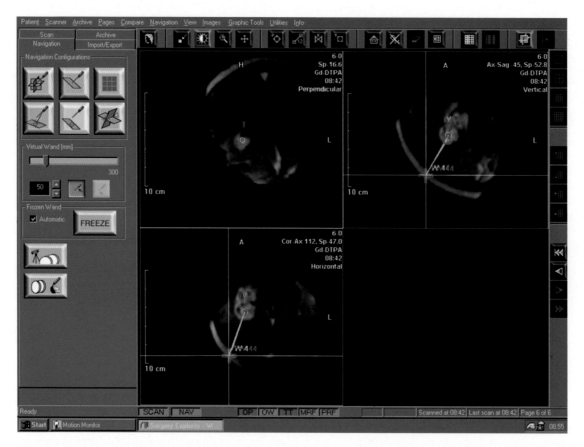

Fig. 1.4 Navigation screen from PoleStar (Medtronic Navigation, Inc., Louisville, CO) platform. A trajectory has been planned and depth obtained for stereotactic biopsy in a patient with a right parietal mass.

I Background

◆ Room Shielding

An OR must be properly shielded for iMRI use, as is the case for a dMRI unit. Shielding has to prevent magnetic interference from outside the room, and prevent the magnetic field from affecting equipment or patients elsewhere. An advantage of a low-field-strength iMRI is the rapid fall-off of the magnetic field. In the case of the PoleStar N20, the 5 gauss (G) line is 2.2 m from between the magnet poles. Thus no special magnetic shielding of the OR is necessary.

More complicated is the need to shield the room from radiofrequency interference (RFI) by unfiltered electrical alternating current, the noise from which will cause serious degradation of the images. This is especially a concern with low-field-strength iMRI because the comparatively lower signal means that the signal to noise ratio (SNR) will be heavily dependent on the avoidance of noise. The most common method of isolating electrical current is by shielding the OR itself, thus enclosing the magnet and everything else in a Faraday cage.[12] Copper typically is used to create the shield. Imaging inside the shield requires that all unfiltered electrical sources need to be turned off and unplugged. Some operating rooms may have a shield already installed, to prevent RFI during intracranial recording for functional neurosurgery. When this is not the case, a new shield can be installed by creating a "room within a room."[14]

If the original OR is large enough this will not have an adverse affect on workflow.

As many electrical sources as possible should have noise filters placed so that they need not be unplugged during imaging. This can be facilitated by running multiple power lines through booms or other common outlets in the room. The process of shutting down, unplugging, and turning devices on again does add several minutes to each imaging session.

◆ Local Shield

Another option is to use a local RFI shield – one that surrounds the patient and magnet. The advantages of this approach include avoiding the need to construct a room shield, an expensive and possibly unreliable solution; the ability to leave electrical equipment turned on while imaging; and allowing staff to enter and exit the OR during imaging without concern for external RFI. Disadvantages are that while imaging, the patient is not in complete view; special care must be taken to avoid contaminating the surgical field when the shield is closed; and the OR table must be carefully positioned over the base of the shield. The PoleStar system includes a local RFI shield that has been described by Levivier et al.[15] It is kept "collapsed" at the foot of the OR table most of the time, and

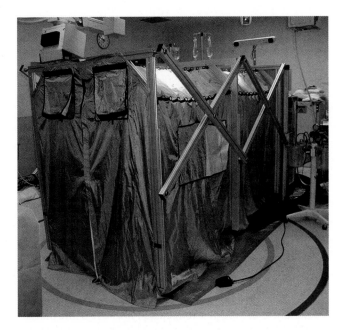

Fig. 1.5 Local radiofrequency interference shield closed during imaging with the PoleStar N20 (Medtronic Navigation, Inc., Louisville, CO).

opened to surround the magnet and the patient's head for image acquisition (**Fig. 1.5**). Room construction for use of this "StarShield" should take into account where the base plate should be positioned in relation to overhead lights, the alignment of the room, etc. **Table 1.1** provides a comparison between the different shielding solutions.

◆ Control Room

Any iMRI is a complex device, and the PoleStar N20 is no less so despite its compact design. While mobile within the OR, the system is not truly portable. The computer and gradients that connect to the magnet are housed in an adjacent control room. Most likely this will be a preexisting storage room converted for this use, but of course a new OR construction can build a dedicated control room. This space will also

contain a chiller that maintains the magnet at the required temperature and a penetration panel, through which connections to the magnet in the OR will pass. If a room RFI shield is chosen, this panel must be carefully installed to avoid electrical noise creation in the OR. The control room should have enough room for the staff to comfortably enter and work as needed. It should be properly air-conditioned to keep the computer rack from overheating.

◆ Operating Room Layout

Designing the OR for a PoleStar N20 installation requires some other considerations. The magnet must be tethered to the above-mentioned control room with a cable that connects to the computer and gradient rack, and to the chiller. This ~15-cm-thick cable should be long enough to allow for flexibility in magnet positioning, and ideally lie in a manner that will minimize the risk of staff tripping over it. The most practical solution is to use a boom that reduces the length and weight of the exposed cable. The viewing stand and keyboard will be connected with their own, smaller cable via the penetration panel. The infrared-emitting navigation cameras will also need to be connected to an outlet on the OR side of the penetration panel. This cable is ~1-cm thick and allows the cameras to be positioned anywhere in the room. **Figure 1.6** provides a schematic diagram of a typical OR layout for a PoleStar N20, with a dedicated room shield for RFI prevention.

◆ Other Considerations in Low-Field-Strength iMRI

The PoleStar was conceived from the beginning to be operated by the neurosurgeon or his designee among the medical or OR staff. No dedicated technical staff is needed to operate the system, such as radiology technologists. Some facilities have staff that are in charge of various image guidance tools and/or participate in clinical research related to them. Having this sort of person on staff makes the neurosurgeon's life easier, but is not essential. Because the PoleStar is operated by controls in the OR itself, the adjacent

Table 1.1 Room versus Local Shielding for Low-Field Intraoperative Magnetic Resonance Imaging (iMRI)

Factor	Room Shield	Local Shield
Need to shut down electronics during imaging	Yes	No
Need to keep room doors shut during imaging	Yes	No
Ability to observe patient during imaging	Yes	Yes, but limited
Infection risk	No	Possible
Setup for surgery	None needed	Position OR table, bring IV, ventilator lines thru the shield
Cost	Upfront only – about $150,000	$50,000 – but may need to replace copper drapes

Abbreviations: OR, operating room; IV, intravenous.

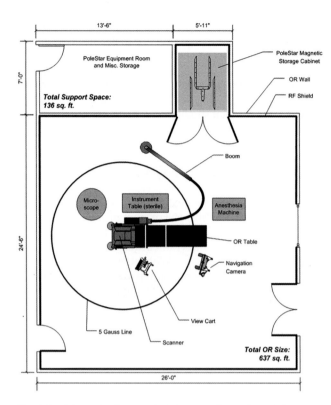

Fig. 1.6 Schematic diagram showing room layout for PoleStar N20 (Medtronic Navigation, Inc., Louisville, CO) intraoperative magnetic resonance imaging, with dedicated room shielding. (Courtesy of Medtronic Navigation.)

I Background

control room need not be large enough to accommodate a technician sitting at a console.

As noted above, the 5 G line of the PoleStar N20 is only 2.2 m from the center of the magnet poles. This means that such equipment as computers and other devices that could be harmed by exposure to a magnetic field can be safely operated in the room. Credit cards, ID cards, watches, etc., can be brought into the room, although the surgical team should remove them from their persons, as they will be in direct contact with the magnet. Few special surgical tools are needed to work in the PoleStar environment. In practice, ferromagnetic hand tools (e.g., periosteal elevators) can be brought within 25 cm of the magnet without noticeable attraction. Because surgery is done with the magnet lowered below the operating field, this is never a concern. More complex instruments such as high-speed drills, operating microscopes, and ultrasonic aspirators can be used in a routine fashion. The only exception is the rare occasion when surgery is done through the raised magnet poles, such as in stepwise resection of a low-grade glioma. In these instances the surgeon may alternate surgery with serial imaging until the goals have been reached. Tools brought between the magnet poles must be MRI-safe; in addition, having an MRI-compatible ultrasonic aspirator (Selector, Integra Radionics, Burlington MA) is convenient in this situation. It also is helpful to have a limited number of MRI-compatible retractors, including those for the scalp, the brain, and a nasal speculum for transnasal approaches. Note that a liquid

crystal display (LCD) monitor is not subject to magnetic interference as is a cathode ray tube screen.[22] If iMRI-assisted endoscopic surgery is planned then an LCD monitor will be very useful.

Although as noted the PoleStar will not interfere with the function of electromagnetic devices in the OR, a standard policy is that all life-support equipment – the anesthetic machine, ventilator, and monitor – should be MRI-compatible. Many centers have such equipment for use in dMRI acquired under anesthesia and are familiar with its use. Several vendors supply MRI-compatible anesthetic units. Any OR that is considering iMRI installation (at any field strength) should take this requirement into account.[23]

◆ Surgery with the PoleStar N20

Workflow with the PoleStar system ideally should follow neurosurgical routine, or close to it. The OR table is reversed to ensure that the magnet can be parked underneath. While the patient is being anesthetized and lines are being placed, the iMRI is turned on and moved into the OR, using the pneumatic-assist mechanism. A QA test is done to confirm basic functioning of the device. When the patient is ready for positioning, the head is fixed in the proprietary, MRI-compatible headholder. When possible, the flexible, disposable receive coil should be placed around the patient's head so that it can be included under the sterile drapes. This way, there will be no need for coil replacement when imaging is repeated during surgery. The patient reference frame is attached to the headholder, and the infrared cameras are positioned.

The magnet is brought into its "parked" (under the OR table) position by two people, and adjusted so that the magnet poles and gantry will not collide with the table side rails or the headholder once it is raised to imaging position. When the patient position is finalized, unfiltered electrical sources are turned off and unplugged (or the StarShield is closed over the patient). The magnet is raised and centered as much as possible around the surgical site. A typical imaging session will include an 8 second "esteady" (reverse fast imaging with steady state precession [PSIF]) sequence to confirm positioning and low noise levels; a T1-weighted (T1W) 1 minute scan without contrast; and a 6.5 minute sequence with single-dose gadolinium enhancement. The magnet is then lowered below the table. The navigation wand is used to confirm accurate tracking, and to mark the incision if necessary.

A sterile prep and drape is done, using a clear plastic orthopedic isolation drape so that the magnet position can be tracked during intraoperative scanning. Surgery then begins in a standard fashion, using regular instruments, Mayo stands, and back tables as needed. When the surgeon decides, scanning is repeated. This process is the same as the preoperative imaging session; in addition, ferromagnetic instruments are removed from the surgical field, which should also be covered appropriately to ensure sterility. After imaging is completed, the magnet is again lowered and surgery continues. Navigation may be done immediately, using the new scan, without the need for registration. Closure is

8

done in the routine fashion, and an image may be repeated to rule out hematoma, pneumocephalus, or other concerns.

In my series of 403 iMRI-guided surgeries an average of three imaging sessions were done per case, so that typically an intraoperative image was acquired that had the potential to affect the surgery. In 29% of the operations additional surgery (most often tumor removal) was done based on intraoperative scans), and in 10% additional dissection was avoided by confirming that the surgical goals had been reached. Most operations were for resection of mass lesions, with 43 of 403 done for stereotactic biopsy or catheter placement. These and related data are summarized in **Table 1.2**. Insertion of electrodes for deep brain stimulation (DBS) has been described in a high-field MRI environment (using a diagnostic scanner).[24] DBS has not been routinely possible with the PoleStar N20, as this system has not been tested to ensure complete safety of imaging with DBS electrodes in place (as per the manufacturer, Medtronic Navigation, Inc., Louisville, CO). If and when this is done, the vertical gap design of the magnet should allow for DBS to be done, as opposed to the horizontal gap of other low-field systems (see next section). The PoleStar images will not be sufficient for direct targeting of such structures as the subthalamic nucleus, but indirect targeting from third ventricular anatomy will be possible. In practice, DBS in this iMRI could be done by registering preoperative, high-field dMRI images to the images acquired in the OR. Imaging during surgery can then be performed to ensure correct electrode placement, rule out hematoma, etc.

◆ Other Low-Field iMRI Designs

The vertically oriented PoleStar N20 is not the only possible low-field iMRI solution. Units with a horizontal magnet gap remain an important option in contemporary image guidance.[25–27] The Magnetom Open (SiemensAG, Erlangen, Germany), a 0.2 T system, was first adapted as an iMRI by neurosurgeons in Germany.[25,26] They developed the "twin operating theater" concept, wherein complex surgery was performed in a room separate from the scanner ("Site A"). Some relatively routine operations could be performed in the iMRI room, outside of the magnet ("Site B"), with minor interventions being possible in the magnet gap itself ("Site C"). The main advantage of this system is that the image quality is near-diagnostic. The major disadvantages are the need for patient transport into the magnet in nearly all cases, from either Site A or Site B, with the concomitant disruption to surgical routine and the potential for infections (although none have been reported); the location of the imaging suite outside of the main OR; and the separate construction required.

A similar concept was used at the University of Cincinnati, where an iMRI suite was created based on a 0.3 T horizontal gap MRI (Hitachi Airis, Hitachi Medical Corp., Tokyo, Japan).[27] Likewise, in this setup, operating sites where defined in their relation to the magnet center, with a separate OR for "complex intracranial procedures such as craniotomy for tumor resection." Surgery requiring fewer

Table 1.2 Patient and Technical Data for Use of Low-Field-Strength Intraoperative Magnetic Resonance Imaging (iMRI)

Diagnosis	
Tumor	342
Inflammatory	21
Epilepsy	9
Hydrocephalus	8
CSF leak	6
Miscellaneous	11
Total	403
Tumor diagnoses	
High-grade glioma	114
Low-grade glioma	28
Pituitary macroadenoma	88
Pituitary microadenoma	11
Meningioma	59
Skull base carcinoma	11
Schwannoma	8
Craniopharyngioma	6
Colloid cyst	5
Metastatic tumor	6
Epidermoid	4
Hemangioblastoma	1
CP papilloma	1
Total	342
Procedure	
Craniotomy	250
Transsphenoidal	110
Biopsy, catheter placement	43
Time added by iMRI (hours)	
Range	0.25–4
Mean	1.0
Number of scanning sessions per surgery	
Range	1–9
Mean	3.0

Abbreviations: CSF, cerebrospinal fluid; CP papilloma, choroid plexus papilloma.

instruments, such as transsphenoidal operations, could be done in Site A, where a relatively small movement of the MRI-compatible OR table was needed to bring the patient into scanning position.[28] Only minimally invasive procedures such as biopsies could be done in the magnet isocenter. The need for patient transport and separate suite construction were similar with this design as with the Siemens Magnetom. The major difference (and from

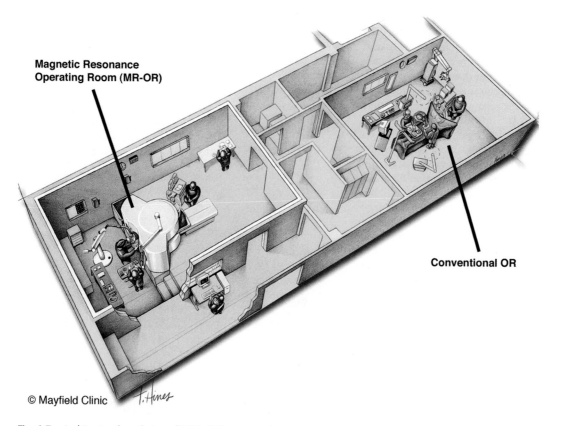

Magnetic Resonance
Operating Room (MR-OR)

Conventional OR

© Mayfield Clinic   T. Hines

Fig. 1.7 Architectural rendering of 0.3 tesla intraoperative magnetic resonance imaging "shared-resource" suite at the University of Cincinnati, Ohio. (Courtesy of Dr. Ronald Warnick, printed with permission of Mayfield Clinic.)

the PoleStar design as well) was the ability to use the MRI for diagnostic imaging, a so-called shared-resource imaging unit (**Fig. 1.7**). During the first 18 months of the imager's operation, 82 neurosurgical procedures were done—but 962 diagnostic MRIs were acquired on both inpatients and outpatients. This option also has been described in 1.5 T iMRI systems[29] and has the important advantage of making the iMRI a profit center for the hospital (when used for outpatient imaging) as opposed to a cost center. This is hardly a trivial consideration when one is planning construction of a suite that will cost several million dollars. (Image quality of the PoleStar N20 will not support routine diagnostic use, but the cost of this system is closer to $1,000,000, with relatively few operating costs.)

◆ The Future of Low-Field iMRI

There has already been some degree of convergence in the world of iMRI. The development of the PoleStar N20 itself represented some small compromise with the notion of a very small iMRI. Similarly, the commercial abandonment of the pioneering Signa iMRI was a bow to practical considerations. High-field iMRI has evolved by making these systems more "user friendly." This has been done by allowing for surgery to be done in the fringe fields,[30] by moving them in and out of the OR,[31] or by moving the scanners out of the

OR completely.[9,11] With the development of MR imagers with ever-higher field strengths,[32,33] will there be an "arms race" to move these more powerful magnets into the OR? Will concerns regarding patient safety limit enthusiasm for these changes,[34] or will the increasing expense and likely complexity of more-powerful MRI call into question the added surgical benefit of such devices?

At the other end of the spectrum, there is a limit to how much field strength can be added before a low-field system is no longer "low." In the case of the PoleStar N20, more magnet power will mean a larger and heavier system. This might yield a larger FOV and more diagnostic-like images, but at a cost of decreased mobility, a larger footprint, and no doubt less willingness by surgeons to use the system. The future of this system probably lies in making it yet easier to use, for instance, by making it more mobile or even portable, so it can travel between rooms, increasing the magnet gap if possible, improving receiving coil technology, and the like. At the same time, low field iMRI of the Magnetom or Airis types described above may continue to find a place as shared-resource devices that can be used for outpatient diagnostic imaging. Modifying these systems so that surgery can routinely be done in the same room as the magnet, and providing practical solutions for patient positioning, instrumentation, etc., may make these devices more popular among neurosurgeons.

◆ Conclusion

Low-field strength iMRI, in the form of the PoleStar system, can be used as a workhorse for most image-guided neurosurgical applications. This is due to the unit's small size, mobility, and installation in a regular neurosurgical OR that requires few modifications. Other low-field units are useful as shared resource devices that can pay their own way. High-field iMRI systems will play an important role, most likely as tools for select neurosurgical applications, and to push the envelope of intraoperative imaging. For the foreseeable future, low-field strength iMRI will continue to make this critical point: for iMRI to be useful, it has to be used.

References

1. Damadian R. Tumor detection by nuclear magnetic resonance. Science 1971;171(976):1151–1153

2. Lauterbur PC. Progress in n.m.r. zeugmatography imaging. Philos Trans R Soc Lond B Biol Sci 1980;289(1037):483–487

3. Edelstein WA, Hutchison JM, Smith FW, Mallard J, Johnson G, Redpath TW. Human whole-body NMR tomographic imaging: normal sections. Br J Radiol 1981;54(638):149–151

4. Black PM, Moriarty T, Alexander E III, et al. Development and implementation of intraoperative magnetic resonance imaging and its neurosurgical applications. Neurosurgery 1997;41(4):831–842, discussion 842–845

5. Mittal S, Black PM. Intraoperative magnetic resonance imaging in neurosurgery: the Brigham concept. Acta Neurochir Suppl 2006;98:77–86

6. Fahlbusch R, Ganslandt O, Nimsky C. Intraoperative imaging with open magnetic resonance imaging and neuronavigation. Childs Nerv Syst 2000;16(10-11):829–831

7. Hall WA, Martin AJ, Liu H, et al. High-field strength interventional magnetic resonance imaging for pediatric neurosurgery. Pediatr Neurosurg 1998;29(5):253–259

8. Sutherland GR, Kaibara T, Louw D, Hoult DI, Tomanek B, Saunders J. A mobile high-field magnetic resonance system for neurosurgery. J Neurosurg 1999;91(5):804–813

9. Matsumae M, Koizumi J, Fukuyama H, et al. World's first magnetic resonance imaging/x-ray/operating room suite: a significant milestone in the improvement of neurosurgical diagnosis and treatment. J Neurosurg 2007;107(2):266–273

10. Pamir MN, Peker S, Ozek MM, Dincer A. Intraoperative MR imaging: preliminary results with 3 tesla MR system. Acta Neurochir Suppl 2006;98:97–100

11. Jankovski A, Francotte F, Vaz G, et al. Intraoperative magnetic resonance imaging at 3-T using a dual independent operating room-magnetic resonance imaging suite: development, feasibility, safety, and preliminary experience. Neurosurgery 2008;63(3):412–424, discussion 424–426

12. Hadani M, Spiegelman R, Feldman Z, Berkenstadt H, Ram Z. Novel, compact, intraoperative magnetic resonance imaging-guided system for conventional neurosurgical operating rooms. Neurosurgery 2001;48(4):799–807, discussion 807–809

13. Schulder M, Liang D, Carmel PW. Cranial surgery navigation aided by a compact intraoperative magnetic resonance imager. J Neurosurg 2001;94(6):936–945

14. Kanner AA, Vogelbaum MA, Mayberg MR, Weisenberger JP, Barnett GH. Intracranial navigation by using low-field intraoperative magnetic resonance imaging: preliminary experience. J Neurosurg 2002;97(5):1115–1124

15. Levivier M, Wikler D, De Witte O, Van de Steene A, Balériaux D, Brotchi J. PoleStar N-10 low-field compact intraoperative magnetic resonance imaging system with mobile radiofrequency shielding. Neurosurgery 2003;53(4):1001–1006, discussion 1007

16. Black PM, Alexander E III, Martin C, et al. Craniotomy for tumor treatment in an intraoperative magnetic resonance imaging unit. [see comment] Neurosurgery 1999;45(3):423–431, discussion 431–433

17. Nabavi A, Black PM, Gering DT, et al. Serial intraoperative magnetic resonance imaging of brain shift. Neurosurgery 2001;48(4):787–797, discussion 797–798

18. Nimsky C, Ganslandt O, Hastreiter P, Fahlbusch R. Intraoperative compensation for brain shift. Surg Neurol 2001;56(6):357–364, discussion 364–365

19. Unsgaard G, Ommedal S, Muller T, Gronningsaeter A, Nagelhus Hernes TA. Neuronavigation by intraoperative three-dimensional ultrasound: initial experience during brain tumor resection. Neurosurgery 2002;50(4):804–812, discussion 812

20. Clatz O, Delingette H, Talos IF, et al. Robust nonrigid registration to capture brain shift from intraoperative MRI. IEEE Trans Med Imaging 2005;24(11):1417–1427

21. Salas S, Brimacombe M, Schulder M. Stereotactic accuracy of a compact intraoperative MRI system. Stereotact Funct Neurosurg 2007;85(2-3):69–74

22. Schwartz TH, Stieg PE, Anand VK. Endoscopic transsphenoidal pituitary surgery with intraoperative magnetic resonance imaging. Neurosurgery 2006;**58**(1, Suppl)ONS44–ONS51, discussion ONS44–ONS51

23. Berkenstadt H, Perel A, Ram Z, Feldman Z, Nahtomi-Shick O, Hadani M. Anesthesia for magnetic resonance guided neurosurgery: initial experience with a new open magnetic resonance imaging system. J Neurosurg Anesthesiol 2001;13(2):158–162

24. Martin AJ, Larson PS, Ostrem JL, et al. Placement of deep brain stimulator electrodes using real-time high-field interventional magnetic resonance imaging. Magn Reson Med 2005;54(5):1107–1114

25. Steinmeier R, Fahlbusch R, Ganslandt O, et al. Intraoperative magnetic resonance imaging with the Magnetom open scanner: concepts, neurosurgical indications, and procedures: a preliminary report. Neurosurgery 1998;43(4):739–747, discussion 747–748

26. Wirtz CR, Bonsanto MM, Knauth M, et al. Intraoperative magnetic resonance imaging to update interactive navigation in neurosurgery: method and preliminary experience. Comput Aided Surg 1997;2(3-4):172–179

27. Bohinski RJ, Kokkino AK, Warnick RE, et al. Glioma resection in a shared-resource magnetic resonance operating room after optimal image-guided frameless stereotactic resection. Neurosurgery 2001;48(4):731–742, discussion 742–744

28. Bohinski RJ, Warnick RE, Gaskill-Shipley MF, et al. Intraoperative magnetic resonance imaging to determine the extent of resection of pituitary macroadenomas during transsphenoidal microsurgery. Neurosurgery 2001;49(5):1133–1143, discussion 1143–1144

29. Hall WA, Martin AJ, Liu H, Nussbaum ES, Maxwell RE, Truwit CL. Brain biopsy using high-field strength interventional magnetic resonance imaging. Neurosurgery 1999;44(4):807–813, discussion 813–814

30. Fahlbusch R, Nimsky C. Intraoperative MRI developments. Neurosurg Clin N Am 2005;16(1):xi–xiii

31. Kaibara T, Saunders JK, Sutherland GR. Advances in mobile intraoperative magnetic resonance imaging. Neurosurgery 2000;47(1):131–137, discussion 137–138

32. Novak P, Novak V, Kangarlu A, Abduljalil AM, Chakeres DW, Robitaille PM. High resolution MRI of the brainstem at 8 T. J Comput Assist Tomogr 2001;25(2):242–246

33. Xu D, Cunningham CH, Chen AP, et al. Phased array 3D MR spectroscopic imaging of the brain at 7 T. Magn Reson Imaging 2008;26(9):1201–1206

34. Shrivastava D, Hanson T, Schlentz R, et al. Radiofrequency heating at 9.4T: in vivo temperature measurement results in swine. Magn Reson Med 2008;59(1):73–78

2

Mid-Field Suite Design

Nicolas Foroglou and Peter M. Black

In the history of neurosurgery, the introduction of the surgical microscope and neuronavigation systems stand out as watershed moments that enabled more accurate and effective surgery for tumors. Neuronavigation systems started as framed stereotaxy, evolved to frameless stereotaxy, and more recently, evolved to incorporate image registration and fusion systems that guide the neurosurgeon through the phases of craniotomy, picket-fencing of the tumor, and surgical resection. On a macroscopic scale, such systems afford greater accuracy to the surgeon. That said, however, navigation systems have several potential sources of error. Registration may be inaccurate because of scalp movement, images may have geometrical distortion, and the brain may shift relative to the cranium between the time of scanning and the time of surgery.

Brain shift results from fluid shifts, tumor resection, and leakage of cerebrospinal fluid (CSF) following dural incision. Brain shift greater than 10 mm has been documented as soon as 1 hour after opening the dura. With fluid loss and introduction of air, the brain settles dependently, away from the surgeon. Such shift may be on the order of a millimeter or two, or more than a centimeter. The error induced by this type of shift may be accentuated in the presence of preoperative hydrocephalus or loss of parenchymal volume. Owing to these sources of error, the usefulness of navigation quickly diminishes during the surgical procedure.[1–8] With the development of intraoperative magnetic resonance (MR)-guided neurosurgery, such neuronavigation systems could be updated periodically, allowing for accommodation of brain shift. Although various methodologies have been proposed, what they have in common is postcraniotomy imaging. The three-dimensional (3D) slicer, for instance, used at the Brigham and Women's Hospital, afforded very rapid updating and reregistration of prior volumetric imaging.

The first intraoperative MR imaging (iMRI) system, a mid-field system, was General Electric's so-called double-doughnut Signa SP system (General Electric Medical Systems, Waukesha, WI), developed at the Brigham and Women's Hospital (Boston, MA) and installed in 1994 (**Fig. 2.1**). It was a 0.5 tesla (0.5 T) system that tried to reach a balance between the otherwise competing goals of surgical accessibility and image quality. It allowed real-time imaging during surgery, real-time navigation, immediate assessment of such complications as hemorrhage, and verification of planned resection. The first brain tumor extirpation guided by intraoperative magnetic resonance was in 1996 in this magnet.[1] Similar systems were installed at Stanford (California), Heidelberg (Germany), and University College (London) and developed important early concepts.

Since the Brigham solution, many alternative iMRI systems have been developed. Such systems have offered variations on the initial theme, including differences in surgical access, magnetic field strength, fixed versus mobile nature of the patient, the scanner, or both. Multiplanar imaging, high tissue discrimination, and absence of ionizing radiation have been fundamental to nearly all subsequent systems; a few efforts have included x-ray imaging within or near the MRI scanner.

Image quality depends on many factors, including system field strength homogeneity and stability of the static and gradient magnetic fields, and coil design. The optimal design of a magnet with regard to field homogeneity would be a complete sphere, without an opening.[9] However, as access to a patient is a prerequisite for surgery and monitoring, design of further intraoperative systems necessarily involves compromises between the generally mutually exclusive nature of image quality and surgical access.[1,10–18]

Among the many unique features of the mid-field GE system was that the MRI suite by necessity functioned as, and therefore was inherently designed as, a neurosurgical operating room with positive pressure and surgical sterility throughout. The Signa SP was an MRI scanner sited within an environment in which neurosurgical procedures could be performed under full anesthetic monitoring; the device became the operating room and table.

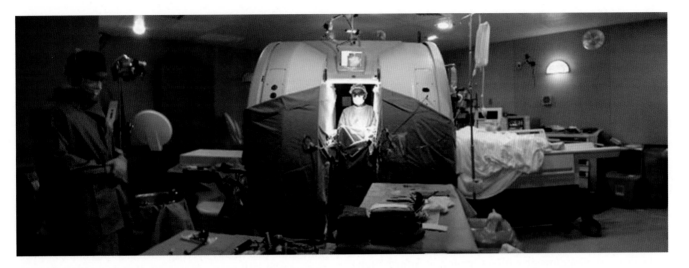

Fig. 2.1 The GE Signa (General Electric Medical Systems, Waukesha, WI) intraoperative magnetic resonance imaging system.

Subsequent systems offered a different balance between spatial constraints necessary for high-quality imaging and the freedom necessary for surgical intervention. At present, low-field systems (0.12–0.2 T) offer the advantage of greater patient access while they are disadvantaged by diminished signal-to-noise ratio and reduced spatial and contrast resolution. High-field (1.5–3 T) systems, on the other hand, restricted surgical access during scanning, but offer a wide range of adjunctive imaging protocols. The ideal configuration of an iMRI-guided neurosurgical suite remains challenging: to enable broad surgical access, yet provide optimal imaging capabilities.

The development of the GE mid-field system also required new surgical cutlery and medical equipment that would be safe to use within the magnetic field. Innovative solutions were required for nearly everything, ranging from surgical instruments, anesthesia equipment, and patient-monitoring devices. The new configurations required new drapes. In-room high-resolution radio frequency-shielded display monitors, new interfaces between optically lined 3D digitizers and the control software of the MRI scanners to update neuronavigation systems all required reengineering.[1,10,11] Additionally, the MRI scanners and adjunctive imaging technologies all required new solutions. Such requirements included higher quality low-noise receiver chains to give lower field systems higher signal-to-noise ratio images and the development of rapid gradient echo pulse sequences to allow adequate tissue contrast in the time frame sufficient for device tracking (0.3–7 s per image). As mentioned earlier, one such critical development was the development of Slicer, an open source image-guided therapy software system developed at the Surgical Planning Laboratory at the Brigham and Women's Hospital (**Fig. 2.2**).[19]

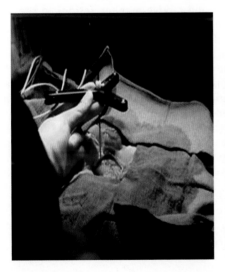

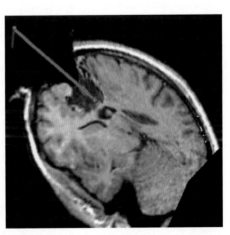

A   B

Fig. 2.2 The Slicer navigation system. **(A)** Hand-held optical tracking device. Note the three light-emitting diodes located at the ends of the arms of the device are used to establish the plane of imaging and the proposed path of the needle or probe that is passed through the center of the device. **(B)** A probe, demonstrated in red, is being used to investigate with imaging a tumor resection cavity for residual disease.

◆ Applications in Surgical Oncology

With the introduction of iMRI-guided neurosurgery at the Brigham and Women's Hospital, new approaches to surgical oncology were needed, including

- ◆ Surgical planning, including multimodality image integration
- ◆ Neurobiopsy
- ◆ Resection guidance
- ◆ Verification of completeness of resection
- ◆ Monitoring for potential complications

◆ Surgical Planning

Conventional neuroimaging offers anatomic information about the location and extent of brain tumors, allowing for preoperative surgical planning, whether by a freehand approach or stereotaxy, either framed or frameless. Such imaging also includes MR and computed tomography angiography (MRA, CTA), which allows for relational information about overlying vascular structures.

More recently, the acquisition of physiologic characteristics of brain tissue and tumors by MRI has become routine. Such imaging includes diffusion-, perfusion- and susceptibility-weighted imaging (SWI), allowing for potential differentiation of types of tissues and fluids. As well, functional MRI (fMRI) and diffusion tensor imaging (DTI) and fiber tracking (tractography) reveal tumoral relationships to eloquent cortices and critical underlying and subjacent white matter tracks. Today, it is now possible to differentiate invasive tumors from those that deviate, but do not invade, these white matter tracts, thus allowing for more appropriate planning and prognostication. At the Brigham program, many of these features were anticipated and incorporated into the Signa SP scanner, even at mid-field strength.

In addition to changes in the approach to the surgical resection of brain tumors, the advent of live MRI allowed for much smaller craniotomies; feedback on the substance and location of remaining tumor; and accommodation of brain shift secondary to fluid loss, brain swelling, or tumor resection, or a combination of these factors, allowed for much more accurate resections. Coupling this new information with fMRI or electroencephalography enabled surgery on tumors otherwise thought to be inoperable due to potential involvement of eloquent cortex.

◆ Neurobiopsy

Looking back over the history of neurobiopsy, what initially involved freehand approaches subsequently progressed to skull-mounted trajectory guides. Such systems were employed in the setting of biplane fluoroscopy, the trajectories aligned in orthogonal planes toward markings on orthogonal views of plain film x-rays. Lesions identified on pneumoencephalography were targeted and biopsied. Unfortunately,

from the beginning, both approaches were limited by brain shift and by the blind nature of the approach, such that no valuable information was available about adjacent structures either along the trajectory or at the target. Needless to say, although tumors that were large and in relatively isolated areas, such as the frontal or parietal lobes, could be easily accessed with little collateral injury, the same could not be said of pineal region tumors where adjacent venous structures offered significant opportunities for injury and potentially fatal intracranial hemorrhage.

Subsequent developments of frame-based stereotactic biopsy offered the advantage of being very accurate, but could not overcome the potential risks to the patient. Rather, with the advent of the CT scanner, the neurosurgeon would finally be able to carefully plan a safe trajectory, avoiding critical vascular and other structures. Nevertheless, brain shift could potentially override such planning and complications could still occur. Moreover, frame-based techniques were and are compromised by significant patient discomfort during frame placement, the need of preoperative imaging and associated delays from the time of imaging to the time of the procedure, and the persistent "blind" nature of the procedure, as the needle passes through the brain.

With the introduction of frameless stereotaxy, at least the invasive nature of the stereotactic frame would be obviated. Other disadvantages, however, persisted. Thus it would not be until the advent of true intraoperative imaging, initially by ultrasound, subsequently by CT, and most recently, by MRI, that surgeons would be able to "see" what they are doing real-time or in near real-time. Finally, surgeons were offered the potential to overcome the potential inaccuracies created by brain shift.

iMRI-guided brain biopsy in the GE mid-field system, in particular, presented several advantages.[20] First, with the ability to visualize both the target and the biopsy needle (by its signal void), the frame and/or frameless fiducial markers could be obviated. Surgeons could finally directly visualize the lesion, the needle, and the trajectory. In addition, for the first time, in an interactive manner, lesions in the brain could be sampled in real time, with direct observation of the biopsy needle entering the target, in orthogonal planes, ensuring accurate localization. Tissue sampling from the target could be confirmed by visual inspection of the needle. Upon biopsy needle withdrawal, MRI now offered immediate feedback to the surgeon with regard to potential biopsy-induced tumoral hemorrhage. Finally, pathophysiologic imaging (i.e., MR spectroscopy) offered surgeons the opportunity to sample tissue based on the ratio of phosphocholine/creatinine and N-acetylaspartate (NAA) levels in the most aggressive areas of the tumor, thus avoiding misdiagnosis due to internal heterogeneity of gliomas.[21] iMRI biopsy has proved to be safe and accurate.

◆ Resection Guidance

Although iMRI-guidance simplified and enhanced the safety of neurobiopsy, it was with respect to surgical guidance of tumor resection that the new mid-field system and subsequent systems truly offered a quantum leap. In the mid-field system, the neurosurgeon could visualize intraoperative changes that may occur in the cortex, white matter, or deep-seated structures in relation to the lesion.[22,23] Whether by freehand or by use of adjunctive frameless stereotaxy, surgeons now had the opportunity to update their geographic understanding of their progress and the location of residual tumor. Surgeon after surgeon, upon learning to operate in the MR environment, came to understand and rely on the probability of residual tumor by MR signature when their own visual inspection had suggested a complete resection. This was a truly revolutionary and "eureka" moment for neurosurgeons, and iMRI-guided neurosurgery had rightfully claimed its place as a defining moment in the history of neurosurgery.

Progression of surgery could now be followed objectively by the surgeon,[1] and the global status of the brain could now be assessed for potential intraoperative complications, such as intracerebral hemorrhage, cerebral edema, hydrocephalus, etc. Auxiliary adjuncts of iMRI such as perfusion MRI, diffusion MRI, MRA, and MR venography (MRV) were added to various systems, depending on field strength, and were able to demonstrate intraoperative vascular ischemia. iMRI thus not only reflected surgical anatomy, it also yielded information about the functional integrity and dynamic changes in the course of surgery, allowing the surgeon to alter his or her surgery accordingly.

◆ Establishing Degree of Resection

As noted earlier, the most important advance of mid-field (MRI) in neuroncologic surgery was in its potential to reveal to the neurosurgeon the degree of tumor resection at any point during the surgery. In particular, surgeons came to understand that resection of gliomas based only on direct visualization, even if assisted by the operating microscope, is usually incomplete.[24,25] The tumor contour is irregular. In the case of high-grade glioma, the adjacent brain is often invaded by tumor, making complete resection difficult at best. In the case of low-grade glioma, as is well known to neurosurgeons, the definition of tumor from normal brain becomes indistinct. Additionally, surgeons and patients would come to benefit from the ability to overcome brain shift, as iMRI could reveal tumoral rests allowing for more complete resection. Finally, with improvements in multimodality image registration during iMRI-guided tumor resection, tumors situated on or adjacent to eloquent cortices could be approached with improved safety.

Intraaxial Neoplasms

Although there is no class I evidence yet, several recent articles[25–32] suggest that the degree of resection of both high- and low-grade gliomas correlates with both progression-free and overall survival rates. Lacroix et al have suggested that the degree of resection of glioblastomas should be greater than 98% to have a significant survival advantage.[29] In another glioblastoma study,[32] a residual volume of less than 10 cm^3

represented a significant factor influencing the 1-year survival rate. Concerning low-grade gliomas, the extent of resection was found to be a statistically significant predictive factor in two recent prospective studies[33,34] and three retrospective studies.[35–37] The same may be true for predictive patients harboring low-grade gliomas,[38] and for adult patients with brain metastases.[39]

Real-time intraoperative information regarding the surgical fields offers valuable information to the surgeon concerning residual tumor. iMRI, as confirmed from all published series, improves the degree of resection of intraaxial tumors and is optimized when coupled with intraoperatively updated neuronavigation.[1,40–42]

Patient selection for intraaxial resection under iMRI guidance is based on

1. The location and nature of the lesion
2. Relationship to eloquent brain cortices
3. Deep white matter or nuclei location for which the trajectory of the approach needs to be optimized
4. Small lesions that might be difficult to locate accurately
5. Anticipated macroscopic appearance difficult to distinguish from normal brain

iMRI-guided tumor resection also mandated a new level of collaboration between neurosurgeons and neuroradiologists. Whereas preoperative and delayed postoperative MRI is typically fairly straightforward at distinguishing tumor from normal brain, iMRI presented two new diagnostic challenges: (1) differentiation of tumor from operative changes due to local operative hemorrhage; and (2) with imaging often taking place in a delayed fashion relative to contrast administration, MR signatures on turbo fluid attenuation inversion recovery (turboFLAIR) and contrast administration would become more complicated. In particular, local imbibition of contrast would pose such a significant diagnostic dilemma that the administration of contrast would be avoided until absolutely necessary. Thus the interpretation of intraoperative control of tumor resection now differed substantially from that of standard diagnostic imaging.

As noted above, surgical resection in and around eloquent cortices under local anesthesia can be performed within the iMRI setting safely with direct cortical and subcortical stimulation. At the Brigham and Women's Hospital, ~40% of tumor cases have been completed under intravenous sedation anesthesia.

Extraaxial Neoplasms

Although the benefits of iMRI-guidance are easy to understand in the setting of intraaxial neoplasm, such benefits have not been intuitively obvious with regard to extraaxial tumors. These benefits are more intangible, related to improved surgical planning, intraoperative monitoring of brain alterations, degree of resection, and potential complications. Additionally, iMRI has been of particular value in the transsphenoidal approach for pituitary surgery and in some skull base approaches.

In transsphenoidal surgery, surgeons are faced with the decision, "when is enough." As the standard transsphenoidal approach does not permit complete visualization of suprasellar and parasellar spaces, surgeons must hope that any suprasellar components will fall into the field of view with the progress of surgery. Regrettably, often after initial resection, some tumor remnants can be difficult to identify. In particular, as a result of collapse and folding of the tumor, the pseudocapsule may collapse and/or fold on itself. Similarly, intratumoral fibrous septations may also compromise visual understanding of the tumor.

With the advent of the mid-field and other systems, iMRI has demonstrated its record of safety. In particular, during transsphenoidal surgery, surgeons now can objectively assess the extent of their resection of pituitary adenoma.[11,13,43–47] In fact, iMRI has revealed that residual tumor is visible and would have otherwise not been recognized in ~40% of cases. A combination of endoscopy or extended transsphenoidal approach with iMRI may further advance the efficiency and safety of transsphenoidal surgery.

In the case of skull base tumors, iMRI offers the surgeon information on the distance from the tip of a surgical instrument to the tumor border, as well as the extent of residual tumor. Moroever, with the accommodation of intraoperative brain shift, iMRI allows for more rapid and safer tumor debulking of meningiomas and other skull base tumors that frequently extend around or displace major vessels and cranial nerves.

◆ Monitoring Complications

Lastly, at the end of the procedure, final imaging control can be performed in situ, to exclude immediate operative and perioperative complications. These include the development of diffuse cerebral edema, intracerebral hemorrhage, acute hydrocephalus, and cerebral ischemia. A tailored exam with dedicated MR pulse sequences such as gradient echo or susceptibility-weighted imaging, in particular, is helpful to identify procedural hemorrhage. Diffusion-weighted imaging is also generally diapositive of questions regarding cerebral infarction. Additionally, the final round of iMRI obviates the need for postoperative imaging as a routine practice prior to hospital discharge. Although not the most significant component of the patient's care model, imaging immediately upon completion of the surgery is likely to expedite hospital discharge, and with it, minimize hospital costs in the face of diagnosis-related group (DRG) driven reimbursements.

◆ Conclusions

The GE Signa system was the pioneering mid-field iMRI system that essentially turned the MR suite into an operating room. Because of its relatively low-field strength it allowed real-time navigation, immediate confirmation of result, and multiple updates. Many important contributions were made by multiple investigators using this system. However, the field of iMRI was developed on multiple platforms; ultimately, the field appears to have bifurcated into very low-field systems – typically more ergonomic relative to the patient and the surgeon, yet constrained by MR rules of image signal to noise ratio, hence image quality, relative to field strength – and high-field systems that afford advanced imaging despite the physical constraints of such systems.

References

1. Black PM, Moriarty T, Alexander E III, et al. Development and implementation of intraoperative magnetic resonance imaging and its neurosurgical applications. Neurosurgery 1997;41(4):831–842, discussion 842–845

2. Hill DL, Maurer CR Jr, Maciunas RJ, Barwise JA, Fitzpatrick JM, Wang MY. Measurement of intraoperative brain surface deformation under a craniotomy. Neurosurgery 1998;43(3):514–526, discussion 527–528

3. Maurer CR Jr, Hill DL, Martin AJ, et al. Investigation of intraoperative brain deformation using a 1.5-T interventional MR system: preliminary results. IEEE Trans Med Imaging 1998;17(5):817–825

4. Hata N, Nabavi A, Wells WM III, et al. Three-dimensional optical flow method for measurement of volumetric brain deformation from intraoperative MR images. J Comput Assist Tomogr 2000;24(4):531–538

5. Nimsky C, Ganslandt O, Hastreiter P, Fahlbusch R. Intraoperative compensation for brain shift. Surg Neurol 2001;56(6):357–364, discussion 364–365

6. Nabavi A, Black PM, Gering DT, et al. Serial intraoperative magnetic resonance imaging of brain shift. Neurosurgery 2001;48(4):787–797, discussion 797–798

7. Reinges MH, Nguyen HH, Krings T, Hütter BO, Rohde V, Gilsbach JM. Course of brain shift during microsurgical resection of supratentorial cerebral lesions: limits of conventional neuronavigation. Acta Neurochir (Wien) 2004;146(4):369–377, discussion 377

8. Hartkens T, Hill DL, Castellano-Smith AD, et al. Measurement and analysis of brain deformation during neurosurgery. IEEE Trans Med Imaging 2003;22(1):82–92

9. Hinks RS, Bronskill MJ, Kucharczyk W, Bernstein M, Collick BD, Henkelman RM. MR systems for image-guided therapy. J Magn Reson Imaging 1998;8(1):19–25

10. Tronnier VM, Wirtz CR, Knauth M, et al. Intraoperative diagnostic and interventional magnetic resonance imaging in neurosurgery. Neurosurgery 1997;40(5):891–900, discussion 900–902

11. Steinmeier R, Fahlbusch R, Ganslandt O, et al. Intraoperative magnetic resonance imaging with the Magnetom open scanner: concepts, neurosurgical indications, and procedures: a preliminary report. Neurosurgery 1998;43(4):739–747, discussion 747–748

12. Hall WA, Liu H, Martin AJ, Pozza CH, Maxwell RE, Truwit CL. Safety, efficacy, and functionality of high-field strength interventional magnetic resonance imaging for neurosurgery. Neurosurgery 2000;46(3):632–641, discussion 641–642

13. Lewin JS. Interventional MR imaging: concepts, systems, and applications in neuroradiology. AJNR Am J Neuroradiol 1999;20(5):735–748

14. Chu RM, Tummala RP, Hall WA. Intraoperative magnetic resonance image-guided neurosurgery. Neurosurg Q 2003;13(4):234–250

15. Hall WA. The safety and efficacy of stereotactic biopsy for intracranial lesions. Cancer 1998;82(9):1749–1755

16. Albayrak B, Samdani AF, Black PM. Intra-operative magnetic resonance imaging in neurosurgery. Acta Neurochir (Wien) 2004;146(6):543–556, discussion 557

17. Bohinski RJ, Kokkino AK, Warnick RE, et al. Glioma resection in a shared-resource magnetic resonance operating room after optimal image-guided frameless stereotactic resection. Neurosurgery 2001;48(4):731–742, discussion 742–744

18. Hadani M, Spiegelman R, Feldman Z, Berkenstadt H, Ram Z. Novel, compact, intraoperative magnetic resonance imaging-guided system for conventional neurosurgical operating rooms. Neurosurgery 2001;48(4):799–807, discussion 807–809

19. Hata N, Piper S, Jolesz FA, et al. Application of open source image guided therapy software in MR-guided therapies. Med Image Comput Comput Assist Interv 2007;10(Pt 1):491–498

20. Mittal S, Black PM. Intraoperative magnetic resonance imaging in neurosurgery: the Brigham concept. Acta Neurochir Suppl 2006;98:77–86

21. Hall WA, Martin AJ, Liu H, Nussbaum ES, Maxwell RE, Truwit CL. Brain biopsy using high-field strength interventional magnetic resonance imaging. Neurosurgery 1999;44(4):807–813, discussion 813–814 Review

22. Ganslandt O, Steinmeier R, Kober H, et al. Magnetic source imaging combined with image-guided frameless stereotaxy: a new method in surgery around the motor strip. Neurosurgery 1997;41(3):621–627, discussion 627–628

23. Jolesz FA, Kikinis R, Talos IF. Neuronavigation in interventional MR imaging. Frameless stereotaxy. Neuroimaging Clin N Am 2001;11(4):685–693, ix ix.

24. Albert FK, Forsting M, Sartor K, Adams HP, Kunze S. Early postoperative magnetic resonance imaging after resection of malignant glioma: objective evaluation of residual tumor and its influence on regrowth and prognosis. Neurosurgery 1994;34(1):45–60, discussion 60–61

25. Berger MS, Deliganis AV, Dobbins J, Keles GE. The effect of extent of resection on recurrence in patients with low grade cerebral hemisphere gliomas. Cancer 1994;74(6):1784–1791

26. Daneyemez M, Gezen F, Canakçi Z, Kahraman S. Radical surgery and reoperation in supratentorial malignant glial tumors. Minim Invasive Neurosurg 1998;41(4):209–213

27. Devaux BC, O'Fallon JR, Kelly PJ. Resection, biopsy, and survival in malignant glial neoplasms. A retrospective study of clinical parameters, therapy, and outcome. J Neurosurg 1993;78(5):767–775

28. Keles GE, Lamborn KR, Berger MS. Low-grade hemispheric gliomas in adults: a critical review of extent of resection as a factor influencing outcome. J Neurosurg 2001;95(5):735–745 Review

29. Lacroix M, Abi-Said D, Fourney DR, et al. A multivariate analysis of 416 patients with glioblastoma multiforme: prognosis, extent of resection, and survival. J Neurosurg 2001;95(2):190–198

30. Laws ER, Shaffrey ME, Morris A, Anderson FA Jr. Surgical management of intracranial gliomas—does radical resection improve outcome? Acta Neurochir Suppl (Wien) 2003;85:47–53

31. Mäurer M, Becker G, Wagner R, et al. Early postoperative transcranial sonography (TCS), CT, and MRI after resection of high grade glioma: evaluation of residual tumour and its influence on prognosis. Acta Neurochir (Wien) 2000;142(10):1089–1097

32. Keles GE, Lamborn KR, Chang SM, Prados MD, Berger MS. Volume of residual disease as a predictor of outcome in adult patients with recurrent supratentorial glioblastomas multiforme who are undergoing chemotherapy. J Neurosurg 2004;100(1):41–46

33. Pignatti F, van den Bent M, Curran D, et al; European Organization for Research and Treatment of Cancer Brain Tumor Cooperative Group; European Organization for Research and Treatment of Cancer Radiotherapy Cooperative Group. Prognostic factors for survival in adult patients with cerebral low-grade glioma. J Clin Oncol 2002;20(8):2076–2084

34. Shaw E, Arusell R, Scheithauer B, et al. Prospective randomized trial of low- versus high-dose radiation therapy in adults with supratentorial low-grade glioma: initial report of a North Central Cancer Treatment Group/Radiation Therapy Oncology Group/Eastern Cooperative Oncology Group study. J Clin Oncol 2002;20(9):2267–2276

35. Hanzély Z, Polgár C, Fodor J, et al. Role of early radiotherapy in the treatment of supratentorial WHO Grade II astrocytomas: long-term results of 97 patients. J Neurooncol 2003;63(3):305–312

36. Jeremic B, Milicic B, Grujicic D, et al. Hyperfractionated radiation therapy for incompletely resected supratentorial low-grade glioma: a 10-year update of a phase II study. Int J Radiat Oncol Biol Phys 2003; 57(2):465–471

37. Lo SS, Hall WA, Cho KH, Orner J, Lee CK, Dusenbery KE. Radiation dose response for supratentorial low-grade glioma—institutional experience and literature review. J Neurol Sci 2003;214(1-2):43–48

38. Pollack IF, Claassen D, al-Shboul Q, Janosky JE, Deutsch M. Low-grade gliomas of the cerebral hemispheres in children: an analysis of 71 cases. J Neurosurg 1995;82(4):536–547

39. Lagerwaard FJ, Levendag PC, Nowak PJ, Eijkenboom WM, Hanssens PE, Schmitz PI. Identification of prognostic factors in patients with brain metastases: a review of 1292 patients. Int J Radiat Oncol Biol Phys 1999;43(4):795–803 Review

40. Wirtz CR, Knauth M, Staubert A, et al. Clinical evaluation and follow-up results for intraoperative magnetic resonance imaging in neurosurgery. Neurosurgery 2000;46(5):1112–1120, discussion 1120–1122

41. Nimsky C, Ganslandt O, von Keller B, Fahlbusch R. Preliminary experience in glioma surgery with intraoperative high-field MRI. Acta Neurochir Suppl (Wien) 2003;88:21–29

42. Bergsneider M, Sehati N, Villablanca P, McArthur DL, Becker DP, Liau LM. Mahaley Clinical Research Award: extent of glioma resection using low-field (0.2 T) versus high-field (1.5 T) intraoperative MRI and image-guided frameless neuronavigation. Clin Neurosurg 2005; 52:389–399

43. Sutherland GR, Kaibara T, Louw D, Hoult DI, Tomanek B, Saunders J. A mobile high-field magnetic resonance system for neurosurgery. J Neurosurg 1999;91(5):804–813

44. Bernstein M, Al-Anazi AR, Kucharczyk W, Manninen P, Bronskill M, Henkelman M. Brain tumor surgery with the Toronto open magnetic resonance imaging system: preliminary results for 36 patients and analysis of advantages, disadvantages, and future prospects. Neurosurgery 2000;46(4):900–907, discussion 907–909

45. Kaibara T, Saunders JK, Sutherland GR. Advances in mobile intraoperative magnetic resonance imaging. Neurosurgery 2000;47(1):131–137, discussion 137–138

46. Schwartz RB, Hsu L, Wong TZ, et al. Intraoperative MR imaging guidance for intracranial neurosurgery: experience with the first 200 cases. Radiology 1999;211(2):477–488 Review

47. Fahlbusch R, Ganslandt O, Buchfelder M, Schott W, Nimsky C. Intraoperative magnetic resonance imaging during transsphenoidal surgery. J Neurosurg 2001;95(3):381–390

3

High-Field Suite Design

Charles L. Truwit, Yogesh Kumar, and Walter A. Hall

Since its inception in 1994, intraoperative magnetic resonance imaging-guided (iMRI-) neurosurgery has emerged from its multifaceted beginnings into an accepted approach benefitting patients suffering from brain tumors as well as those requiring functional neurosurgery. Although iMRI suites are not yet commonplace, they have been implemented in many centers, with dozens more in the planning and building stages. In the early years of the mid-1990s a variety of suites were conceived; with them, a variety of MR field strengths, ranging from 0.12 to 1.5 T. More recently, 3 T suites have been implemented. In this chapter, considerations around suites operating at 1.5 T and 3.0 T will be presented.

Fundamental to any such consideration is the issue of what one is trying to achieve. Specifically, if the intraoperative MR scanner is to be used largely for monitoring tumor resection, for updating surgical guidance systems, and for post-operative tumor and tumor bed assessment, the MR scanner, suite geometry, and patient accessibility are less important. In these scenarios, either the tabletop of the surgical table or the entire surgical table itself must be MR-compatible. The surgical-patient interaction is handled outside the 5 Gauss line, and either the patient is moved into the scanner or the scanner is moved over the patient in order to image during surgery.

An alternative scenario affords surgery within the 5 Gauss line, typically, immediately adjacent to the scanner, but also within the confines of the scanner. In such a configuration, all of the procedures enabled in the first scenario are still possible. In addition, however, minimally-invasive procedures driven by real-time MR imaging, rather than periodically updated frameless stereotaxy, become a major component of the workload. Nevertheless, there are tradeoffs: scanner access dictates few degrees of freedom for the surgical table and the use of strictly MR-compatible surgical instruments becomes mandatory.

A variation of both scenarios puts not only the MR suite adjacent to the surgical suite, but houses additional imaging equipment, such as a PET-CT or a biplane angiography suite. These set-ups blur the distinction between the first and second scenarios because the MR-suite is enabled to perform surgery and minimally-invasive procedures as in scenario 2.

iMRI-guided neurosurgery started at the Brigham and Women's Hospital in 1994 using the Signa SP (General Electric Medical Systems, Waukesha, WI).[1] That system involved two cylindrical magnets to create inversely overlapping external magnetic fields between the two magnets, such that an imaging volume was created between the two magnet bores. The system's principal advantage rested with the patient and surgeon's hands being situated within the imaging volume, allowing for "real-time" and "continuous" MR imaging during the surgery (**Fig. 3.1**). The GE Signa SP was the only such system ever developed, until the very low-field PoleStar (now owned by Medtronic Surgical Navigation, Inc., Louisville, CO) system, which theoretically allowed for similar access.[2] The original PoleStar included an MRI-compatible, but otherwise essentially standard surgical table, and two mobile magnets that could be elevated from the floor to the lateral head position (**Fig. 3.2**). Although the scanner operated at very low field (0.12 T), limited field of view imaging was possible. All subsequent systems have focused on moving the patient in and out of the scanner or moving the scanner in and out of the surgical theater.[3-12]

At the University of Minnesota, in conjunction with Philips Healthcare (Andover, MA), the first comprehensive clinical approach to iMRI at high field strength (1.5 T) was undertaken; that suite opened in late 1996.[6,7] To date, over 1,100 neurosurgeries have been performed. The Minnesota suite consists of an MR diagnostic and surgical suite that combines the capabilities of a 1.5T scanner and C-arm DSA unit with the strict requirements of a neurosurgical suite (**Fig. 3.3**). In short, in the morning, a brain tumor resection can be undertaken, and in the afternoon, routine diagnostic MR imaging can be performed.

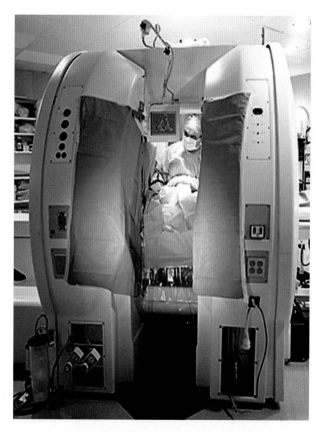

Fig. 3.1 GE Signa SP (double donut; General Electric Medical Systems, Waukesha, WI) was installed in 1994 as the first intraoperative magnetic resonance imaging scanner, operating at 0.5 tesla. Note the neurosurgeon standing between the two poles of the magnet. Patient is draped such that surgical access can be achieved from either side.

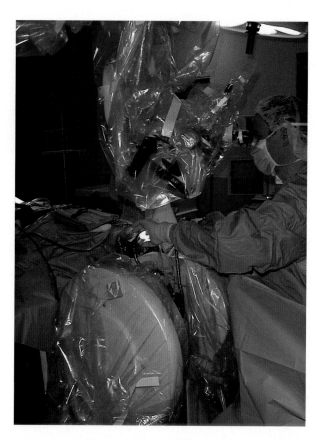

Fig. 3.2 Medtronic (Medtronic Surgical Navigation, Inc., Louisville, CO) PoleStar low-field MRI scanner operates at 0.12 tesla. Note the neurosurgical access from above the patient's head.

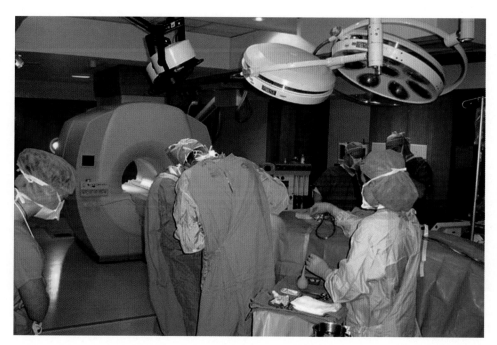

Fig. 3.3 **(A)** Philips Intera 1.5 tesla scanner intraoperative magnetic resonance imaging suite at the University of Minnesota. Surgery can be performed safely outside the 5 gauss line. Patient can be shuttled into the scanner by means of a tabletop transfer from the surgical side of the suite to the MRI table and into the scanner. (*Continued on page 20*)

A

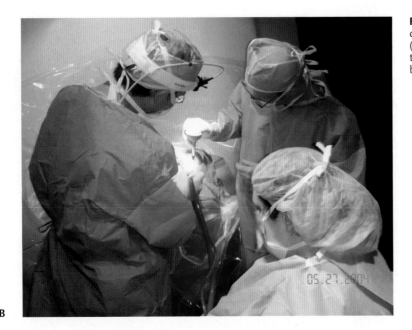

B

Fig. 3.3 (*Continued*) **(B)** Alternatively, procedures can be performed from the rear of the scanner (Philips 3.0T Intera), with direct neurosurgical access to the patient's head. The patient can be introduced back into the scanner for imaging.

At the University of Minnesota Center for MR-guided Therapy, a range of neurosurgeries are possible, including full craniotomy for tumor resection (**Fig. 3.4**), neurobiopsy (**Fig. 3.5**), neurostimulator, depth electrode (**Fig. 3.6**), and Ommaya reservoir placement. Over the past 12 years, advanced neuroimaging has been introduced to varying degrees at the Minnesota site and at other 1.5 T sites, including diffusion tensor fiber tracking, functional brain MR imaging, MR spectroscopy (**Fig. 3.7**), and MR angiography.[13] These advances have afforded more specific approaches, including

MR spectroscopic-targeted biopsy (**Fig. 3.8**) and intraoperative surgical planning to avoid white matter injury when resecting tumors.

At the Foothills Hospital in Calgary, in partnership with Interventional MR Imaging Systems (IMRIS, Winnipeg, Manitoba, Canada), another 1.5 T program was initiated, contemporaneous to that of the University of Minnesota. In Calgary, a neurosurgical suite was built in which an ancillary MR room was created to garage a mobile 1.5 T scanner.[4] The IMRIS approach was one of a fixed patient and a mobile

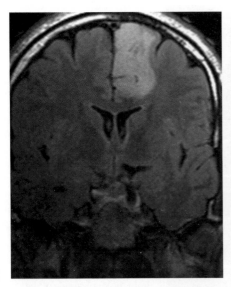 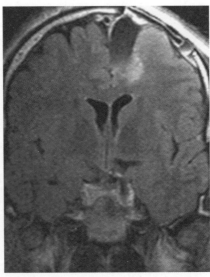 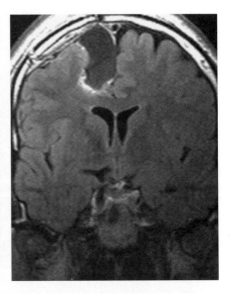

A–C

Fig. 3.4 **(A)** Preoperative coronal turbo fluid attenuation inversion recovery magnetic resonance image (turbo FLAIR MRI) of a low-grade glioma of the left superior frontal gyrus. **(B)** Intraoperative image reveals residual tumor left along inferolateral aspect of tumor bed. **(C)** Postoperative image shows complete tumor resection.

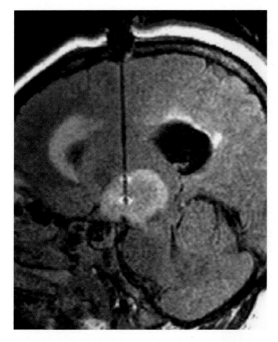

Fig. 3.5 Sagittal turbo fluid attenuation inversion recovery magnetic resonance image (turbo FLAIR MRI) obtained with patient at isocenter of the scanner bore. Note thin signal void of needle apparently within the tumor bed. Orthogonal image (not shown) confirms successful intratumoral placement. Needle artifact it minimized by placement of needle along main magnetic field (B_0) and by reversing the read gradient against the direction of B_0. Typical artifact at needle tip confirms such orientation.

scanner (**Fig. 3.9**), much like a rad/fluoro unit, suspended from the ceiling. Initially, the IMRIS system used a proprietary scanner with a third-party front end. This has evolved over time, such that today, the IMRIS system is installed with either a short-bore 1.5 T Espree (SiemensAG, Erlangen, Germany) or a 3 T Trio (Siemens, at one site).

Common to nearly all sites undertaking iMRI is an emphasis on minimally invasive surgical access. This emphasis has been addressed along two pathways. First, by the development of MRI-compatible optical tracking systems (frameless stereotaxy) to perform surgical targeting and track surgical instruments, surgeries can be performed with nearly real-time imaging. In this scenario, frameless stereotaxy datasets can be obtained nearly ad hoc, allowing for intraoperative updating of the datasets to overcome issues of brain shift. This approach has offered a relatively painless entry into iMRI for sites entering this field.

A second approach focuses on the next level of surgical access: truly prospective MRI-guidance. Two major approaches to this concept emerged. The first, pioneered at the Brigham and Women's Hospital in Boston, involved merging prospective (real-time) data with retrospective data. That incredibly novel approach led to the development of the three-dimensional (3D-) slicer (**Fig. 3.10**) that rapidly imports a real-time localizer (three cross-secting planes) into the previously obtained frameless stereotactic volume.[14] Immediate reregistration of optical or other frameless stereotaxy is automated. Thus surgeons can operate and watch their dataset update at the same time.

The second approach, developed at the University of Minnesota, was entirely prospective.[15] Uniquely, this approach employed the actively acquired MR image to create and align a surgical trajectory. No extra hardware or software was required, as it could be performed using almost any imaging sequence. Since time ultimately became a rate-limiting factor, a HASTE or a very rapid T1-weighted image (if contrast was needed) sequence was employed, with image acquisition at one to two frames per second. Prospective stereotaxy required the use of an MR-visible pen or stylus, which in the

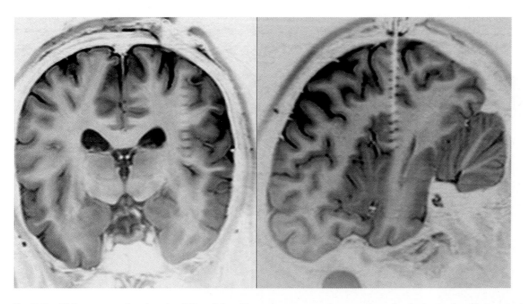

Fig. 3.6 Oblique coronal and sagittal T1-weighted inversion recovery images show depth electrode with terminal centimeter within posterior aspect of heterotopic gray matter. Metal artifact is well-contained by working largely parallel to the Bolton point.

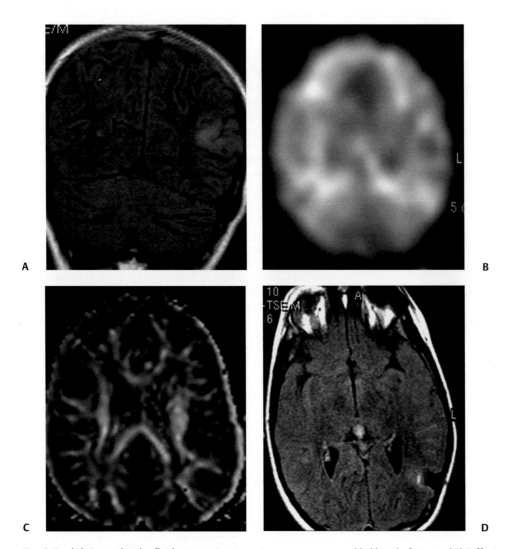

Fig. 3.7 **(A)** Coronal turbo fluid attenuation inversion recovery magnetic resonance image (turbo FLAIR MRI) reveals abnormal hyperintensity of left superior temporal gyrus. **(B)** Corresponding hyperintensity on choline map of MR spectroscopy exam confirms likelihood of tumor. **(C)** Diffusion tensor image shows relative displacement of U-fibers, suggesting a less invasive nature of the tumor. **(D)** Postoperative axial turboFLAIR MRI shows complete resection of low-grade astrocytoma.

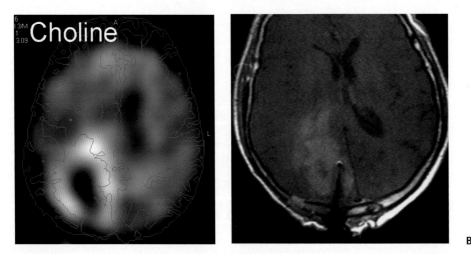

Fig. 3.8 **(A)** Choline map of patient with right occipital lesion shows hyperintensity peripherally. **(B)** Note medial placement of needle within area corresponding to choline hyperintensity. Biopsy revealed recurrent glioma.

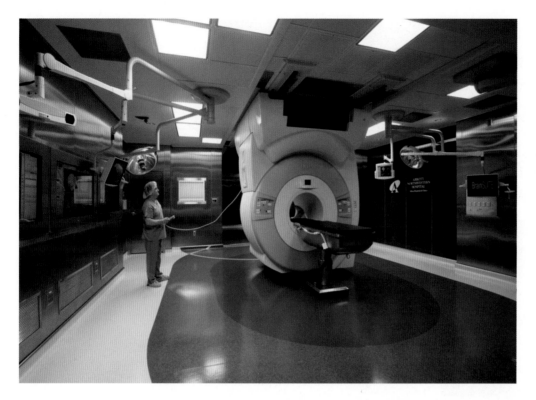

Fig. 3.9 IMRIS suite (IMRIS, Winnipeg, Manitoba, Canada). Note scanner suspended from ceiling rails. (Courtesy of Abbott/NW Hospital, Minneapolis, MN.)

Minnesota suite was performed with the use of the Navigus (Medtronic-IGN, Melbourne, FL), also developed at the University of Minnesota.[16] The Navigus is a skull-mounted ball-and-socket device that is entirely MR-compatible and whose alignment stem is MR-visible.

Beyond neurobiopsy and routine minimally-invasive procedures, functional neurosurgeries, such as cingulotomy, capsulotomy, depth electrode placement, and most notably, neurostimulator placement for the treatment of tremor and Parkinson's disease, have been performed under MR-guidance.[17] With the introduction of the Navigus, cingulotomy and depth electrode placement have become simple and efficient procedures.

Deep brain stimulation (DBS) of the thalamic ventral intermediate nucleus (VIM) and subthalamic nuclei (STN) have become acceptable clinical options for the treatment of essential tremor and Parkinson's disease, respectively. In general, DBS placement is a safer and more controlled therapy than irreversible thermal ablation. Neurosurgeons at the University of Minnesota were the first to report success in iMRI-guided neurostimulator placement, initially in the thalamus for amelioration of essential tremor, and subsequently, into the subthalamus for the treatment of Parkinson's disease. Those cases were the first to demonstrate the benefits of imaging for targeting *after* placement of burr hole(s) to allow for potential brain shift prior to targeting.

Subsequently, investigators at the University of California, San Francisco successfully implanted DBS leads entirely under MRI-guidance.[17,18] Using a next generation Navigus, thus eliminating the cumbersome stereotactic frame and making this procedure considerably less time-intensive, neurosurgeons perform the procedure entirely at the "back end" of, and inside, the MRI scanner (**Fig. 3.13**). This accomplishment effectively demonstrated the potential "disruptive technology" nature of iMRI as the driver of the procedure and opened the door to additional minimally invasive therapies, such as MRI-guided targeted drug delivery procedures.

Another important development regarding high-field iMRI suites (including the Minnesota Suite, the IMRIS suite of suites, and minimally invasive procedures at the back end of the scanner) was the introduction of higher-field suites at 3 T. At the National Institutes of Health, investigators successfully performed prostate ablation under MRI-guidance, using a Philips 3 T system. Shortly thereafter, in 2004, the Minnesota team introduced its second, modified iMRI-guided neurosurgery suite, outfitted with a Philips 3 T MRI scanner.[19,20] Subsequent 3 T neurosurgical systems were introduced in 2006 (NIH – Philips, Barrow Institute – GE) and 2008 (Foothills – IMRIS).

Over the first 15 years, iMRI has seen many approaches and has been performed at many field strengths. Today, the primary evolutionary process has largely ended. In 2009, thus, high-field iMRI is available at both 1.5 T and 3 T using cylindrical, short-bore MRI scanners. Three principal suites are now commercially available from Philips, General Electric,

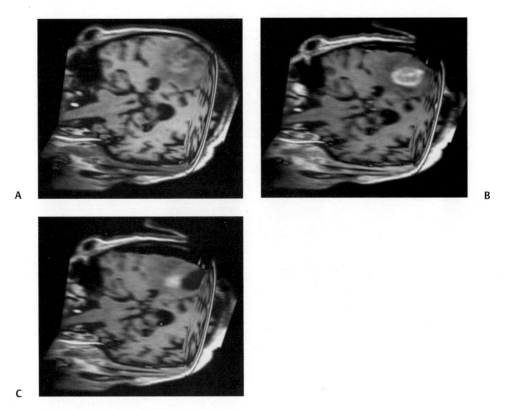

Fig. 3.10 Three-dimensional slicer. **(A)** Cross-sectional reference scans are spliced into preoperative volume scan for purposes of registration. Updated reference scans demonstrate progressive brain shift following **(B)** opening of dura and **(C)** subsequent dural closure.

and Siemens. The latter is primarily available through IM-RIS, although Siemens will outfit a suite without IMRIS, and IMRIS will apparently offer a Philips or General Electric scanner if requested. Philips offers its suite in partnership with BrainLab.

No further substantive efforts are being made at mid-field strength, although a few legacy Signa-SP and other systems are still in operation. At low field, however, the Medtronic PoleStar system continues to provide a lower cost alternative.

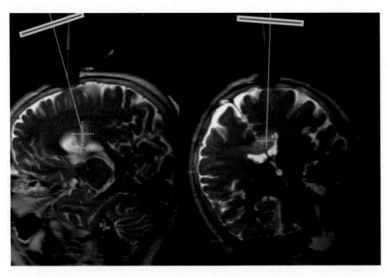

Fig. 3.11 Prospective stereotaxy: starting at the biopsy site, a targeting line is drawn out through a pivot point of the Navigus (Image-Guided Neurologics, Melbourne, FL) trajectory guide. Note that the alignment stem is not yet aligned in either the oblique **(A)** sagittal or **(B)** coronal plane. Image plane (*yellow* in **[A,B]**) is set normal to trajectory lines.

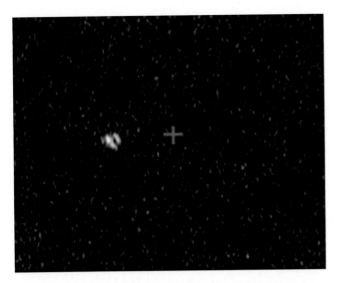

c

Fig. 3.11 (*Continued*) **(C)** reveals the cross section of the alignment stem and the proposed targeting point. The alignment stem is repositioned prospectively using live magnetic resonance (MR) imaging. The trajectory is then set, the trajectory guide locked, and a confirmatory scan performed. Biopsy can then be performed either under MR guidance to watch the needle reach the target, or it can be performed at measured depth. (Courtesy of Medtronic-IGN, Melborne, FL.)

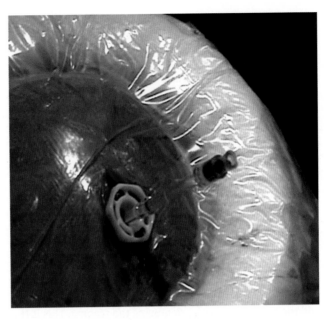

Fig. 3.12 Navigus (Medtronic-IGN, Melbourne, FL) is a skull mounted trajectory guide that uses a saline (or contrast-enhanced saline) filled stem for alignment with intended surgical pathway. Navigus may be inserted into a burr hole, as shown, or an external configuration, on the skull surface for use with twist drill. (Courtesy of Medtronic-IGN, Melbourne, FL.)

At high field, regardless of the scanner manufacturer, still under discussion is the question of the moving patient or the moving magnet. The latter is the approach first reported by the Calgary group. This concept derived from the neurosurgeon's desire to add imaging to the operating room without impacting the environment and more importantly, without moving the positioned surgical patient. To date, 10 such IMRIS systems have been installed; 10 more are due to be installed in 2009 and 2010. Clearly, the IMRIS approach has gained traction among neurosurgeons.

Although the initial installation was somewhat cumbersome, subsequent upgrades to the Siemens Espree (1.5 T) and Verio (3 T) systems and improvements in shimming technology have afforded relatively rapid deployment of the scanner so as to minimize the impact on the duration of surgery. These systems afford full functionality MR imaging in a 70 cm bore. As the scanner is suspended from a ceiling mounted rail system, when not in use, the scanner is garaged away from the surgical field, thus permitting full operating room capabilities, including the use of non-MRI safe surgical cutlery and electrical devices. When needed for intraoperative or postoperative scanning, the patient is cleared of all ferromagnetic material, the magnet ferried into the operative field and over the patient's previously positioned head (or spine), and images obtained. Once completed, the scanner is again ferried to the magnet garage.

Reports to date address the value of the IMRIS approach in surgical planning, monitoring of tumor resection, and assessing for surgical complications. Given the full functionality of the newer scanners, advanced imaging including diffusion tensor imaging and MR angiography (MRA) is available. Not yet reported, however, is the potential value of the IMRIS approach in functional neurosurgery and other minimally invasive surgeries. With the introduction of the new, 70 cm, short-bore Espree scanner, one can easily envision a range of such minimally invasive neurosurgeries in the IMRIS suites.

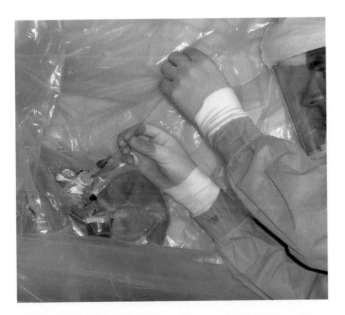

Fig. 3.13 Neurostimulator placement at the back end of a 1.5 tesla scanner: a neurosurgeon introduces a neurostimulator under sterile conditions through a skull-mounted access device. (Courtesy of Medtronic-IGN, Melbourne, FL.)

Fundamental to the IMRIS approach, of course, is the fact that positioned patients undergoing neurosurgery cannot, and should not be moved during the surgery.[4] This assumption further holds that patient safety is optimized as the patient is never moved. Although this may be intuitively obvious to some, there is a significant population of surgeons who do not necessarily subscribe to this tenet. Such dissenters could argue that surgeons often reposition patients in Trendelenburg and reverse Trendelenburg, as well as often roll (tilt) patient tables (and their patients) during surgical procedures, both to optimize surgical exposure and to alter cerebral blood flow dynamics. This does not seem substantively different from operating at the rear of the scanner (Philips) and sliding the patient into the bore ~1 to 3 feet to obtain an intraoperative MR image, or even from the various approaches of surgery beyond 5 gauss: in-line (Philips), rotating table (Siemens), and separate, mobile table (GE).[21–23]

Thus a second school of thought suggests it may be acceptable to move the patient a short distance rather than add the time and expense of moving the scanner. This is the approach taken initially in Minnesota and subsequently Los Angeles, California, Cleveland, Ohio, Erlangen, Germany (all initially at 0.2 T and subsequently at 1.5 T), and elsewhere. To date, these sites have reported considerable success without complications.

That said, the original equipment manufacturers (OEMs) have been reluctant to create an iMRI "product." Instead, during iMRI's first 15 years, only three such products have been sold: first, the GE Signa SP, which has been discontinued, involved a fixed magnet and a fixed patient. Second, IMRIS sold, and still sells, a ceiling-mounted high-field scanner that shuttles in and out of the surgical theater as needed. Finally, the very low-field (0.12 T) Medtronic Polestar system affords iMRI-guided intracranial procedures. All other systems have largely been shaped by the local investigators using off-the-shelf MRI scanners. Each OEM has developed system modifications that allow their off-the-shelf scanners to be used for iMRI, although nearly each site has slightly different such modifications.

The first of such OEM-modified systems was the Minnesota suite of 1996. That approach, described above, involved a 1.5 T short-bore scanner with an in-line surgical pedestal. To transfer the surgical patient from the surgical field (outside the 5 gauss line), the table was extended maximally toward the scanner, whereupon the table engaged the scanner couch and a mobile table top is shuttled toward, into, and occasionally partially out the back end of the scanner. The initial system utilized an angiography pedestal and a modified table top that satisfied both x-ray and MRI requirements. The principal weakness of this approach was that the pedestal and table offered neither significant Trendelenburg or reverse Trendelenburg positioning nor any lateral tilt (roll) potential. Regrettably, neither Philips, nor any third-party partner stepped forward to fulfill this need. Although several such systems were installed, and continue to be used today, the system remains at heart a noncommercial system.

What the Minnesota approach revealed, however, was that a fixed scanner and a mobile patient was feasible, and the safety of patients and surgical staff could be ensured. This revelation led to multiple similar approaches, most important of which was the Siemens rotating table approach for both 0.2 T and 1.5 T. That system involved a specially designed surgical pedestal placed just beyond the 5 gauss line. This pedestal allowed for much more positioning flexibility: Trendelenburg, reverse Trendelenburg positioning, and lateral tilt were now possible. In other words, a much more familiar surgical environment was available. Rapidly, these systems replaced earlier Siemens versions at the University of Erlangen and UCLA (Los Angeles, CA). Other, 0.2 T systems (Case Western, Cleveland, OH) also benefitted from the addition of the new surgical table. In Erlangen, the replacement of their 0.2 T system with a 1.5 T system afforded an entirely new level of imaging: not only high resolution and rapid scanning was possible with the 1.5 T system, now MRA, diffusion tractography, and fMRI became a routine part of intraoperative imaging.[13]

Finally, some investigators raised the bar again. Would it be possible for the full functionality of surgical tables to be implemented? Specifically, as in conventional operating theaters, would it be possible introduce tables that flex? Both GE and Philips did accept this challenge, teaming up with third-party surgical table vendors to develop variations on the earlier Minnesota-Philips in-line approach. Implementations of high-field suites with these tables have been seen in Rochester, Minnesota (GE) and Tokai, Japan (Philips).

Alternatively, the potential of operating completely at the back end of the scanner remains incompletely investigated. Despite success in Minnesota performing both minimally invasive procedures and full craniotomies at the back end, both at 1.5 T and 3 T (**Fig. 3.14**), few sites have challenged the OEMs either to standardize or to improve upon this approach. Strangely, an improved solution is possible, especially with newer wide-bore scanners, such as the Siemens Espree 1.5 T system. In principle, there is no substantive barrier to changing the MRI table insert to accommodate both a surgical head holder and table tilt. Potentially, in such wider-bore systems, a modest degree of Trendelenburg or reverse Trendelenburg positioning is also possible.

Despite these improvements, the OEMs have not fully embraced iMRI-guided neurosurgery. Indeed, by 2006, despite investigator enthusiasm, the market for this field appeared to be waning. For various reasons, this did not occur. Most significantly, with the introduction of the Siemens Espree, and its adoption by IMRIS as the flagship scanner, a rapid increase in sales of IMRIS systems has occurred. As noted above, over 20 such systems are either installed or being installed as of early 2009, leaving the OEMs scrambling to enter – or reenter – the iMRI market.

The IMRIS approach has evolved from its early implementation in Calgary. Today, five distinct surgical suites are offered. All include either one magnet bay that services various combinations of one or two operating rooms (ORs) to one OR and one MRI suite or one MRI suite (instead of a magnet bay) that services one or two ORs. The various

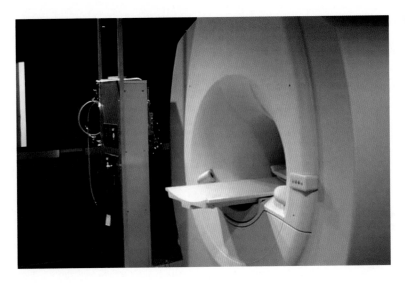

Fig. 3.14 Rear access to a 3.0 tesla Philips (Philips Healthcare, Andover, MA) Intera magnetic resonance imaging scanner. Note the table extension which gives neurosurgical access to patient. An anesthesia column sits just to left of the scanner.

configurations all include integrated audio and video, allowing for communications among the various team members, as well as recording and routing of audio-video sources, allowing for display of not only the MRI scans, but also the video feed from the surgical microscope, as well as hands-free telephone and intercom functions. What the IMRIS team offers is similar to that of the early GE Signa SP: a relatively complete package. Moreover, IMRIS has sought out MRI-compatible partners in lighting and displays that give their suites the feel of futuristic OR theaters.

iMRI-guided neurosurgery is now an accepted standard of care in some communities. In the Minnesota Greater Twin Cities region, for instance, there are, as of 2009, six high-field (1.5–3 T) installed and functional systems. Patients with infiltrating, intraaxial brain tumors can reasonably expect that their surgeries will be performed using MRI-guidance. Notwithstanding the economic downturn, it is not unreasonable to anticipate that such will become the standard in other communities. It will be interesting to see which approach – fixed patient with mobile scanner or fixed scanner with mobile patient – will emerge as the preferred solution.

References

1. Schenck JF, Jolesz FA, Roemer PB, et al. Superconducting open-configuration MR imaging system for image-guided therapy. Radiology 1995;195(3):805–814
2. Hadani M, Spiegelman R, Feldman Z, Berkenstadt H, Ram Z. Novel, compact, intraoperative magnetic resonance imaging-guided system for conventional neurosurgical operating rooms. Neurosurgery 2001;48(4):799–807, discussion 807–809
3. Black PM, Moriarty T, Alexander E III, et al. Development and implementation of intraoperative magnetic resonance imaging and its neurosurgical applications. Neurosurgery 1997;41(4):831–842, discussion 842–845
4. Sutherland GR, Kaibara T, Louw D, Hoult DI, Tomanek B, Saunders J. A mobile high-field magnetic resonance system for neurosurgery. J Neurosurg 1999;91(5):804–813
5. Fahlbusch R, Ganslandt O, Buchfelder M, Schott W, Nimsky C. Intraoperative magnetic resonance imaging during transsphenoidal surgery. J Neurosurg 2001;95(3):381–390
6. Hall WA, Martin AJ, Liu H, et al. High-field strength interventional magnetic resonance imaging for pediatric neurosurgery. Pediatr Neurosurg 1998;29(5):253–259
7. Hall WA, Liu H, Martin AJ, Pozza CH, Maxwell RE, Truwit CL. Safety, efficacy, and functionality of high-field strength interventional magnetic resonance imaging for neurosurgery. Neurosurgery 2000;46(3):632–641, discussion 641–642
8. Bohinski RJ, Kokkino AK, Warnick RE, et al. Glioma resection in a shared-resource magnetic resonance operating room after optimal image-guided frameless stereotactic resection. Neurosurgery 2001;48(4):731–742, discussion 742–744
9. Tronnier VM, Wirtz CR, Knauth M, et al. Intraoperative diagnostic and interventional magnetic resonance imaging in neurosurgery. Neurosurgery 1997;40(5):891–900, discussion 900–902
10. Steinmeier R, Fahlbusch R, Ganslandt O, et al. Intraoperative magnetic resonance imaging with the Magnetom open scanner: concepts, neurosurgical indications, and procedures: a preliminary report. Neurosurgery 1998;43(4):739–747, discussion 747–748
11. Martin AJ, Hall WA, Liu H, et al. Brain tumor resection: intraoperative monitoring with high-field-strength MR imaging-initial results. Radiology 2000;215(1):221–228
12. Rubino GJ, Farahani K, McGill D, Van De Wiele B, Villablanca JP, Wang-Mathieson A. Magnetic resonance imaging-guided neurosurgery in the magnetic fringe fields: the next step in neuronavigation. Neurosurgery 2000;46(3):643–653, discussion 653–654
13. Nimsky C, Ganslandt O, Fahlbusch R. 1.5 T: intraoperative imaging beyond standard anatomic imaging. Neurosurg Clin N Am 2005;16(1):185–200, vii
14. Nabavi A, Gering DT, Kacher DF, et al. Surgical navigation in the open MRI. Acta Neurochir Suppl (Wien) 2003;85:121–125
15. Truwit CL, Liu H. Prospective stereotaxy: a novel method of trajectory alignment using real-time image guidance. J Magn Reson Imaging 2001;13(3):452–457
16. Hall WA, Liu H, Martin AJ, Maxwell RE, Truwit CL. Brain biopsy sampling by using prospective stereotaxis and a trajectory guide. J Neurosurg 2001;94(1):67–71
17. Martin AJ, Larson PS, Ostrem JL, et al. Placement of deep brain stimulator electrodes using real-time high-field interventional magnetic resonance imaging. Magn Reson Med 2005;54(5):1107–1114
18. Starr PA, Martin AJ, Ostrem JL, Talke P, Levesque N, Larson PS. Subthalamic nucleus deep brain stimulator placement using high-field interventional magnetic resonance imaging and a skull-mounted aiming device: technique and application accuracy. J Neurosurg 2009 Aug 14. [Epub ahead of print]

19. Hall WA, Galicich W, Bergman T, Truwit CL. 3-tesla intraoperative MR imaging for neurosurgery. J Neurooncol 2006;77(3):297–303
20. Truwit CL, Hall WA. Intraoperative magnetic resonance imaging-guided neurosurgery at 3-T. Neurosurgery 2006; 58(4, Suppl 2)ONS-338–ONS-345
21. Lewin JS, Nour SG, Meyers ML, et al. Intraoperative MRI with a rotating, tiltable surgical table: a time use study and clinical results in 122 patients. AJR Am J Roentgenol 2007;189(5):1096–1103
22. Nimsky C, Ganslandt O, Von Keller B, Romstöck J, Fahlbusch R. Intraoperative high-field-strength MR imaging: implementation and experience in 200 patients. Radiology 2004;233(1):67–78
23. McPherson CM, Bohinski RJ, Dagnew E, Warnick RE, Tew JM. Tumor resection in a shared-resource magnetic resonance operating room: experience at the University of Cincinnati. Acta Neurochir Suppl (Wien) 2003;85:39–44

4

Optimal Pulse Sequences

Gurpreet Singh Sandhu, Jonathan S. Lewin, and Sherif Gamal Nour

The spectrum of intraoperative use of magnetic resonance imaging (MRI) in neurosurgery covers a wide range of applications including anatomic, functional, metabolic, and interventional imaging. No single-pulse sequence can provide such a large variety of information single-handedly; different pulse sequences have to be employed depending upon the goal of imaging, patient's anatomy, and imaging characteristics of pathologic lesions. A pulse sequence for intraoperative MRI (iMRI) should be able to provide valid and consistent information about a particular structure, event, or a physiologic phenomenon as per the neurosurgeon's requirement, keeping affect of other confounding factors to a minimum, in the shortest possible time interval. A group of available MR parameters are modified to make a specific pulse sequence for a specific purpose.

Pulse sequences for intraoperative use in neurosurgery can be broadly classified into three main categories. The first category consists of conventional general purpose imaging sequences such as T1-, T2-, and proton-density weighted imaging sequences, inversion recovery sequences, contrast-enhanced imaging, and so on. The second category includes sequences for physiologic and functional mapping such as diffusion tensor imaging (DTI), MR spectroscopy (MRS), functional MRI (fMRI), and perfusion MRI. The third category consists of faster imaging sequences used for guidance of biopsy needles and interventional devices and various temperature mapping techniques for the monitoring of thermal ablation procedures. Susceptibility-weighted imaging (SWI) is another emerging technique that is increasingly being employed intraoperatively.

In the following sections, a brief overview of the fundamentals of MR image formation is given. This is followed by basic information about the various pulse sequences employed for the acquisition of images with different types of contrasts. Applications of these pulse sequences for minimally invasive and open MRI-guided neurosurgical procedures are then described. In the final section, various imaging techniques employed for the purposes of mapping of pathologic lesions on brain images are explained.

◆ Basic Principles of Magnetic Resonance Imaging

MR image formation is based upon electromagnetic activity of atomic nuclei with odd numbered nucleons (protons + neutrons), with hydrogen nuclei most often exploited due to their natural abundance in the human body.[1] Each nucleus induces a magnetic field in its vicinity by rotating around its own axis. Exposure to an external magnetic field causes the nuclei to wobble or precess around the axis of magnetic field with a frequency called *Larmor frequency*.[2]

When a patient is placed inside the bore of the MRI scanner, a small fraction of the hydrogen nuclei in the body align themselves along the magnetic field to attain the lowest energy state level producing a net magnetization vector (called *equilibrium magnetization*) in the direction of the magnetic field (*z-axis*). Application of an excitation pulse redirects a portion of the equilibrium magnetization into a plane perpendicular to it (the *xy-plane*). As the system returns to equilibrium, magnetization in the xy-plane precesses around the main magnetic field and induces current in a receiver coil. This current becomes the MR signal. Disappearance of magnetization in xy-plane and recovery of magnetization in z-axis are two different processes. Realignment of net magnetization to equilibrium state occurs through the process of T_1 *recovery* and is characterized by longitudinal relaxation time (T_1). At the same time, magnetization in xy-plane disappears by two different processes called T_2 *decay* and T_2^* decay. These are characterized by spin-spin relaxation times (T_2 and T_2^*, respectively). T_1 Recovery occurs as the spinning nuclei release energy into the environment. Dephasing of transverse magnetization due to interaction between the spinning nuclei and their magnetic fields forms the basis of T_2 decay. In addition to interaction between spinning nuclei and their magnetic fields, magnetic field inhomogeneities also contribute to dephasing of transverse magnetization in T_2^* decay. Different tissues possess different values of T_1, T_2, and T_2^* depending upon arrangements at cellular and subcellular levels. T_1 and T_2 values of compact tissues are lower than those of fluid tissues such as blood and CSF. However, T_2^* for all the tissues is much lower than their corresponding T_2 values.[2–4]

To form the final MR image, the imaging volume of interest is divided into subdivisions called *voxels* (volumetric regions) by using gradient coils in three different directions (x-, y-, and z-axes). Dimensions of the individual voxels in an imaging area depend upon the strength of gradients applied. A *gradient* is a linear variation of the magnetic field strength in a selected region. Precession frequency is also changed along with this change in magnetic field strength. A *slice selection gradient* (Gs) selects the cross-section of the patient to be imaged. A *phase-encoding gradient* (Gp) results in phase shift in the spinning protons. A *frequency encoding gradient*, also called a *readout gradient* (Gr), shifts the frequency of the spinning protons. Coordinates provided by these three gradients aid in exact localization of signal to a particular voxel and this information is stored in what is called *k-space*.[3] K-space is a matrix in which the acquired data are stored. To acquire a complete image, different voxels are excited and data are collected. The magnitude of Gp and Gr need to be changed to acquire data from different voxels. Fourier transform of this data are then performed to get the final image. Data in the central portion of k-space provide more contribution to the gross appearance of the image, whereas the peripheral portions of the k-space carry information relating to the sharp transitions in the image (small structures, edges, etc.).

The time interval between the application of the excitation RF pulse and the peak of the corresponding detected signal is called *echo-time* (TE). To obtain signal from all voxels, the excitation pulse is applied many times to obtain a complete image. The time interval between the applications of two successive excitation RF pulses is called *repetition time* (TR).[2] By varying values of TR and TE of pulse sequences, different weightings can be provided to the acquired MR images. T2-Weighted images (T2WIs) are obtained using longer values of TE and TR. T1WIs are obtained using shorter values of TR and TE. Proton density-weighted images are obtained by using longer values of TR and shorter values of TE.

◆ Pulse Sequences: An Overview

An introduction to various types of MR pulse sequences is provided in this section. These sequences can be used for navigation purposes as well as functional neuroimaging with or without some modifications. MR pulse sequences can broadly be divided into two main groups depending on the application of a 180-degree refocusing pulse: *spin-echo* (SE) and *gradient-echo* (GRE) sequences.

Spin Echo Sequences

SE is the most commonly used pulse sequence in neuroimaging.[5] Magnetization, after flipping into the transverse plane by application of 90-degree radiofrequency (RF) pulse, starts to dephase due to T_2 and T_2^* relaxation. A 180-degree pulse is applied after time TE/2, which reverses the polarity of rotating spins. Hence spins that were previously dephasing start to rephase again to produce an echo at time TE, which is acquired as a signal. This is followed by a long interval, TR so that longitudinal magnetization recovers fully before the next excitation pulse is applied. This process is repeated for each voxel to acquire complete data. Values of TR and TE are varied to obtain various types of contrasts as described in the previous section.

Acquisition time for most conventional SE sequences is very long (up to 10 minutes). Multiecho SE pulses (called by various names such as turbo-SE or TSE, fast-SE or FSE, and rapid acquisition with relaxation enhancement or RARE) are employed to counter this problem. In these sequences, several echoes are acquired after an RF excitation pulse by application of several 180-degree refocusing pulses. The length of this "echo-train" indicates the factor of acceleration. With improvement in gradient strengths and bandwidth, it is now feasible to acquire data for the entire k-space using FSE in a single excitation. Further decrease in data acquisition time can be attained by implementing various techniques such as partial k-space acquisition algorithms, parallel imaging, and partial Fourier.[4] Half Fourier acquisition single-shot turbo spin-echo (HASTE) is a single shot TSE in which an initial preparation pulse is applied for contrast enhancement and produces highly T2WIs.

SE sequences may be modified to form SE-echo planar imaging (SE-EPI) and SE-inversion recovery (SE-IR) pulse sequences. SE-EPI pulse sequence is a fast imaging sequence in which all of the k-space lines are acquired in a single TR (single-shot EPI) or in two or more TRs (multishot EPI). SE-EPI is considered the imaging technique of choice for diffusion-weighted imaging. In the SE-IR pulse sequence, an inversion pulse is applied before the application of a conventional pulse sequence to flip the magnetization vector upside down. After the inversion pulse ceases, spinning nuclei start recovering longitudinal magnetization and pass through the transverse plane (called *null point*). Depending upon their respective inherent T_1 relaxation times, different tissues possess different null points. When a 90-degree excitation pulse for SE is applied at the null point of a specific tissue, SE signal for that tissue gets suppressed. One application of IR pulse sequences, fluid-attenuated inversion-recovery (FLAIR) pulse sequences is particularly useful in suppressing signal from cerebrospinal fluid (CSF) to detect hyperintense lesions in periventricular areas of the brain.[3]

Gradient Echo Sequences

GRE sequences are significantly faster than SE sequences with the primary difference in sequence design being the absence of the 180-degree refocusing pulse. Instead, gradients are used for phase reversal and echo formation. Additionally, the RF excitation pulse of smaller angle (less than 90 degrees) decreases the time required for magnetization recovery and hence subsequent excitation pulses can be applied at shorter time intervals (i.e., TR is decreased). Therefore, significant reduction in scan time is attained; however, at the expense of image quality. A magnetization preparation pulse can be applied at the beginning of GRE pulses to improve the image quality.[5] Gradients do not refocus magnetic field inhomogeneities. Therefore, GRE sequences are generally more $T2^*$-weighted when compared with the true T2-weighting produced by SE sequences. Furthermore, GRE sequences are sensitive to magnetic susceptibility differences between different tissues. This results in the formation of signal voids at tissue interfaces. These attributes of GRE sequences – rapid acquisition and sensitivity to magnetic susceptibility – impact their utility for intraoperative use. During procedure guidance, rapid acquisition permits near-real-time image updates of the location and orientation of interventional devices. Sensitivity to magnetic susceptibility contributes to artifactual widening of interventional devices, which can complicate targeting of small tumors or navigating within areas of complex anatomy particularly during high-field interventions.[3]

Depending on the method of gradient application, GRE sequences are further classified into three categories: *coherent or partially refocused, fully refocused,* and *spoiled* GRE. Partially refocused GRE sequences use one rewind gradient to rephase the $T2^*$ magnetization and therefore preserve $T2^*$ effects. These sequences are particularly useful for intraoperative hemorrhage detection. Fully refocused GRE sequences differ from partially refocused GRE sequences in that gradients in all the three directions are refocused and the phase of the RF pulse is also alternated between 0 degrees and 180 degrees between successive excitations. Steady-state free precession (SSFP), also called fast imaging with steady precession (FISP), a time inversed version of FISP (PSIF) and an FISP with balanced gradients in all spatial directions (TrueFISP, also called FIESTA) are examples of this category. Sequences of this category produce images with T2W/T1W contrast in a very short acquisition time and are particularly useful for interventional device tracking. In *spoiled GRE*, a spoiler gradient or RF pulse is used to eradicate any remaining magnetization after each echo. This produces a similar effect to T1W- or proton density-weighted MRI. This is particularly useful for contrast-enhanced MRI.[3] Values of TR and TE can also be employed to vary image contrast as explained in the section "Basic principles of MRI." Similar to SE pulse sequences, GRE pulse sequences are also used to construct EPI and IR sequences.

Contrast-enhanced MRI is performed by injecting paramagnetic contrast agents intravenously to shorten T_1, which renders brain tumors brighter and therefore readily detectable as a result of preferential contrast distribution due to the broken blood–brain barrier (BBB) within the tumor tissue.[3]

◆ Pulse Sequences for Intraoperative Magnetic Resonance Imaging

Monitoring of neurosurgical procedures by employing iMRI is helpful for the guidance of minimally invasive procedures such as brain biopsy, deep brain stimulator placement, and thermotherapy procedures and for the monitoring of open neurosurgical procedures such as tumor resection and temporal lobectomy. Depending on surgical requirements, two-dimesional (2D) or three-dimensional (3D) images with different contrasts can be obtained to guide a neurosurgical procedure. 3D images for intraoperative use are often acquired preoperatively due to their longer acquisition times; 2D images can be acquired intraoperatively with continuous image updates. Functional, metabolic, and tractology data obtained from fMRI, MRS, and DTI can be integrated into these image datasets as detailed below in the Pulse Sequences for Functional Neuronavigation section.

T1W fast imaging may be performed using spoiled-GRE sequences such as fast-low angle shot sequence (FLASH), spoiled gradient echo sequence (SPGR), and T1W fast field echo sequence (FFE) or FISP. Magnetization preparation may be added to improve image contrast. T2W fast imaging may be performed by using single-shot TSE sequences such as HASTE, single-shot-FSE (SS-FSE), SS-TSE, RARE, and PSIF. An orthogonal HASTE sequence is commonly used to determine the trajectory to target lesions during biopsy.[6] An axial RARE sequence is often used to localize voxels for performance of MRS.[7] FISP and PSIF are commonly used for real-time navigation of interventional devices.[8] TrueFISP provides a mixed T1W/T2W contrast with a high contrast-to-noise ratio at near real-time fast imaging.[9] 3D T1WIs are often obtained by employing a magnetization-prepared rapid gradient echo (MP-RAGE) sequence, which employs magnetization preparation to provide better image contrast. Due to longer image acquisition time, 3D images are typically obtained prior to the actual neurosurgical procedure, after the head is already fixed in an MRI-compatible head holder.[10]

An intraoperative intracranial hemorrhage, if it occurs, is a severe complication that may put the patient's life in jeopardy. The diamagnetic nature of hemoglobin present in hyperacute hemorrhage is difficult to detect on MRI.[11] Therefore, "hemorrhage scans" consisting of HASTE, $T2^*$-weighted GRE, and FLAIR are performed to exclude intraoperative hemorrhage during minimally invasive as well as open neurosurgeries.[12] Preoperative images are acquired using these three sequences as baseline. These sequences are repeated intraoperatively at any stage as per the neurosurgeon's discretion and are compared with the baseline images to detect intraoperative hemorrhage.[13] HASTE is a heavily T2W, high-speed sequence in which data are acquired after an initial preparation pulse for contrast enhancement with the use of a very long echo train (single-shot TSE). The hallmark of a hyperacute hemorrhage on GRE images is a rim of hypointense signal that surrounds an isointense core. FLAIR provides a hyperintense appearance to hyperacute intraparenchymal hemorrhages.[14,15]

Minimally Invasive Procedures

To perform minimally invasive procedures, faster pulse sequences are used to obtain 2D images in near-real time for device navigation as well as monitoring of various interventional procedures. Imaging is further helpful to exclude intraoperative complications.

Interactive MR Imaging Guidance

Various techniques are available for interactive near-real-time guidance of interventional devices. These can be broadly classified into four categories: freehand techniques, stereotactic techniques, augmented reality techniques, and image fusion techniques,[16] with stereotactic techniques being particularly useful for image-guided minimally invasive neurosurgical procedures such as biopsy, deep brain stimulator (DBS) placement, cyst aspiration, and thermal ablation. Guiding these procedures under low-field MRI is performed using continuous imaging with FISP (TR/TE/FA/NSA: 17.8 ms/8.1 ms/90 degree/1–3, acquisition time: 1.7–4 s/frame) or PSIF (TR/TE/FA/NSA: 19.4 ms/9.5 ms/ 35 degree /2, acquisition time: 5 s/frame).[8] Continuous imaging at high-field MRI is performed by employing T2W HASTE (TR/TE: 1000–5000 ms/90 ms; echo-train length [ETL]: 92; matrix: 192 × 256; field of view [FOV]: 160–250 mm) and T1W GRE sequences (TR/TE/FA: 10 ms/6.4 ms/10 degree; matrix: 128 × 128; FOV: 100 mm).[17,18] HASTE is free of geometric image distortion due to local static field inhomogeneity, which makes it suitable for MRI-based near-real-time guidance (**Fig. 4.1**).[17] High-field guidance is commonly performed using the prospective stereotaxy technique described below.[19-21] In prospective stereotaxy, image guidance is commonly performed using insertion scans consisting of a three-dimensional (3D) T2W TSE sequence (e.g., TR/TE/FA/ETL: 2000 ms/92 ms/90 degree /56, acquisition time: 1 min 22 s) by employing snapshot images acquired in two orthogonal planes at increments as the needle is advanced.[21] A fluoroscopic acquisition (fluoro-scan; TR/TE/FA: 6.0 ms/3.0 ms/60 degree; FOV: 128 mm; matrix: 128 × 128; slice thickness: 10 mm; 200 ms/frame)

is also described for alignment of trajectory guide in prospective stereotaxy and biopsy guidance.[18,21]

Stereotactic techniques are classified into *frame-based* and *frameless* stereotaxy. Frame-based stereotactic systems employ MRI-compatible external stereotactic frames to calculate the target location based upon Cartesian coordinates and allow needle advancement along a predetermined trajectory. They are, however, limited by application of cumbersome frames, inability to navigate beyond fixed trajectories, and inability to compensate for intraoperative brain shift. Frameless stereotactic techniques offer the accuracy of a measured stereotactic approach while maintaining the liberty of freehand technique and allowing unlimited trajectories. However, they involve additional equipment and sometimes make procedures more complex. *Frameless stereotaxy* includes *optically linked stereotaxy, active tracking,* and *prospective stereotaxy. Optically linked stereotaxy* is based on actively coupling the scan plane to the orientation of the interventional device by mounting light-emitting diodes (LEDs) or small reflective balls to the interventional device and installing an infrared camera that continuously monitors the emitted or reflected light. The data acquired by the infrared camera, is constantly fed into a 3D digitizer resulting in near-real-time update of the spatial information of the device. This information is shared with measurement control of the MRI scanner to enable automatic scan plane positioning along the new orientation of the interventional device. This system was first described as a component of the double-donut system (SIGNA SP; General Electric Medical Systems, Waukesha, WI) and has also been applied for guidance of image acquisition on C-arm systems (developed in collaboration with Radionics, Burlington, MA and SiemensAG,

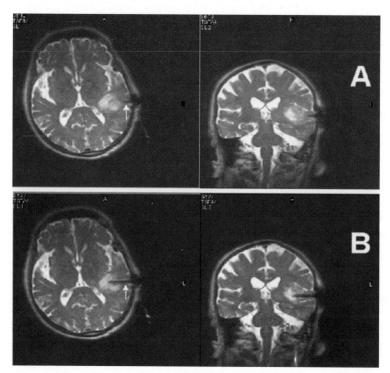

Fig. 4.1 Intraoperative image-based monitoring of needle introduction at near-real-time rate by employing HASTE (half-Fourier acquisition single-shot turbo spin echo) sequence. Axial (*left*) and coronal (*right*) images obtained at the **(A)** initial and **(B)** final time points of the biopsy needle introduction process are shown. The biopsy needle appears as a dark line on these magnetic resonance images. (From Liu H, Hall WA, Truwit CL. Remotely-controlled approach for stereotactic neurobiopsy. Computer Aided Surgery 2002;7:245. Reprinted with permission.)

Erlangen, Germany).[22–25] *Active tracking* is another technique for automatic scan plane readjustment that is based on the same idea of actively linking the image plane to the orientation of the interventional device. The link, however, does not employ infrared light as in the optical tracking system and thereby eliminates the need for expensive stereotactic cameras and other added equipment. Rather, this system replaces the hardware equipment with a software interface that serves to link the measurement unit of the imager with prototype wireless fiducial markers tuned to the resonance frequency of the scanner and mounted to biopsy needles or to other interventional devices. The method has also been effectively used to drive image acquisition during intravascular flexible catheter and coil tracking under MRI.[26] No clinical data are yet available using this system. An "adaptive image parameters" software has also been reported,[27,28] which can be used in conjunction with active tracking to allow automated intraoperative adjustments of imaging parameters other than scan plane position and/or orientation, such as FOV, temporal resolution, and tissue contrast. *Prospective frameless stereotaxy* is a technique that has widely been used for neuronavigation and works in reverse order to that of optically linked and adaptive tracking methods.[29] It starts by locating the target, which is then aligned with a pivot point, where a trajectory guide (Navigus; Image-Guided Neurologics, Melbourne, FL) is secured to the patient's skull. The needle trajectory is subsequently aligned on a virtual line in the space along the extension of these two points: the intracranial target and the skull pivot point (**Fig. 4.2**). Once the needle is aligned along the correct

trajectory, the pivot is locked and repeated fluoroscopic MRI scans can be obtained to monitor needle advancement toward the target in near real-time.[30,31]

Image fusion methods aim at maximizing the information content provided to the interventionalist during the interventional procedure by integrating functional and/or metabolic data into the usual anatomic images, while the latter are being interactively updated to reflect the temporal position of the interventional device and its relation to vital structures.[32–34] The freehand and stereotactic techniques of guidance are applicable using these methods. The ability to register data from various brain mapping techniques to the corresponding anatomic volume during neuronavigation can clearly contribute to a more favorable procedure outcome by enabling the salvage of critical areas (e.g., eloquent cortex).

Biopsy Needle/Interventional Device Visualization

While performing minimally invasive procedures, proper visualization of the operative instrument such as a biopsy needle is essential. Various factors that can affect the accuracy of positioning of MR-guided biopsy and aspiration needles can be broadly classified into *pulse sequence-dependent* and *needle-dependent* factors. Magnetic field strength, sequence design, pulse sequence acquisition bandwidth, and direction of frequency encode direction comprise the category of pulse sequence-dependent factors. Sensitivity to magnetic susceptibility is the most important pulse sequence issue. The commonly used GRE sequences (FISP, TrueFISP, and PSIF) are

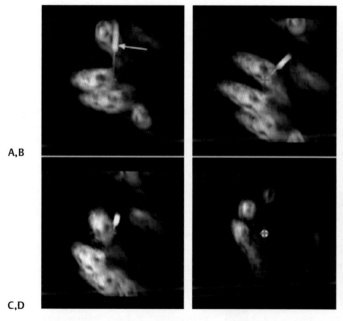

A,B

C,D

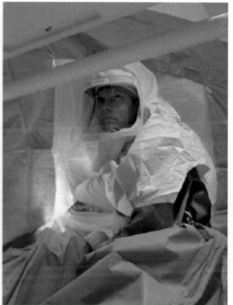

E

Fig. 4.2 The procedure for aligning the trajectory guide is shown. **(A–D)** A fluoroscopic magnetic resonance sequence that is orthogonal to, and centered on, the desired trajectory is run at a level external to the patient's head. **(E)** The surgeon reaches into the bore during scanning and manipulates the trajectory guide until the distal tip of the guide is centered in this image (indicated by a *cross*). This process requires an in-room monitor for the surgeon to view the fluoroscopic images. Individual frames from this fluoroscopic sequence **(A–D)** reveal the linear alignment indicator (*arrow* in **[A]**) and the surgeon's hand. When properly aligned, the alignment indicator is completely superimposed at the center of the image **(D)**. (From Martin AJ, Hall WA, Roark C, Starr PA, Larson PS, Truwit CL. Minimally invasive precision brain access using prospective stereotaxy and a trajectory guide. J Magn Reson Imaging 2008; 27(4): 739. Reprinted with permission.)

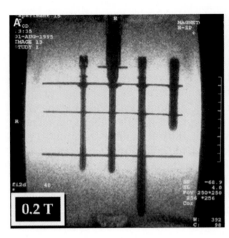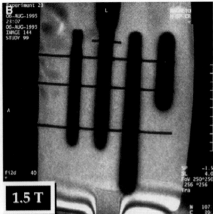

Fig. 4.3 Effect of magnetic field strength on needle visualization. Magnetic resonance imaging scans of the same set of various needles were taken at **(A)** 0.2 T and **(B)** 1.5 T by employing fast imaging with steady-state free precession (FISP) sequence with the shafts of needles perpendicular to the static magnetic field. Note the marked artifactual widening of the needles caused by the higher magnetic field strength in **(B)**. (From Lewin JS, Duerk JL, Jain VR, et al. Needle localization in MR-guided biopsy and aspiration: effects of field strength, sequence design, and magnetic field orientation. AJR Am J Roentgenol 1996;166(6):1337–45. Reprinted with permission.)

associated with more prominent susceptibility artifacts from needles than are the relatively slower spin echo (SE) or turbo spin echo (TSE) sequences. Therefore, to reduce artifactual needle widening, the use of TSE imaging for position confirmation or primary guidance should be strongly considered when needle placement within 5 mm of major neurovascular structures is contemplated rather than relying on the more rapid GRE sequences for guidance of the entire procedure.[35] The higher the magnetic field strength, the larger the apparent width of the needles and other interventional devices is.[36] On the low-field (0.2 T) system, the apparent needle width under GRE image guidance ranges from ~4 mm for smaller gauges to 9 mm for larger gauges (**Fig. 4.3**).[35] The degree of artifactual widening can be reduced to half by using a TSE pulse sequence. Artifactual needle widening can also be decreased by using higher sampling bandwidth, however, at the expanse of some degree of spatial malpositioning.[35] Needle artifact is wider when the frequency-encode direction is perpendicular to the long axis of the needle during image acquisition. A reduction or increase in the apparent needle width by a factor of 0.33 to 2.5 can be obtained by swapping the frequency- and phase-encoding axes relative to the needle shaft (**Fig. 4.4**).[35] This effect can be used to decrease the apparent needle width when the needle artifact obscures adjacent anatomic structures by setting the frequency-encode axis parallel to the needle shaft.[22,23] Needle-dependent factors affecting the apparent needle width are the needle composition, and its orientation with respect to the main magnetic field of the MRI scanner. Materials such as high-nickel and high-chromium stainless steel may be adequate at 0.2 T, but may give rise to unacceptable artifact at 1.5 T. On the other hand, small-caliber needles constructed from low-artifact materials, such as titanium, may be difficult to identify in certain clinical settings at low-field strength.[35] The apparent needle width on MRI is highest when it is aligned perpendicular to the axis of the main magnetic field (**Fig. 4.5**).[35] When the needle is perpendicular to the main magnetic field, the distortion of needle appearance is observed along the entire needle. On the other hand, when the needle is parallel to the field, a distortion of needle appearance occurs mostly at the tip and hub and, to a lesser extent, along the needle shaft.[35]

Intraoperative MRI-Guided Thermotherapy

MRI is also used for real-time monitoring of LASER thermal therapies of highly anaplastic brain tumors such as glioblastoma multiforme. Continuous temperature mapping during LASER therapy is performed by a software package based on the temperature-dependent phase shift of the MRI signal.

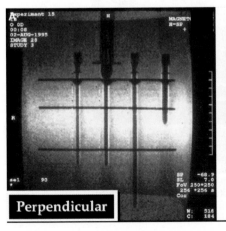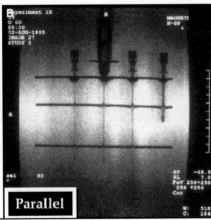

Fig. 4.4 Effect of frequency-encoding direction on needle visualization. Spin echo images of the same set of needles as in Fig. 4.3 were obtained with the frequency-encoding direction **(A)** perpendicular to needle shafts and **(B)** parallel to needle shafts. The sequence used in **(A)** resulted in more artifactual needle widening than that used in **(B)** yet rendered the needle tip more visible. (From Lewin JS, Duerk JL, Jain VR, et al. Needle localization in MR-guided biopsy and aspiration: effects of field strength, sequence design, and magnetic field orientation. AJR Am J Roentgenol 1996;166(6):1337–45. Reprinted with permission.)

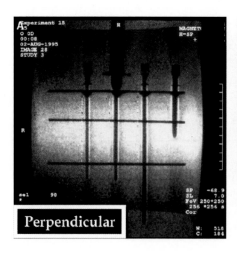

Perpendicular

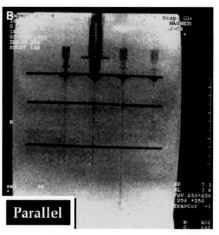

Parallel

Fig. 4.5 Effect of needle orientation relative to the main magnetic field. Spin echo magnetic resonance imaging scans of the same set of needles were obtained with needle shafts **(A)** perpendicular and **(B)** parallel to a static magnetic field at 0.2 T. Note the marked reduction in artifactual needle widening when needles are parallel to the static magnetic field. This effect can render smaller needles invisible during interventions. (From Lewin JS, Duerk JL, Jain VR, et al. Needle localization in MR-guided biopsy and aspiration: effects of field strength, sequence design, and magnetic field orientation. AJR Am J Roentgenol 1996;166(6):1337–45. Reprinted with permission.)

Fast GRE sequences are employed for phase data acquisition. Prior to the start of LASER therapy, a high-resolution image is acquired, which depicts the pathology selected for thermal treatment. This image is loaded onto a real-time image processor and is used as a background image for calculated thermal maps. Two regions, area for thermal treatment and another area away from actual site of the thermal therapy, are selected as regions of interest on this image. The sequence for temperature mapping is started with LASER therapy. The phase of the first complex data area is taken as the starting phase and each following phase image is subtracted from the starting phase, which in turn is converted into a temperature map.[37]

Open Neurosurgery

iMRI is often employed for brain tumor resection, pituitary operations, skull base tumor resections, and excision of refractory epileptic areas. Previous reports document that additional surgical resection is required in 27.5 to 92% of neurosurgical procedures based on information provided by intraoperative imaging (72.8% at our institution).[8] Conventional imaging techniques such as T1W and T2W, and FLAIR are typically used for anatomic assessment of brain lesions. FLAIR images are especially useful for detection of periventricular white matter lesions (where bright signal from CSF makes it otherwise difficult).[38] However, it is less sensitive than T2WIs in detecting posterior fossa lesions. Double inversion-recovery (DIR) pulse sequence employs two different inversion pulses attenuating signal from CSF as well as from white matter and has advantage over FLAIR in detecting infratentorial lesions and lesions with poor contrast on T2WIs.[39] T2WIs are also used for calculation of T2 and volume ratios of the hippocampus for diagnosis of hippocampal sclerosis in patients with temporal lobe epilepsy. It predicts the risk of postoperative amnesia in candidates for temporal lobe epilepsy surgery.[40] DTI and fMRI images can be further employed to obtain information regarding white matter tracts and eloquent cortical areas, respectively.[41] MRS is employed to obtain metabolic information

so as to properly localize the boundary between a pathologic lesion and normal brain tissue. The basics of these sequences and their applications for intraoperative use are discussed below in the Pulse Sequences for Functional Neuronavigation section.

Three sets of scans are often acquired for tumor resection: the first set is acquired before the start of surgery. The second set is acquired to evaluate the extent of resection when the surgeon believes resection is complete or when resection is too close to eloquent cortex or essential tracts. The final set of scans is acquired after completion of craniotomy to exclude the presence of hematoma developed during surgical closure. Conceivably, modifications to these depend on the overall surgeon's preference and on the specific circumstances of individual surgical procedures. Similarly, the specific batteries of pulse sequences comprising these sets of scans vary between different groups. The T1W MP-RAGE sequence has widely been used to obtain a 3D reference image for navigation purposes after fixation of the head with an MRI compatible head-holder.[10] Hemorrhage scans consisting of HASTE, FLAIR, and T2*W GRE are obtained just before the start of the operative procedure and are repeated at various stages after tumor resection and after closure of craniotomy to detect operative hemorrhage.[12,13] Diffusion-weighted imaging (DWI) scans can be added to hemorrhage scans if suspicion for an ischemic infarct arises during surgery. Each set of images prolongs surgery by ~10 to 15 minutes.[12] The SWI technique described later in this chapter is an emerging technique for the evaluation of intraoperative hemorrhages.

Our group uses FISP, PSIF, 2D and 3D T1W FLASH, T1W SE, T2W TSE, and TSE-FLAIR for various purposes in iMRI-guided neurosurgery on low-field MRI scanners (**Table 4.1**). Imaging time for these sequences vary from 1.7 seconds to 8 minute 31 seconds at low field (0.2 T) MRI to acquire 3 to 19 sections (thickness: 3–5 mm thick; FOV: 20–25 cm; matrix: 128–256 × 256). Mean total scan time for performance of an iMRI-guided neurosurgical procedure on low-field MRI at our institution is 35 minutes 17 seconds. FISP and PSIF are employed for real-time tracking of interventional devices. We use contrast-enhanced T1W FLASH in all three orthogonal directions

Table 4.1 Various Sequences Employed for Intraoperative Magnetic Resonance Imaging at 0.2 T and Their Parameters

Sequence	TR (ms)	TE (ms)	α (°)	TI (ms)	ETL	Acquired Signals	Imaging Time
FLAIR	6,000	91-93		1,840	7	1-3	4 min 19 s–8 min 31 s
FLASH	286–418	90	90	-	-	2	2 min 28 s– 4 min 30 s
FISP	17.8	8.1	90	-	-	1-3	1.7–4s/image
PSIF	19.4	9.5	35	-	-	2	≈ 5 s/image
T1-weighted SE	432	26	90	-	-	2-5	3 min 54 s–6 min 58 s
T2-weighted TSE	3,500–7,000	102	90	-	7-17	1-3	2 min 57 s–5 min 2 s

Abbreviations: ETL, echo-train length; FISP, fast imaging with steady precession; FLAIR, fluid-attenuated inversion recovery; FLASH, fast low-angle shot; PSIF, reverse fast imaging with steady-state free precession; SE, spin-echo; TSE, turbo spin-echo; TE, echo time; TI, inversion time; TR, repetition time; α, flip angle.

Source: Lewin JS, Nour SG, Meyers ML, et al. Intraoperative MRI with a rotating, tiltable surgical table: a time–use study and clinical results in 122 patients. AJR Am J Roentgenol 2007; 189: 1099. Reprinted with permission.

along with optional T2WIs for craniotomies. Baseline scans are obtained after craniotomy and before the start of surgical resection. These scans are repeated during surgery to evaluate the extant of resection (**Fig. 4.6**). Coronal and sagittal T2WIs and 3D coronal T1WIs are employed for transsphenoidal surgery.[8] Similar scans are also acquired for

iMRI-guided skull base surgeries.[42] Another group also uses T1W SE (coronal and sagittal), and optional T2W TSE (coronal and sagittal) for transsphenoidal surgery and repeats T1W SE after contrast administration for craniopharyngiomas surgery.[43] For glioma surgery, that group uses inversion recovery sequence (repeated after contrast administration), dark blood

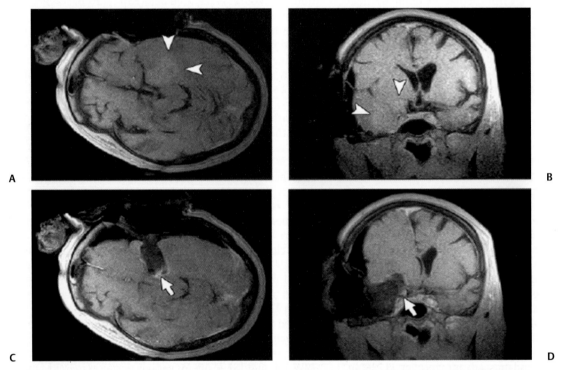

Fig. 4.6 Low-field (0.2 T) intraoperative magnetic resonance imaging during open neurosurgery: Contrast-enhanced two-dimensional fast-low angle shot sequence (FLASH) images (flip angle: 90 degrees; number of signals averaged: 2) in a 71-year-old woman during resection of temporal lobe glioblastoma. **(A)** Axial (repetition time/ echo time [TR/TE]: 418/9; acquisition time: 3 minutes 36 seconds) and **(B)** coronal (TR/TE: 330/9; acquisition time: 2 minutes 30 seconds) images obtained after craniotomy show faintly enhancing partially ill-defined lesion (*arrowheads*) involving left-sided mesial temporal lobe and extending superiorly into inferior aspect of ipsilateral lentiform nucleus. Adjacent edema is responsible for mass effect exerted on left lateral ventricle, sylvian fissure, and overlying cortical sulci. **(C)** Axial (TR/TE: 418/9; acquisition time: 3 minutes 36 seconds) and **(D)** coronal (TR/TE: 330/9; acquisition time: 2 minutes 30 seconds) images obtained after resection show minimal residual enhancement along deep aspect of resection bed and small nodule (*arrows*) medially, denoting residual neoplastic tissue. Further resection was subsequently performed based on these intraoperative imaging findings. (From Lewin JS, Nour SG, Meyers ML, et al. Intraoperative MRI with a Rotating, Tiltable Surgical Table: A Time–Use Study and Clinical Results in 122 Patients. AJR Am J Roentgenol 2007;189: 1100. Reprinted with permission.)

Table 4.2 Various Sequences Employed for Intraoperative Magnetic Resonance Imaging at 1.5 T and Their Parameters

Sequence	Slice Thickness (mm)	TR (ms)	TE (ms)	FOV (mm)	In Plane Resolution (mm)	No. of Acquisitions	Imaging Time
T1-weighted TSE	4	6,490	98	230	0.44 × 0.74	3	5 min 39 s
FLAIR	4	10,000	103	230	0.44 × 0.74	1	6 min 2 s
T1-weighted SE	4	525	17	230	0.89 × 0.89	2	3 min 59 s
MP-RAGE	1	2,020	4,038	250	0.49 × 0.49i	1	8 min 39 s
MRS CSI	10	1,600	135	160	6.7 × 6.7	2	12 min 45 s
fMRI	3	1,580	60	192	3 × 3	1	3 min 13 s
DTI	1.9	9,200	86	240	1.87 × 1.87	5	5 min 31 s
HASTE	5	1,000	89	230	-	5	25 s
Fluid suppressed EPI	5	9,000	85	230	-	1	1 min 2 s

Abbreviations: CSI, chemical shift imaging; DTI, diffusion tensor imaging; EPI, echo planar imaging; FLAIR, fluid- attenuated inversion recovery; fMRI, functional magnetic resonance imaging; FOV, field of view; HASTE, half Fourier acquisition single-shot turbo spin echo; MP-RAGE, magnetization-prepared rapid acquisition gradient echo; MRS, magnetic resonance spectroscopy; SE, spin echo; TE, echo time; TR, repetition time; TSE, turbo spin-echo; EPI, echo-planar imaging. (*Source:* Nimsky C, Ganslandt O, Buchfelder M, Fahlbusch R. Intraoperative visualization for re-section of gliomas: the role of functional neuronavigation and intraoperative 1.5 T MRI. Neuro Research 2006; 28: 483; Nimsky C, Ganslandt O, Keller BV, Romstöck J, Fahlbusch R. Intraoperative high-field-strength MR imaging: implementation and experience in 200 patients. Radiology 2004; 233: 67–78. Adapted with permission.)

sequence, and 3D T1W FLASH for glioma surgery.[43] For epilepsy surgery and for resection control in cavernomas and nongliomatous brain tumors, they use 3D T1W FLASH, and optional T2W TSE. 3D T1W FLASH is repeated after contrast administration for lesions showing contrast enhancement on preoperative images.[43]

A recognized advantage of intraoperative imaging at high-field strengths is the higher contrast- and signal-to-noise ratios obtainable, and therefore the ability to achieve sufficient image quality in a time-efficient manner for surgical decisions to be reliably made. Additionally, high-field scanners enjoy a full armamentarium of functional mapping capabilities as detailed in the next section. For iMRI on high-field (1.5 T) MRI scanners, one group uses T2W TSE, FLAIR, T1W SE, 3D MP-RAGE, MRS, fMRI, and DTI (**Table 4.2**). T2W TSE, FLAIR, and T1W SE sequences are used to obtain different cross-sectional images at various stages of the surgery to assess the completeness of the tumor resection (**Fig. 4.7**). MRS, fMRI, and DTI are employed for the purpose of functional neuronavigation to obtain metabolic information

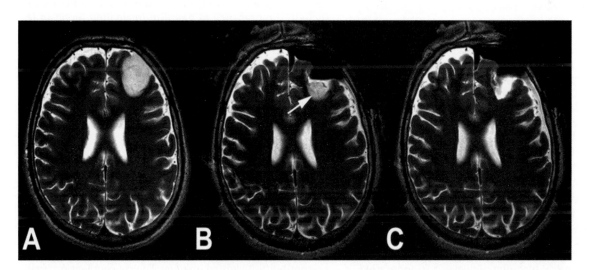

Fig. 4.7 High-field (1.5T) intraoperative magnetic resonance imaging (MRI) during open neurosurgery: 38-year-old male patient with a left frontal WHO grade III astrocytoma. Intraoperative T2-weighted imaging revealed a distinct tumor remnant (*white arrow*) that could be further removed, resulting in a completion of the resection, which was confirmed by repeated intraoperative imaging: **(A)** preoperative, **(B)** the first intraoperative, and **(C)** the second intraoperative MRI. (From Nimsky C, Ganslandt O, Buchfelder M, Fahlbusch R. Intraoperative visualization for resection of gliomas: the role of functional neuronavigation and intraoperative 1.5 T MRI. Neuro Research. 2006; 28:484. Reprinted with permission.)

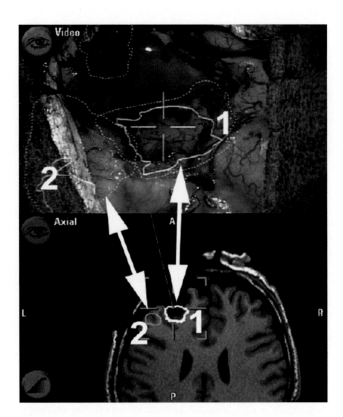

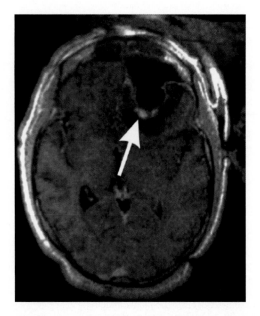

Fig. 4.9 Intraoperative magnetic resonance image (MRI) during resection of a left frontal astrocytoma (WHO grade III) acquired on 0.2 T MRI scanner shows contrast media enhancement at the resection border (*arrow*). Intraoperative reinvestigation revealed a small blood clot at this position. (From Nimsky C, Ganslandt O, Tomandl B, Buchfelder M, Fahlbusch R. Low-field magnetic resonance imaging for intraoperative use in neurosurgery: a 5-year experience. Eur Radiol 2002; 12:2698. Reprinted with permission.)

Fig. 4.8 The same patient as in Fig. 4.7. Intraoperative magnetic resonance image data were used for updating the navigation system; upper part: intraoperative view with superimposed contours depicting the tumor remnant (1) and the preoperative localized adjacent Broca area (2); lower part: corresponding navigation screen depicting the T1-weighted axial slice (please note that the left–right orientation was changed in the axial display, so that the correspondence to the intraoperative view is visible more easily). (From Nimsky C, Ganslandt O, Buchfelder M, Fahlbusch R. Intraoperative visualization for resection of gliomas: the role of functional neuronavigation and intraoperative 1.5 T MRI. Neuro Research 2006; 28:485. Reprinted with permission.)

about the tumor and to localize adjacent eloquent brain areas (**Fig. 4.8**).[10] The transsphenoidal pituitary surgery protocol of this group consists of coronal and sagittal HASTE images and T1W SE images for initial preliminary scans followed by high-resolution T2W TSE images. Glioma surgery protocol of this group includes T2W TSE, FLAIR, T1W SE, and fluid-suppressed EPI imaging. If contrast enhancement is seen on preoperative MR images, a contrast-enhanced T1W SE image is acquired. This is followed by acquisition of a 3D MP-RAGE image as a reference image for navigation purposes. If intraoperative imaging shows residual tumor, imaging is repeated after further resection and before closure of the craniotomy. However, they do not advocate repeating the contrast-enhanced imaging at that time.[44]

Contrast-enhanced MRI is valuable for preoperative tumor assessment and surgical planning. However, intraoperative contrast administration changes the relaxation parameters in its distribution and affects the contrast on subsequent imaging sequences. Various groups adopt different strategies for the use of gadolinium during iMRI. The general consensus is, however, to minimize contrast administration in the

intraoperative setting. Hall et al generally reserve intravenous contrast administration until the tumor has been resected to prevent diffusion of contrast into the edematous brain region around the tumor site, where the BBB is already disrupted or surgically breached.[12] Other factors that may potentially complicate the interpretation of intraoperative contrast-enhanced MRI scans and mimic residual tumors include the presence of gadolinium-loaded blood in the resection cavity (**Fig. 4.9**) and the enhancement of hemostyptic material applied at the resection border (**Fig. 4.10**).

MRA can be used to delineate vascular structures whenever required. The time-of-flight (ToF) method is very useful for this purpose. The phase-contrast method can be used to calculate flow rates. The contrast-enhanced method is less desirable for intraoperative purposes due to the reasons explained above.

Susceptibility-Weighted Imaging

Magnetic susceptibility is the degree of magnetization induced when a substance or tissue is placed within an external magnetic field and results in local distortion of the uniform external field. The local field inhomogeneities translate into phase differences in MRI and form the basis of susceptibility-weighted imaging. The concept was originally introduced in the work published by Reichenbach et al[45] in 1997, who described the use of the paramagnetic property of intravascular deoxyhemoglobin to obtain MR venograms. In that work, a method was developed to filter phase artifacts while preserving the local phase of interest. This

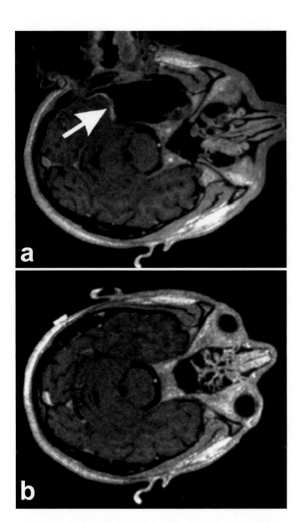

Fig. 4.10 Intraoperative magnetic resonance image **(A)** acquired on 0.2 T MRI scanner shows contrast enhancement at the temporal resection border, caused by hemostyptic material placed on the resection border (*arrow*). This enhancement is not visible in the preoperative image **(B)**. (From Nimsky C, Ganslandt O, Tomandl B, Buchfelder M, Fahlbusch R. Low-field magnetic resonance imaging for intraoperative use in neurosurgery: a 5-year experience. Eur Radiol 2002; 12:2698. Reprinted with permission.)

allowed the design of new SWIs by combining the filtered phase images with magnitude images. Subsequently, the concept was increasingly used for hemorrhage detection because most blood products, including deoxyhemoglobin, methemoglobin, and hemosiderin are paramagnetic substances that are highly visible on MR images that emphasize the loss of signal intensity associated with rapid spin dephasing.[46]

With the development of parallel imaging, it became possible to obtain SWIs of the entire brain in a time-efficient manner. For example, a typical imaging protocol for SWI of the brain on a 1.5 T MRI scanner using a 3D velocity compensated GRE sequence (TR/TE/FA: 48 ms/ 40 ms/20 degree; FOV: 240 × 240; matrix; 512 × 256; slice thickness 2 mm; 56 slices) can be implemented in 2.58 minutes using an acceleration factor of 2. The resulting data are processed online to obtain magnitude and phase images.[47] SWI can be

better performed at 3 T as compared with 1.5 T scanners due to the ability to use shorter echo time (TE) and to obtain a higher signal-to-noise ratio (SNR). This allows the acquisition of faster scans, increased slice coverage, and the acquisition of isotropic in-plane resolution.[48]

SWI can exploit the susceptibility differences of various tissues; therefore, it has been found to provide relevant information in a variety of disorders including cerebral infarctions, neoplasms, and neurodegenerative disorders associated with intracranial calcification or iron deposition.[49] However, the major application of SWI has been its use for the evaluation of various forms of cerebral hemorrhage/blood products including petechial shearing hemorrhages associated with traumatic diffuse axonal injury (DAI), other cerebral microbleeds associated with hypertensive encephalopathy and cerebral vasculitis, subarachnoid hemorrhage and pial siderosis, and small low-flow vascular malformations such as venous angiomas, telangiectasias, and cavernomas.[50] Several studies have shown that SWI is more sensitive than conventional T2*W gradient-echo sequences in detecting the size, number, and distribution of hemorrhagic lesions in DAI.[46,51,52]

Reports on the value of SWI have been largely derived from routine diagnostic scans. The concept does appear to be potentially helpful for hemorrhage detection in the intraoperative setting as well. A potential limitation for the use of SWI intraoperatively is the susceptibility artifact arising at the air–tissue interface at the craniotomy site, which may interfere with detecting subtle superficial hemorrhage. Other susceptibility effects may also be related to operative bed debris or operative devices. These should be readily identified and removed from the field. Preexisting sources of susceptibility effects in the imaged field such as cerebral or tumor calcifications, areas of preexisting tumor hemorrhage or necrosis, or areas of cerebral iron deposition should also be accounted for by careful preoperative review of the diagnostic scans.

◆ Pulse Sequences for Functional Neuronavigation

The integration of functional data into neuronavigation systems is known as functional neuronavigation: it helps in minimizing the odds of postoperative morbidity by preventing surgical injury to eloquent brain areas while maximizing the chances of resection of pathologic lesions.[53,54] In addition to MRI methods such as fMRI, DTI, MRS, and perfusion MRI, data from positron emission tomography (PET) and magnetoencephalography has also been employed for functional neuronavigation in iMRI.[10,53,54] Information provided by these techniques is particularly helpful to localize the tumor margins, assess tumor cell differentiation, differentiate between malignant tumors and necrosis, and obtain information regarding white matter tracts and eloquent cortex close to pathologic lesions. Data from functional mappings is registered onto anatomic MR images for intraoperative purposes. Using newly developed registration systems, which restore initial patient registration data after successive updates, a time delay of ~1 minute is added to the surgical procedure.[10] Preoperative functional images are also often used intraoperatively for functional neuronavigation. One group has used preoperative functional images acquired just before neurosurgery, registered onto intraoperatively acquired 3D datasets for functional neuronavigation (Vector Vision Sky, BrainLab, Heimstetten, Germany). The authors used a fiducial-based corresponding point technique for image registration. They employed this method for fMRI, DTI, and MRS techniques.[54-56] Images, after registration, can be displayed side by side or in an overlay mode. A grid scale can also be applied using Amira 3.0 software (Indeed Visual Concept, Berlin, Germany) to measure the displacement of pre- and intraoperative position of the pathology so that the surgeon can account for the actual location of white matter tracts and modify the strategy accordingly.[55] Preoperatively acquired functional maps are susceptible to inaccuracies induced by intraoperative brain shift. In a study consisting of 38 patients in whom DTI images were acquired pre- and intraoperatively, this brain shift ranged from an inward shift of 8 mm to an outward shift of 15 mm (**Fig. 4.11**).[54,55] This signifies the value of intraoperative imaging in neurosurgery, where a small misplacement of excision can significantly impact the final outcome in terms of functional capability and overall patient's quality of life. Continuous updates of the neuronavigation system with intraoperative image data are employed to account for inaccuracies caused by intraoperative brain shift. Unfortunately, it results in a loss of previously obtained functional information about eloquent cortices acquired by fMRI. A nonrigid registration algorithm is employed to register previous functional data with sequentially acquired DTI images.[55,57] Nonlinear elastic registration and pattern recognition techniques allow for matching of images with various degrees of brain shifts.[55]

Functional MRI

This method of functional neuronavigation is especially useful to analyze the location of eloquent areas close to pathologic lesions so as to attain minimum postoperative morbidity and hence best functional outcome. Blood oxygen-level dependent (BOLD) method is most often used to obtain fMRI images. Upon neural excitation in particular brain areas, blood flow through the local capillaries increases and outstrips the increase in oxygen demand in individual brain areas. The resulting local increase in the ratio of oxy-hemoglobin (oxy-Hb) to deoxy-hemoglobin (deoxy-Hb) is detected using T2*W GRE sequences. A resulting BOLD map is usually superimposed on a T1W image. A typical fMRI protocol on 1.5 T MRI scanner is a single-shot EPI (TR/TE: 3000 ms/40 ms; FOV: 210 mm; matrix: 64 × 64; slice thickness: 7 mm; intersection gap: 1 mm; repetitions: 72) with a scan time of ~4 minutes.[12,58]

For intraoperative acquisition of fMRI images, individual brain areas are stimulated using area-specific passive stimulation techniques or by making the patient perform a specific task by controlled awakening from anesthesia. Passive stimulation paradigms involve electrical stimulation of tibial and median nerves. A block design of passive stimulation paradigms, in which blocks of neural stimulation are alternated by those of rest, is commonly employed.[59] Passive stimulation methods suffer from the disadvantage that information regarding supplementary motor areas may be missed. Anesthesia regimen of propofol and fentanyl, which is commonly employed for MR-guided neurosurgery, reduces the cortical response to electrical stimulation employed for fMRI data acquisition. Therefore, the intensity of electrical stimulation required for the same degree of cortical stimulation in anesthetized patients is higher than that

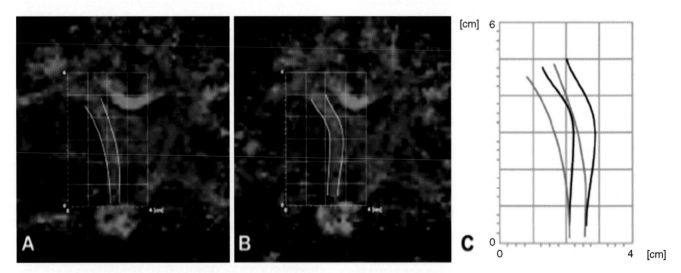

Fig. 4.11 Images obtained in a 61-year-old woman with a grade IV right temporal glioblastoma. A 6-mm inward shift of the pyramidal tract occurred after tumor resection. **(A)** Preoperative and **(B)** intraoperative coronal color-encoded fractional anisotropy maps obtained with diffusion tensor imaging (DTI) after the head was fixed in a horizontal position. Imaging parameters were as follows: repetition time/ echo time [TR/TE]: 9200/86 and high *b* value of 1000 s/mm²; one null image and six diffusion-weighted magnetic resonance images were obtained. **(C)** Overlay of the segmented pyramidal tract. Red and black lines indicate pre- and postoperative measurements, respectively. (From Nimsky C, Ganslandt O, Hastreiter P, et al. Intraoperative diffusion-tensor MR imaging: Shifting of white matter tracts during neurosurgical procedures–initial experience. Radiology 2005;234: 222. Reprinted with permission.)

required for awake patients.[60] However, propofol is still regarded as the best anesthetic agent for intraoperative fMRI acquisition as it does not inhibit stimulus-evoked cortical activity below the limit of the fMRI data acquisition.[59] The controlled awakening method employs temporary awakening of the patient from anesthesia so as to perform a specific task to activate the corresponding eloquent area. This method enables the identification of eloquent areas that cannot be passively stimulated. However, this procedure requires a complex anesthesia regimen and is a time-consuming process.[59] In one study, by employing passive paradigm based on electrical stimulation of the median and tibial nerves, the authors were able to intraoperatively identify the somatosensory cortex and validate the results with functional information obtained with the somatosensory evoked potential (SEP) phase reversal method.[59]

Established functional mapping techniques such as phase reversal require extensive exposure of the brain area and hence undue increase in the size of the craniotomy. Unlike phase reversal and surface mapping, which can only be performed after craniotomy, fMRI data can also be acquired before surgery to optimize the craniotomy position. Furthermore, fMRI data are of a digital nature and can be directly available for neuronavigation immediately after data acquisition; time-consuming offline analysis is not required. An intraoperative combination of fMRI and DTI provides highly valuable information for neurosurgery. fMRI data provide seed points for fiber tracking algorithms to delineate white matter tracks (**Fig. 4.12**). Combined information is particularly helpful during excision of large centrally located tumors with extensive brain shift.[59] A combination of an electroencephalogram (EEG) and fMRI can also be used as an alternative to electrode recording for localization of areas of interictal spikes.[61]

Intraoperative fMRI acquisition is challenged by susceptibility artifacts from fixation hardware and vacant space created by removal of a tumor mass. The artifact created by the vacant space can be avoided by filling the empty space with saline and by applying field mapping for MR imaging.[59] To avoid susceptibility artifacts, head holders made of glass fiber-reinforced plastic are now available.[44] Vascular lesions such as arteriovenous malformations and large blood vessels can also result in signal artifacts.

Diffusion Tensor Imaging

Diffusion tensor imaging (DTI) is used to detect anisotropic water diffusion (diffusion in which one direction is preferred). Because diffusion of water molecules is greatest along the longitudinal direction of neural sheaths,[4] the direction and degree of anisotropy detected provides information regarding the position, orientation, and integrity of white matter tracts with respect to adjacent tumors. Two gradient pulses (with equal strength, but opposite polarity; gradient strength is denoted as *b-value*) are applied before image acquisition in six different directions. For nuclei with zero net diffusion motion, spins dephased by the first gradient are rephased again by the second gradient. Hence high-signal intensity is observed on the subsequent image. On the other hand, if there is a net diffusion movement, the second gradient will not be able to rephase the spins once dephased by the first gradient, resulting in lower signal intensity on the subsequent image.[3,55] A typical protocol for DTI data acquisition on 1.5 T MRI scanner is single-shot diffusion weighted EPI (TR/TE: 9200 ms/86 ms; matrix: 128×128; FOV: 240 mm; 60 sections; section thickness: 1.9 mm; bandwidth: 1502 Hz; b-value: 1000 s/mm^2; voxel size: $1.9 \times 1.9 \times 1.9$ mm^3; averages: 5) with a scan time of 5 minutes 30 seconds.[55] A balanced diffusion gradient design is employed to strongly minimize eddy-current artifacts as compared with a single refocused design. DTI cards are employed to generate DTI

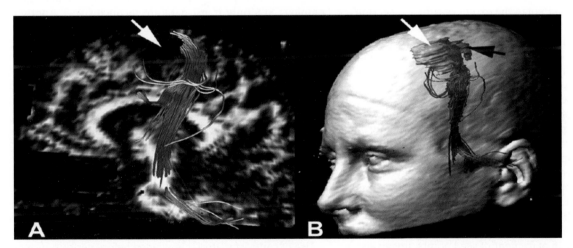

Fig. 4.12 In a patient with a left pre-central WHO grade III oligodendroglioma, diffusion tensor imaging (DTI) data was used to perform fiber tracking to visualize the left pyramidal tract beside the tumor (*white arrow* in [**A,B**]); functional magnetic resonance imaging (fMRI), identifying the motor cortex (*black arrow* in [**B**]), was used as a seed region for fiber tracking ([**A**] fiber tract data visualized together with a sagittal view of the fractional anisotropy maps; [**B**] three-dimensional rendering of the segmented tumor and fMRI activity together with the integrated fiber tract data). (From Nimsky C, Ganslandt O, Buchfelder M, Fahlbusch R. Intraoperative visualization for resection of gliomas: the role of functional neuronavigation and intraoperative 1.5 T MRI. Neuro Research 2006; 28: 486. Reprinted with permission.)

maps.[55] The extent of displacement of proton's position during the time interval between the applications of two gradient pulses determines the degree of signal drop. The greater the displacement; the higher the signal attenuation is. This mechanism allows inference about displacement of water molecules on a spatial scale of 5 to 10 μm.[4] Color-encoded maps of fractional anisotropy are generated to depict white matter tracts. If the patient is lying supine in the MRI scanner with the head straight, white matter tracts with orientation in anterior-to-posterior, left-to-right, and superior-to-inferior direction are coded as green, red, and blue, respectively.[55] These directions of color encoding will, however, change if the head is placed in a tilted position while performing MR imaging. A newer version of DTI task card allows arbitrary section orientations and diffusion gradient direction to be taken into account.[55] A tracking algorithm is usually initiated from user defined seed regions that are often based on a preacquired fMRI (**Fig. 4.12**). It takes less than one minute to track all the fibers passing through a user-defined seed point and an additional 5 minutes for image registration.[55]

DTI is the only method available for 3D visualization of white matter tracts in vivo[62]; it also provides information regarding edema, infiltration, disruption, and displacement of white matter tracts by adjacent pathologic lesions.[63] DTI provides information essential for preoperative planning and surgical risk assessment. It is also valuable in verifying the completeness of resection and in detecting postresection recurrences. In a study comprising 25 patients, DTI findings prompted a change in surgical approach in 16% and impacted the extent of resection during surgery in 68% of patients.[64] Yu et al found the use of DTI to significantly improve the accuracy of tumor resection and postoperative locomotive function.[62] This is particularly valuable with intraoperative (as opposed to preoperative) acquisition to avoid the confounding effect of brain shift associated with resection of deep brain tumors. The ability of DTI to map out the pattern of white matter tract involvement by gliomas is beneficial to plan the extent of tumor resection and to predict the risk of postoperative tumor recurrence.[65,66] As described in the previous section, the combination of fMRI and DTI provides valuable information about eloquent cortical areas as well as deep white matter tracts. The combined use of both techniques helps localize twice as many functional areas as fMRI alone can.[67]

DTI is a user-defined process and results could vary according to the parameters used. Rapid automated or semiautomated methods are desirable for more robust clinical applications. Spatial resolution of DTI images is also a limitation. Small tracts with differing directions within a single voxel will not be imaged secondary to partial volume artifacts. Instead, a low degree of anisotropy will be seen in those voxels, resulting in a misleading average direction.[68]

Various problems faced by intraoperative use of DTI include inaccuracy in placement of seed points, image distortions caused primarily by brain–air interface at the tumor resection bed, and fiber crossings. Various potential solutions such as sensitivity encoding, field map corrections, and nonlinear registration and transformation algorithms can be employed to correct field inhomogeneities.[54–56]

Magnetic Resonance Spectroscopy

Magnetic resonance spectroscopy (MRS) provides metabolic information about the tissues and is performed by obtaining spectra of various NMR sensitive nuclei such as proton (^{1}H), carbon (^{13}C), and phosphorus (^{31}P). Among these techniques, ^{1}H-MRS is most often used for tumor diagnosis in neurosurgery.[69] MRS data can be acquired both preoperatively and intraoperatively. Spectroscopic information obtained from MRS is superimposed upon an anatomic image acquired with the same parameters (voxel size, slice position, etc.) as that of MRS.[69,70] Different sequences such as axial-RARE (TR/TE: 80/3180 ms), inversion-recovery (TR/TE/FA: 4869 ms/ 14 ms/9 degrees) and axial T1W SE (TR/TE: 500 ms/15 ms) have been employed for this purpose.[69–71] Three methods have been employed for intraoperative acquisition of MRS data in neurosurgery: *single voxel spectroscopy* (SVS), *turbo-spectroscopic imaging* (TSI), and *chemical shift imaging* (CSI).[10–12] The SVS method of MRS acquires data from only one voxel and is not able to provide metabolic information from an entire volume of larger brain tumors. On the other hand, by acquiring spectroscopic data from a large number of voxels, TSI and CSI can provide metabolic information from larger volumes. CSI provides metabolic information with better spatial resolution than TSI; however, the former requires more time for data acquisition.[70]

One group uses SVS or TSI or a combination of two techniques under general anesthesia for brain biopsy.[11,12,70] A typical SVS protocol (TR/TE: 136/2000 ms; voxel size: 1.5 × 1.5 × 1.5 cm³, 1 Hz spectral resolution) takes 4.5 minutes for data acquisition from a voxel in the tumor area and a control location in the contralateral hemisphere.[11,12,70] A typical TSI protocol (TE/TR: 272 ms/2000 ms; 32 mm × 32 mm grid of spectra in a single plane; voxel size: 0.66 × 0.66 × 2.0 cm³; spatial resolution: 4.4 Hz; turbo-factor: 3) takes 11 minutes for data acquisition from a single axial slice.[11,12,70] This group employs TSI as the first choice and employs SVS only if TSI data are inconclusive.[70] Another group employs the CSI method for acquisition of spectroscopic data.[10,71] It employs a point resolved spectroscopy (PRESS) volume preselection and chemical shift water suppression slab in the area under investigation. A typical protocol (TR/TE: 1600 ms/35 ms; 24 × 24 circular phase encoding scheme across a 16 cm × 16 cm FOV; slice thickness: 10 cm; voxel size: 0.67 × 0.67 × 1.0 cm³; 50% hamming-filter; number of excitations: 2; spectral bandwidth: 1000 Hz; 1024 complex point acquisition size) takes 13 minutes for MRS data acquisition.[10,71] MRS can also be performed on 3.0 T MRI scanners to obtain spectral resolution and higher SNR.[70] A satisfactory SNR can be obtained with a spatial resolution of less than 0.5 cm³ at 3.0 T with standard head coil.[72] However, no published reports on intraoperative MRS at 3.0 T are available in the literature thus far.

Use of contrast material is avoided before performance of MRS as it alters the spectral data of various metabolites.[11] MRS data from a large volume of the brain can be acquired in one session and a hypothetical voxel can be drawn at any desired position in that volume to analyze the metabolic information in that particular region.[69]

Due to its low sensitivity, MRS detects only those metabolites with a concentration greater than 0.5 mM/l L. Spectral lines of N-acetylaspartate (NAA, at 2.0 ppm), choline (Cho- containing compounds, at 3.2 ppm), total creatinine (Cr, at 3.0), and phosphocreatine (at 3.9 ppm), myoinositol (at 3.6 ppm), lactate (at 1.3 ppm), a mixture of glutamine and glutamate (overlapping multiplates at 2.0–2.5 ppm and 3.75 ppm, respectively), and lipids (broad lines between 0.9–1.3 ppm) can be observed in MRS spectra of brain.[69] NAA reflects neural integrity, creatine is a marker of energy metabolism, and choline is involved in increased membrane and myelin turnover and hence reflects higher cellularity.[71,73] While analyzing MRS data, spectral characteristics of data from the abnormal region are compared with those from the normal parenchyma acquired during the same imaging sequence. Spectral lines of NAA and choline are particularly useful for brain tumor detection, which are characterized by a reduction of signal intensity of NAA and an increase in signal intensity of choline. Tissue necrosis is usually characterized by an abnormally decreased signal intensity of both NAA and choline.[74,75] Lactate is usually not visible in normal brain and is a marker of anaerobic metabolism.[69] Additionally, lipid levels are often increased in some high-grade tumors. Cerebral infarctions and abscesses are characterized by a decrease in signal intensities of choline, creatine, and NAA. Metastases also have an increase in choline, but can be differentiated from high-grade gliomas by their lower lipid levels. Extraaxial tumors are characterized by absence of NAA and a high alanine/creatine ratio.[74,75] MRS spectra are usually read by employing automated spectrum-fitting algorithms (LCModel or VARPRO) and pattern recognition techniques may be used to support a diagnosis.[69]

Metabolic information regarding heterogeneity of glioma is useful for selection of stereotactic biopsy sites, treatment planning, and the assessment of residual tumors. The establishment of the presence of mitotic figures in at least one biopsy site is needed to differentiate grade III from grade II gliomas, two categories with a significant difference in prognosis and treatment planning. Areas with high cell turnover, defined by high intensity from choline, characterize the most aggressive regions to locate optimal biopsy sites (**Fig. 4.13**).[73] MRS has also been shown to help differentiate recurrent tumors from radiation necrosis (sensitivity and specificity of 94.1% and 100%, respectively).[76] Metabolic information provided by 3D MRS can be used to define target volume, dose description, and patient eligibility; to examine treatment response, and to predict sites for posttreatment recurrence for gamma knife radiosurgery in gliomas.[77] MRS can also be used for the localization of epileptic foci (characterized by increase in NAA/choline ratio) and measurement of hippocampal volumes for epilepsy surgery.[78] MRS is also helpful for detecting microscopic tumor extension beyond the margins identified on conventional MRI (**Fig. 4.14**).[70] MRS has also been combined with perfusion imaging (PI) and with diffusion weighted imaging (DWI) for tumor grading, defining tumor margins, and differentiating tumor recurrence from radiation necrosis.[79]

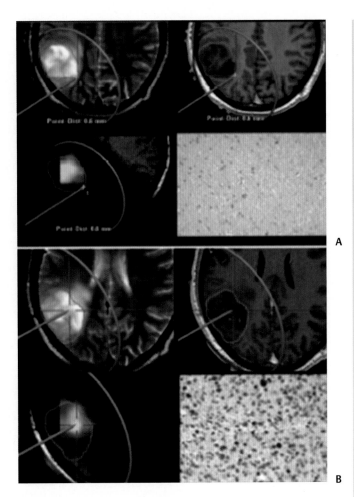

A

B

Fig. 4.13 Illustrative examples of biopsies taken from the center of pathologic metabolite change and from the border zone: T1- and T2-weighted magnetic resonance images and metabolic map are displayed. The right lower images show tumor cell density of each corresponding locus, which was 15% in **(A)** the border zone and **(B)** 100% in the center. (From Ganslandt O, Stadlbauer A, Fahlbusch R, et al. Proton MR spectroscopic imaging integrated into image-guided surgery: correlation to standard magnetic resonance imaging and tumor cell density. Neurosurgery 2005; 56, 2: 295. Reprinted with permission.)

In a retrospective study of 26 patients with MRS coupled with trajectory-guided biopsy, a 100% diagnostic yield was obtained without clinically significant hemorrhage.[11] The authors were able to obtain diagnostic tissue in all 35 first SVS-guided biopsy procedures performed by employing freehand technique. They were also able to obtain diagnostic tissue in all of 40 MRS guided brain biopsies by employing the trajectory guide/prospective stereotaxy technique.[11] TSI has reportedly less diagnostic yield than SVS. The same authors were able to obtain diagnostic tissue in only 13 out of 17 patients (76%) by employing TSI. More spectral contamination is observed in TSI data than in SVS data.[11,70] SVS offers higher SNR and better spectral resolution than TSI.[70] SVS can be employed to obtain confirmatory information in areas where TSI is unable to provide clear metabolic information.[70]

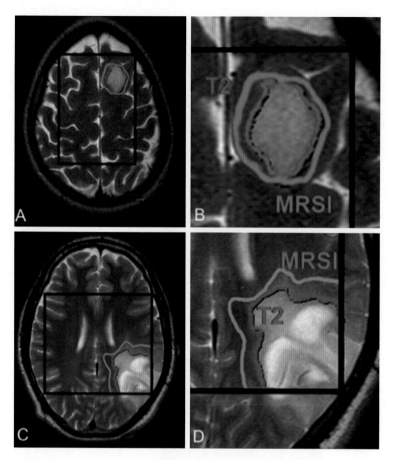

Fig. 4.14 Metabolic information provided by intraoperative magnetic resonance spectroscopy (MRS) helps in the more accurate definition of brain tumor edges than conventional MR images. Tumor margins are often beyond the edge of signal change as depicted on conventional MR images. This difference can be well appreciated from tumor areas manually segmented from T_2 signal changes (*red line*) and tumor areas automatically segmented from MRS data (*green line*) of two patients with **(A,B)** left frontal astrocytoma and **(C,D)** left temporoparietal astrocytoma. The 1H MRS imaging data indicate in each case a larger tumor dimension, which is further verified by stereotactic biopsy. The *black rectangle* represents the position of the point resolved spectroscopy (PRESS) box. (From Ganslandt O, Stadlbauer A, Fahlbusch R, et al. Proton MR spectroscopic imaging integrated into image-guided surgery: correlation to standard magnetic resonance imaging and tumor cell density. Neurosurgery 2005; 56, 2: 295. Reprinted with permission.)

Dynamic Susceptibility-Weighted Contrast-Enhanced Perfusion MRI

Perfusion MRI is commonly performed by dynamic susceptibility-weighted contrast-enhanced perfusion MRI (DSC-MRI) method. DSC-MRI exploits the susceptibility effect of a gadolinium-based contrast agent within an intravascular compartment and allows for measurement of blood flow from desired brain region. In this technique, a set of T1WIs is rapidly acquired from the region-of-interest during the first pass of intravenously injected gadolinium contrast agent. Contrast arrival in the imaging volume leads to a signal drop from arteries and tissues in the T1WIs. Regional trends of the signal from the set of images are used to estimate local contrast agent concentration and hence hemodynamics parameters.[80] DSC-MRI can be performed using any of two sequences: SE-EPI and GRE-EPI. SE-EPI is sensitive to blood signal from vessels of relatively small diameter ($\approx$10 μm) and underestimates the blood volume, whereas GRE-EPI is sensitive to blood signal from vessels of all sizes and provides hemodynamics information with relatively high accuracy.[80] A typical DSC-MRI protocol on 1.5 T MRI using GRE-EPI sequence (TR/TE: 1500 ms/45 ms; FOV: 240 mm; matrix: 128 × 128; slice thickness: 5 mm; interslice gap: 1.5 mm; temporal resolution 1.5 s 48 repetitions) takes ~72 seconds of scan time and requires 0.05 mM/ kg dose of gadolinium contrast.[80] Three perfusion parameters commonly employed in neurosurgery are relative cerebral blood volume (rCBV), relative peak height (rPH), and percentage of signal-intensity recovery (PSR); they indirectly provide information regarding tumor microvascular density, capillary blood volume and capillary permeability (i.e., BBB integrity), respectively.[81]

All the previous applications of perfusion MRI in neurosurgery have been described for preoperative imaging. In principle, perfusion MRI can also be performed intraoperatively. It can be employed to diagnose a small hemorrhage, analyze the regional variations in tumor vascularity, and distinguish between a recurrent tumor and radiation-induced necrosis. Higher rCBV values from more malignant regions of a glioma (due to relatively high cellularity and microvascular density)[82–85] can be exploited for biopsy site localization. A recurrent brain tumor can also be distinguished from tumor necrosis on DSC-MRI.[81,86] The fact of low rCBV values from brain lymphomas can be exploited for their differentiation from other brain tumors.[87,88] Perfusion MRI data has also been combined with that from fMRI and MRS for differentiation of a necrotic tumor from a pyogenic brain abscess with higher accuracy.[89] DSC-MRI has also been employed to differentiate between high-grade gliomas and metastasis.[90]

DSC-MRI requires gadolinium-based contrast agent administration for image acquisition, which changes the relaxation parameters in its distribution and affects the contrast on subsequent imaging sequences. This problem could be circumvented by using another method of perfusion MRI called arterial spin labeling (ASL), which obviates the need for contrast injection and also provides more accurate information about glioma aggressiveness.[91] Unfortunately, lower SNR and temporal resolution, and limitations regarding the region of brain cover in each exam as compared with DSC-MRI limit the practical applications of the ASL method.[92]

◆ Conclusion

Several pulse sequences can be employed for intraoperative imaging during neurosurgery. An MP-RAGE sequence is typically used to acquire 3D images preoperatively. Hemorrhage scans consisting of HASTE, FLAIR, and T2*W GRE are obtained to detect intraoperative hemorrhage. Near-real-time minimally invasive device guidance is performed by employing FISP, PSIF, HASTE, and T1W GRE sequences. Freehand and stereotactic techniques are often used for device tracking purposes to perform MR-guided minimally invasive procedures. Various factors such as magnetic field strength, sequence design, pulse sequence acquisition bandwidth, direction of frequency encode direction, needle composition, and needle orientation with respect to the main magnetic field of the MRI scanner affect the appearance of needle on MR images. FISP, PSIF, FLASH, T1W SE, T2W TSE, and FLAIR sequences are used to monitor open neurosurgical procedures with iMRI. Intraoperative contrast administration should generally be minimized, and is sometimes reserved until the tumor has been resected. Functional neuronavigation is performed by integrating functional and metabolic data acquired by employing fMRI, DTI, and MRS, methods. Image fusion methods are employed to integrate functional and/or metabolic data into the usual anatomic images. EPI sequence is commonly used to perform fMRI and DTI data acquisitions. SVS, TSI, and CSI are employed to obtain metabolic information with MRS.

References

1. Bloch F. Nuclear induction. Phys Rev 1946;70:460–474
2. Curry TS III, Dowdey JE, Murray RC. Fluoroscopic imaging. In: Curry TS III, Dowdey JE, Murray RC, eds. Christensen's Physics of Diagnostic Radiology. 4th ed. Philadelphia: Lea and Febiger; 1990
3. Bitar R, Leung G, Perng R, et al. MR pulse sequences: what every radiologist wants to know but is afraid to ask. Radiographics 2006;26(2):513–537
4. Roberts TP, Mikulis D, Neuro MR. Neuro MR: principles. J Magn Reson Imaging 2007;26(4):823–837
5. Jackson EF, Ginsberg LE, Schomer DF, Leeds NE. A review of MRI pulse sequences and techniques in neuroimaging. Surg Neurol 1997;47(2):185–199
6. Hall WA, Liu H, Martin AJ, Maxwell RE, Truwit CL. Brain biopsy sampling by using prospective stereotaxis and a trajectory guide. J Neurosurg 2001;94(1):67–71
7. Gruber S, Mlynárik V, Moser E. High-resolution 3D proton spectroscopic imaging of the human brain at 3 T: SNR issues and application for anatomy-matched voxel sizes. Magn Reson Med 2003;49(2):299–306
8. Lewin JS, Nour SG, Meyers ML, et al. Intraoperative MRI with a rotating, tiltable surgical table: a time use study and clinical results in 122 patients. AJR Am J Roentgenol 2007;189(5):1096–1103
9. Scheffler K, Lehnhardt S. Principles and applications of balanced SSFP techniques. Eur Radiol 2003;13(11):2409–2418
10. Nimsky C, Ganslandt O, Buchfelder M, Fahlbusch R. Intraoperative visualization for resection of gliomas: the role of functional neuronavigation and intraoperative 1.5 T MRI. Neurol Res 2006;28(5):482–487
11. Hall WA, Truwit CL. 1.5 T: spectroscopy-supported brain biopsy. Neurosurg Clin N Am 2005;16(1):165–172, vii
12. Hall WA, Truwit CL. Intraoperative MR-guided neurosurgery. J Magn Reson Imaging 2008;27(2):368–375
13. Hall WA, Galicich W, Bergman T, Truwit CL. 3-Tesla intraoperative MR imaging for neurosurgery. J Neurooncol 2006;77(3):297–303
14. Kidwell CS, Wintermark M. Imaging of intracranial haemorrhage. Lancet Neurol 2008;7(3):256–267
15. Sohn CH, Baik SK, Lee HJ, et al. MR imaging of hyperacute subarachnoid and intraventricular hemorrhage at 3T: a preliminary report of gradient echo T2*-weighted sequences. AJNR Am J Neuroradiol 2005;26(3):662–665
16. Nour SG, Lewin JS. Percutaneous biopsy from blinded to MR guided: an update on current techniques and applications. Magn Reson Imaging Clin N Am 2005;13(3):441–464
17. Liu H, Hall WA, Truwit CL. Remotely-controlled approach for stereotactic neurobiopsy. Comput Aided Surg 2002;7(4):237–247
18. Hall WA, Martin AJ, Liu H, Nussbaum ES, Maxwell RE, Truwit CL. Brain biopsy using high-field strength interventional magnetic resonance imaging. Neurosurgery 1999;44(4):807–813, discussion 813–814
19. Truwit CL, Liu H. Prospective stereotaxy: a novel method of trajectory alignment using real-time image guidance. J Magn Reson Imaging 2001;13(3):452–457
20. Martin AJ, Hall WA, Roark C, Starr PA, Larson PS, Truwit CL. Minimally invasive precision brain access using prospective stereotaxy and a trajectory guide. J Magn Reson Imaging 2008;27(4):737–743
21. Martin AJ, Larson PS, Ostrem JL, et al. Placement of deep brain stimulator electrodes using real-time high-field interventional magnetic resonance imaging. Magn Reson Med 2005;54(5):1107–1114
22. Lewin JS, Petersilge CA, Hatem SF, et al. Interactive MR imaging-guided biopsy and aspiration with a modified clinical C-arm system. AJR Am J Roentgenol 1998;170(6):1593–1601
23. Lewin JS. Interventional MR imaging: concepts, systems, and applications in neuroradiology. AJNR Am J Neuroradiol 1999;20(5):735–748
24. Schneider JP, Dietrich J, Lieberenz S, et al. Preliminary experience with interactive guided brain biopsies using a vertically opened 0.5-T MR system. Eur Radiol 1999;9(2):230–236
25. Jolesz FA, Kikinis R, Talos IF. Neuronavigation in interventional MR imaging. Frameless stereotaxy. Neuroimaging Clin N Am 2001;11(4):685–693, ix
26. Hillenbrand CM, Elgort DR, Wong EY, et al. Active device tracking and high-resolution intravascular MRI using a novel catheter-based, opposed-solenoid phased array coil. Magn Reson Med 2004;51(4):668–675
27. Elgort DR, Wong EY, Hillenbrand CM, Wacker FK, Lewin JS, Duerk JL. Real-time catheter tracking and adaptive imaging. J Magn Reson Imaging 2003;18(5):621–626
28. Wacker FK, Elgort D, Hillenbrand CM, Duerk JL, Lewin JS. The catheter-driven MRI scanner: a new approach to intravascular catheter tracking and imaging-parameter adjustment for interventional MRI. AJR Am J Roentgenol 2004;183(2):391–395
29. Truwit CL, Liu H. Prospective stereotaxy: a novel method of trajectory alignment using real-time image guidance. J Magn Reson Imaging 2001;13(3):452–457
30. Liu H, Hall WA, Truwit CL. Neuronavigation in interventional MR imaging. Prospective stereotaxy. Neuroimaging Clin N Am 2001;11(4):695–704
31. Samset E, Hirschberg H. Image-guided stereotaxy in the interventional MRI. Minim Invasive Neurosurg 2003;46(1):5–10
32. Rohlfing T, West JB, Beier J, Liebig T, Taschner CA, Thomale UW. Registration of functional and anatomical MRI: accuracy assessment and application in navigated neurosurgery. Comput Aided Surg 2000;5(6):414–425
33. Gering DT, Nabavi A, Kikinis R, et al. An integrated visualization system for surgical planning and guidance using image fusion and an open MR. J Magn Reson Imaging 2001;13(6):967–975
34. Moche M, Busse H, Dannenberg C, et al. [Fusion of MRI, fMRI and intraoperative MRI data. Methods and clinical significance exemplified by neurosurgical interventions]. Radiologe 2001;41(11):993–1000 [in German]

35. Lewin JS, Duerk JL, Jain VR, Petersilge CA, Chao CP, Haaga JR. Needle localization in MR-guided biopsy and aspiration: effects of field strength, sequence design, and magnetic field orientation. AJR Am J Roentgenol 1996;166(6):1337–1345

36. Liu H, Hall WA, Martin AJ, Truwit CL. Biopsy needle tip artifact in MR-guided neurosurgery. J Magn Reson Imaging 2001;13(1):16–22

37. Schwarzmaier HJ, Eickmeyer F, von Tempelhoff W, et al. MR-guided laser-induced interstitial thermotherapy of recurrent glioblastoma multiforme: preliminary results in 16 patients. Eur J Radiol 2006; 59(2):208–215

38. Mikulis DJ, Roberts TPL, Neuro MR. Neuro MR: protocols. J Magn Reson Imaging 2007;26(4):838–847

39. Turetschek K, Wunderbaldinger P, Bankier AA, et al. Double inversion recovery imaging of the brain: initial experience and comparison with fluid attenuated inversion recovery imaging. Magn Reson Imaging 1998;16(2):127–135

40. Wendel JD, Trenerry MR, Xu YC, et al. The relationship between quantitative T2 relaxometry and memory in nonlesional temporal lobe epilepsy. Epilepsia 2001;42(7):863–868

41. Clark CA, Barrick TR, Murphy MM, Bell BA. White matter fiber tracking in patients with space-occupying lesions of the brain: a new technique for neurosurgical planning? Neuroimage 2003;20(3):1601–1608

42. Dort JC, Sutherland GR. Intraoperative magnetic resonance imaging for skull base surgery. Laryngoscope 2001;111(9):1570–1575

43. Nimsky C, Ganslandt O, Tomandl B, Buchfelder M, Fahlbusch R. Low-field magnetic resonance imaging for intraoperative use in neurosurgery: a 5-year experience. Eur Radiol 2002;12(11):2690–2703

44. Nimsky C, Ganslandt O, Von Keller B, Romstöck J, Fahlbusch R. Intraoperative high-field-strength MR imaging: implementation and experience in 200 patients. Radiology 2004;233(1):67–78

45. Reichenbach JR Jr, Venkatesan R, Schillinger DJ, Kido DK, Haacke EM. Small vessels in the human brain: MR venography with deoxyhemoglobin as an intrinsic contrast agent. Radiology 1997;204(1):272–277

46. Tong KA, Ashwal S, Holshouser BA, et al. Hemorrhagic shearing lesions in children and adolescents with posttraumatic diffuse axonal injury: improved detection and initial results. Radiology 2003;227(2):332–339

47. Thomas B, Somasundaram S, Thamburaj K, et al. Clinical applications of susceptibility weighted MR imaging of the brain - a pictorial review. Neuroradiology 2008;50(2):105–116

48. Haacke EM, Mittal S, Wu Z, Neelavalli J, Cheng YC. Susceptibility-weighted imaging: technical aspects and clinical applications, part 1. AJNR Am J Neuroradiol 2009;30(1):19–30

49. Mittal S, Wu Z, Neelavalli J, Haacke EM. Susceptibility-weighted imaging: technical aspects and clinical applications, part 2. AJNR Am J Neuroradiol 2009;30(2):232–252

50. Thomas B, Somasundaram S, Thamburaj K, et al. Clinical applications of susceptibility weighted MR imaging of the brain - a pictorial review. Neuroradiology 2008;50(2):105–116 Review

51. Tong KA, Ashwal S, Holshouser BA, et al. Diffuse axonal injury in children: clinical correlation with hemorrhagic lesions. Ann Neurol 2004; 56(1):36–50

52. Babikian T, Freier MC, Tong KA, et al. Susceptibility weighted imaging: neuropsychologic outcome and pediatric head injury. Pediatr Neurol 2005;33(3):184–194

53. Nimsky C, Ganslandt O, Kober H, et al. Integration of functional magnetic resonance imaging supported by magnetoencephalography in functional neuronavigation. Neurosurgery 1999;44(6):1249–1255, discussion 1255–1256

54. Nimsky C, Ganslandt O, Hastreiter P, et al. Preoperative and intraoperative diffusion tensor imaging-based fiber tracking in glioma surgery. Neurosurgery 2005;56(1):130–137, discussion 138

55. Nimsky C, Ganslandt O, Hastreiter P, et al. Intraoperative diffusion-tensor MR imaging: shifting of white matter tracts during neurosurgical procedures—initial experience. Radiology 2005;234(1):218–225

56. Nimsky C, Grummich P, Sorensen AG, Fahlbusch R, Ganslandt O. Visualization of the pyramidal tract in glioma surgery by integrating diffusion tensor imaging in functional neuronavigation. Zentralbl Neurochir 2005;66(3):133–141

57. Ruiz-Alzola J, Westin CF, Warfield SK, Alberola C, Maier S, Kikinis R. Nonrigid registration of 3D tensor medical data. Med Image Anal 2002;6(2):143–161

58. Hall WA, Truwit CL. Intraoperative MR imaging. Magn Reson Imaging Clin N Am 2005;13(3):533–543

59. Gasser T, Ganslandt O, Sandalcioglu E, Stolke D, Fahlbusch R, Nimsky C. Intraoperative functional MRI: implementation and preliminary experience. Neuroimage 2005;26(3):685–693

60. Gasser TG, Sandalcioglu EI, Wiedemayer H, et al. A novel passive functional MRI paradigm for preoperative identification of the somatosensory cortex. Neurosurg Rev 2004;27(2):106–112

61. Manganotti P, Formaggio E, Gasparini A, et al. Continuous EEG-fMRI in patients with partial epilepsy and focal interictal slow-wave discharges on EEG. Magn Reson Imaging 2008;26(8):1089–1100

62. Yu CS, Li KC, Xuan Y, Ji XM, Qin W. Diffusion tensor tractography in patients with cerebral tumors: a helpful technique for neurosurgical planning and postoperative assessment. Eur J Radiol 2005;56(2):197–204

63. Wei CW, Guo G, Mikulis DJ. Tumor effects on cerebral white matter as characterized by diffusion tensor tractography. Can J Neurol Sci 2007; 34(1):62–68

64. Romano A, Ferrante M, Cipriani V, et al. Role of magnetic resonance tractography in the preoperative planning and intraoperative assessment of patients with intra-axial brain tumours. Radiol Med (Torino) 2007;112(6):906–920

65. Lu S, Ahn D, Johnson G, Cha S. Peritumoral diffusion tensor imaging of high-grade gliomas and metastatic brain tumors. AJNR Am J Neuroradiol 2003;24(5):937–941

66. Price SJ, Jena R, Burnet NG, Carpenter TA, Pickard JD, Gillard JH. Predicting patterns of glioma recurrence using diffusion tensor imaging. Eur Radiol 2007;17(7):1675–1684

67. Ulmer JL, Salvan CV, Mueller WM, et al. The role of diffusion tensor imaging in establishing the proximity of tumor borders to functional brain systems: implications for preoperative risk assessments and postoperative outcomes. Technol Cancer Res Treat 2004;3(6):567–576

68. Reinges MHT, Schoth F, Coenen VA, Krings T. Imaging of posthalamic visual fiber tracts by anisotropic diffusion weighted MRI and diffusion tensor imaging: principles and applications. Eur J Radiol 2004;49(2):91–104

69. Gruber S, Stadlbauer A, Mlynarik V, Gatterbauer B, Roessler K, Moser E. Proton magnetic resonance spectroscopy in brain tumor diagnosis. Neurosurg Clin N Am 2005;16(1):101–114, vi

70. Martin AJ, Liu H, Hall WA, Truwit CL. Preliminary assessment of turbo spectroscopic imaging for targeting in brain biopsy. AJNR Am J Neuroradiol 2001;22(5):959–968

71. Ganslandt O, Stadlbauer A, Fahlbusch R, et al. Proton magnetic resonance spectroscopic imaging integrated into image-guided surgery: correlation to standard magnetic resonance imaging and tumor cell density. Neurosurgery 2005; 56(2, Suppl)291–298, discussion 291–298

72. Gruber S, Mlynárik V, Moser E. High-resolution 3D proton spectroscopic imaging of the human brain at 3 T: SNR issues and application for anatomy-matched voxel sizes. Magn Reson Med 2003;49(2):299–306

73. Stadlbauer A, Gruber S, Nimsky C, et al. Preoperative grading of gliomas by using metabolite quantification with high-spatial-resolution proton MR spectroscopic imaging. Radiology 2006;238(3):958–969

74. Dowling C, Bollen AW, Noworolski SM, et al. Preoperative proton MR spectroscopic imaging of brain tumors: correlation with histopathologic analysis of resection specimens. AJNR Am J Neuroradiol 2001; 22(4):604–612

75. Möller-Hartmann W, Herminghaus S, Krings T, et al. Clinical application of proton magnetic resonance spectroscopy in the diagnosis of intracranial mass lesions. Neuroradiology 2002;44(5):371–381

76. Zeng QS, Li CF, Zhang K, Liu H, Kang XS, Zhen JH. Multivoxel 3D proton MR spectroscopy in the distinction of recurrent glioma from radiation injury. J Neurooncol 2007;84(1):63–69

77. Chuang CF, Chan AA, Larson D, et al. Potential value of MR spectroscopic imaging for the radiosurgical management of patients with recurrent high-grade gliomas. Technol Cancer Res Treat 2007;6(5):375–382

78. Krsek P, Hajek M, Dezortova M, et al. (1)H MR spectroscopic imaging in patients with MRI-negative extratemporal epilepsy: correlation with ictal onset zone and histopathology. Eur Radiol 2007;17(8):2126–2135

79. Zeng QS, Li CF, Liu H, Zhen JH, Feng DC. Distinction between recurrent glioma and radiation injury using magnetic resonance spectroscopy in combination with diffusion-weighted imaging. Int J Radiat Oncol Biol Phys 2007;68(1):151–158

80. Østergaard L. Principles of cerebral perfusion imaging by bolus tracking. J Magn Reson Imaging 2005;22(6):710–717

81. Barajas RF, Chang JS, Sneed PK, Segal MR, McDermott MW, Cha S. Distinguishing recurrent intra-axial metastatic tumor from radiation necrosis following gamma knife radiosurgery using dynamic

susceptibility-weighted contrast-enhanced perfusion MR imaging. AJNR Am J Neuroradiol 2009;30(2):367–372

82. Arvinda HR, Kesavadas C, Sarma PS, et al. Glioma grading: sensitivity, specificity, positive and negative predictive values of diffusion and perfusion imaging. J Neurooncol 2009;94(1):87–96

83. Sadeghi N, D'Haene N, Decaestecker C, et al. Apparent diffusion coefficient and cerebral blood volume in brain gliomas: relation to tumor cell density and tumor microvessel density based on stereotactic biopsies. AJNR Am J Neuroradiol 2008;29(3):476–482

84. Emblem KE, Scheie D, Due-Tonnessen P, et al. Histogram analysis of MR imaging-derived cerebral blood volume maps: combined glioma grading and identification of low-grade oligodendroglial subtypes. AJNR Am J Neuroradiol 2008;29(9):1664–1670

85. Law M, Oh S, Johnson G, et al. Perfusion magnetic resonance imaging predicts patient outcome as an adjunct to histopathology: a second reference standard in the surgical and nonsurgical treatment of low-grade gliomas. Neurosurgery 2006;58(6):1099–1107, discussion 1099–1107

86. Hu LS, Baxter LC, Smith KA, et al. Relative cerebral blood volume values to differentiate high-grade glioma recurrence from posttreatment radiation effect: direct correlation between image-guided tissue histopathology and localized dynamic susceptibility-weighted contrast-enhanced perfusion MR imaging measurements. AJNR Am J Neuroradiol 2009;30(3):552–558

87. Lee IH, Kim ST, Kim HJ, Kim KH, Jeon P, Byun HS. Analysis of perfusion weighted image of CNS lymphoma. Eur J Radiol 2009 Jun 3 [Epub ahead of print]

88. Liao W, Liu Y, Wang X, et al. Differentiation of primary central nervous system lymphoma and high-grade glioma with dynamic susceptibility contrast-enhanced perfusion magnetic resonance imaging. Acta Radiol 2009;50(2):217–225

89. Chiang IC, Hsieh TJ, Chiu ML, Liu GC, Kuo YT, Lin WC. Distinction between pyogenic brain abscess and necrotic brain tumour using 3-tesla MR spectroscopy, diffusion and perfusion imaging. Br J Radiol 2009; 82(982):813–820

90. Law M, Cha S, Knopp EA, Johnson G, Arnett J, Litt AW. High-grade gliomas and solitary metastases: differentiation by using perfusion and proton spectroscopic MR imaging. Radiology 2002;222(3): 715–721

91. Kim MJ, Kim HS, Kim JH, Cho KG, Kim SY. Diagnostic accuracy and interobserver variability of pulsed arterial spin labeling for glioma grading. Acta Radiol 2008;49(4):450–457

92. Liu TT, Brown GG. Measurement of cerebral perfusion with arterial spin labeling: Part 1. Methods. J Int Neuropsychol Soc 2007;13(3):517–525

5

Anesthesia Considerations

Reza Gorji

Anesthesia services have been provided for years to patients having magnetic resonance imaging (MRI). Caring for these patients outside of the operating room in the MRI environment is a significant challenge to any anesthesia provider. Anesthesia services are usually required for patients that cannot cooperate during the process of obtaining MRI scans. Claustrophobia, an altered sensorium, or the inability to remain still and cooperative are common indications for the involvement of anesthesia personnel in the care of these patients.

MRI is an integral part of the various neuronavigational systems that are employed to perform neurosurgery in the modern era. Advances in the fields of neurosurgery and radiology combined with the development of MRI-compatible equipment have led to the development of intraoperative MRI (iMRI)-guided surgery. During an iMRI-guided procedure, the patient is imaged several times with MRI while undergoing surgery. The neurosurgeon benefits by having the ability to view the surgical site on MRI with the cranium open before the conclusion of the procedure. Although the provision of anesthesia for iMRI is similar to that during standard MRI, additional complexities related to the surgical aspect of the procedure exist. During iMRI, MRI is an essential part of the operation. The iMRI provides the surgeon with an intraoperative way to monitor the extent of the tumor resection as well as the ability to compensate for brain shift during microscope-based neuronavigation.[1,2] This MRI environment is clearly different than that encountered with conventional MRI and the anesthetic care of the patient must be adapted to this new circumstance and its unique complexities.

For the past decade, neurosurgeons have used various neuronavigation systems to perform precise and skillful surgical procedures. Surgical applications for iMRI include transsphenoidal resection of pituitary tumors, deep brain stimulation electrode placement for Parkinson's disease,[1] cerebral abscess drainage,[2] tumor removal,[3] and brain biopsy.[4] iMRI allows near-real time three-dimensional imaging of the brain once the cranium is open, unlike static standard MRI of the brain.[5] There is little doubt that the anesthesiologist will become more involved in the care of patients undergoing neurosurgical procedures during an iMRI-guided surgical procedure where the imaging is a crucial part of the surgery. Many anesthesiologists are uncomfortable providing anesthesia in MRI suites because of the technical issues associated with the environment.

With a better understanding of the numerous challenges facing the anesthesia team, an effective plan can be formulated and implemented that will minimize patient risk and reduce procedural morbidity and mortality. The goal of the anesthesiologist should be to provide a safe anesthetic for the patient and further contribute to the completion of surgery in an organized and efficient manner. Although significant challenges and obstacles are present during iMRI-guided surgery, anesthesia care for these patients can be safe and effective by adhering to strict standards.

◆ Issues Associated with MRI and Anesthesia Administration

MRI uses high-powered magnetic fields and radiofrequency (RF) pulses to produce digitalized topographic images. Because MRI does not employ ionizing radiation, there are no known physiologic effects experienced by the patient. Difficulties in providing anesthesia services in the MRI suite result primarily from the magnetic field strength and the narrow cylindrical imaging space of most high-field ($\geq$ 1.5 tesla) MRI scanners.

In general, it is understood and accepted that patients must be closely monitored under anesthesia and during surgery. The guidelines published by the American Society of Anesthesiology for nonoperating room locations where anesthesia is provided were first approved in October of 1994 and last amended in 2003.[6] During MRI and iMRI-guided surgery, physiologic monitors must function properly within the strong magnetic field. For a variety of reasons, standard anesthesia machines cannot be used during MRI. These reasons include changing magnetic fields and RF currents, which will cause interference and/or malfunction of the monitoring equipment. Additionally, there is electrical interference between the physiologic monitoring equipment and the MRI scanner and vice versa. Not only do the monitors function poorly in a magnetic field, the images obtained during MRI can be distorted by the electronics inherent to the monitoring equipment. Any object made of metal that is ferromagnetic can be attracted by the strong magnetic fields. This attraction can cause physical injury to personnel in the room and can result in equipment damage. Most MRI suites have a test magnet for the express purpose of identifying ferromagnetic equipment prior to it entering the room. Nonferromagnetic implants are less problematic, but are not completely without their unique risks. The intermittent RF pulses used during MRI can cause heat generation within a metal object. Conducting wires can arc under certain favorable conditions such as when they are conducting electrical current.

Other Obstacles to Providing Optimal Anesthetic Care in an MRI Environment

1. Patient accessibility and their distance from the anesthesia source
2. The need to move the patient into the MRI scanner
3. The length of the operative procedure
4. The availability of trained personnel to provide assistance during transport from the operating room and postanesthesia care unit
5. The risk of thermal injury and RF interference
6. The migration of ferromagnetic instruments
7. Inability of anesthesia providers to hear acoustic monitor alarms during the scanning process

In general, the goal of the anesthesiologist providing anesthesia during MRI is to provide a safe anesthetic to a quiet, comfortable, and immobile patient. For standard MRI, sedation may be all that is necessary in contrast to the majority of iMRI cases where a general anesthetic is more appropriate. Patient movement during imaging can severely degrade the MR image quality. Only during specific neurosurgical procedures such as an awake craniotomy, should a patient receive sedation alone as their anesthetic.

◆ Contraindications to iMRI

The preoperative anesthesia evaluation for iMRI-guided surgery is similar to the assessment for any neurosurgical patient. The strong magnetic fields used during iMRI-guided surgery can dislodge ferromagnetic objects including those implanted in patients. These include cerebral aneurysm clips as well as metallic intraocular foreign bodies. Safe metals that are not ferromagnetic include titanium,[7] silver, gold, and aluminum.

Special attention should be paid to patients with pacemakers (including automatic implantable defibrillators-pacers) and implanted infusion pumps. Pacers and automatic implanted defibrillators will become inactivated in a magnetic field.[8] Patients with these implanted devices are not good candidates for an iMRI-guided surgical procedure.

In procedures where the patient may be awake or receive monitored anesthesia care, contraindications include those conditions indicated above in addition to patient factors that may influence the overall optimal MR image quality. Factors such as the psychologic make-up of the patient can preclude patient selection for awake procedures using iMRI-guidance. Those patients with anxiety disorders, the inability to be cooperative, a fear of closed spaces or claustrophobia, and the inability to understand or comprehend the expectations that are required of them during the procedure may negate their candidacy for this type of surgery.

◆ Anesthesia Equipment

Every effort must be made to use MRI-compatible equipment when performing iMRI-guided surgery. MRI-compatible equipment has filtered electrical current that does not interfere with the performance of the magnet. Equipment used in an MRI environment must meet the following criteria:

1. It has to function properly.
2. It should pose no danger to patient, personnel, and other equipment in the room.
3. It must allow the MRI scanner to obtain clear and nondistorted images.

The equipment needs for iMRI-guided procedures are the same as that for conventional MRI. However, additional pieces of equipment and monitors may be needed during iMRI-guided surgery.

Because of the need for high magnetic field strength and the infrastructure necessary to create these fields, the iMRI suite is usually separate from the main operating room. Sufficient work space must be available for anesthesia personnel in the iMRI-guided surgery suite to function without being handicapped. Rooms adjacent to the iMRI surgical suite may be necessary for storage of anesthesia equipment and of other utilities. The anesthesia provider should have an adequate supply of drugs, infusion pumps (**Fig. 5.1**), and other equipment with common spare parts to perform a safe anesthetic in the iMRI suite. Common items needed for anesthesia care should be routinely stocked separately and in proximity to the iMRI suite. These items should include a large selection of drugs, intravenous medications, and pumps, as well as airway management equipment in the event that a difficult airway is encountered. Nonanesthesia personnel working at these remote locations are usually not familiar with the unique requirements of providing anesthesia and can be of little assistance if there is an anesthesia-related emergency.

In the past, some have advocated having all equipment outside of the magnetic field. The gauss line or the point where ferromagnetic items are attracted to the magnet is

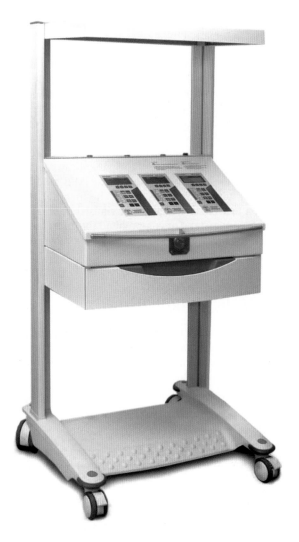

Fig. 5.1 Tesla infusion pumps. (Courtesy of Mammendorfer Institut für Physik und Medizin GmbH.)

between 30 to 50 gauss lines.[9] Image quality is proportional to the magnetic field strength of the scanner. The unit used for quantifying the magnetic field strength is a tesla (T) or 10,000 gauss. Scanners used for iMRI-guided surgery are between 0.12 T and 3 T. To be entirely outside of the magnetic field, the ventilator and monitoring equipment would need to be up to 20 feet away from the scanner. Very long ventilator breathing circuits, intravenous lines, and pressurized monitoring tubing would be necessary.[10]

Monitors that use batteries would need them to be safely secured because they are highly ferromagnetic. To avoid electrical interference from monitoring equipment, it is best to have the iMRI suite powered by filtered electrical current.

Anesthesia Machine

The conventional anesthesia machine in an operating room cannot be used in an MRI suite. The MRI-compatible machine is made of nonferrous materials. There are several MRI-compatible anesthesia machines for the use in the iMRI surgical suite. These machines must be modern and in good working condition. Using older anesthesia machines in the MRI suite is not advisable and will only compound the existing problems of providing anesthesia care in a challenging environment. The gas cylinders located on the anesthesia machine should be nonferrous and the common aluminum tanks are more than adequate.

The option of placing a conventional anesthesia machine outside of the MRI suite and connecting intravenous lines and other equipment to the patient through long hoses and conduits is not practical when providing an anesthetic for an iMRI-guided surgical case. However, this practice is sometimes used when performing a conventional MRI. The unique nature and acuity of an iMRI-guided surgical case is much different than that associated with a conventional MRI. A higher level of vigilance and a more dynamic surgical field exist during iMRI procedures. The immediate presence of an anesthesiologist in the iMRI suite contributes to the added patient safety and favorable outcome of the surgery.

There are several manufacturers of MRI-compatible equipment and anesthesia machines.[11] One such machine is the Draeger Fabius (Draeger Medical, Inc., Telford, PA) MRI machine seen in **Fig. 5.2**. The Fabius MRI-compatible machine is designed for use with 1.5 T and 3.0 T MRI systems. The standard configuration of this machine includes the advanced ventilation modes volume and pressure controlled, pressure support, and synchronous intermittent mechanical ventilation. These ventilator settings are very useful in the care of premature infants, newborns, and adult patients in the intensive care unit.

◆ Airway Management

General anesthesia using an endotracheal tube allows for a secured airway and is preferred in most surgical cases. In the patient undergoing an intracranial procedure, the head and airway will most likely be inaccessible to the anesthesiologist both during the procedure and also when MRI is taking place. A RAE (after the inventors, Ring, Adair, and Elwyn) tube can be very helpful in routing the breathing circuit.[12,13] A laryngeal mask airway (LMA) can be used for very short procedures, but these are very infrequent. Those LMAs and endotracheal tubes that contain ferrous material should be avoided during the MRI portion of MRI-guided surgery. Laryngoscopes must be made of plastic and lithium batteries should be used if available. Plastic laryngoscopes with paper-covered batteries are a viable alternative. Conventional zinc batteries contain ferromagnetic materials and should be avoided. Standard laryngoscopes should not be used in the MRI suite. Alternatively, the airway can be established outside of the critical gauss line.

In cases where a difficult airway is expected many options are available. A safe technique would be to secure the airway outside the MRI suite. In difficult circumstances, it may be best to secure the airway in the main operating room or postoperative care unit, where skilled

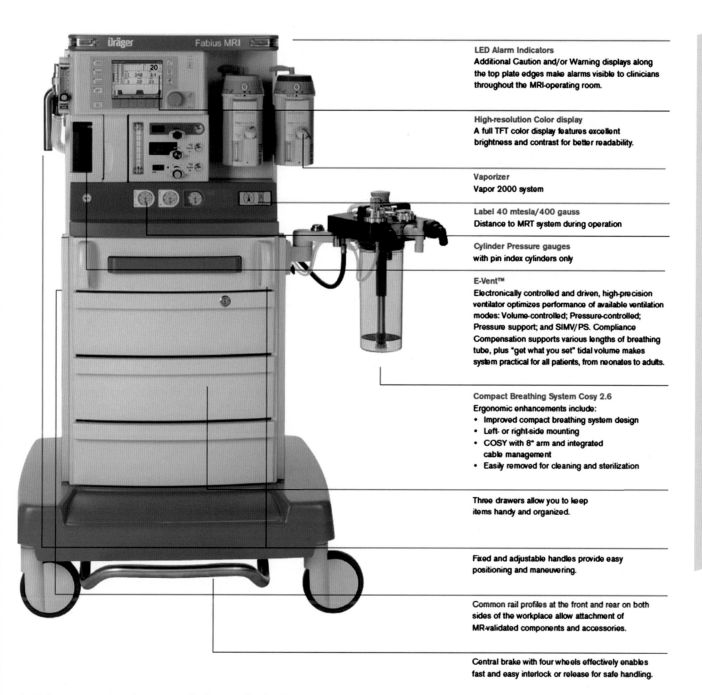

LED Alarm Indicators
Additional Caution and/or Warning displays along the top plate edges make alarms visible to clinicians throughout the MRI-operating room.

High-resolution Color display
A full TFT color display features excellent brightness and contrast for better readability.

Vaporizer
Vapor 2000 system

Label 40 mtesla/400 gauss
Distance to MRT system during operation

Cylinder Pressure gauges
with pin index cylinders only

E-Vent™
Electronically controlled and driven, high-precision ventilator optimizes performance of available ventilation modes: Volume-controlled; Pressure-controlled; Pressure support; and SIMV/PS. Compliance Compensation supports various lengths of breathing tube, plus "get what you set" tidal volume makes system practical for all patients, from neonates to adults.

Compact Breathing System Cosy 2.6
Ergonomic enhancements include:
• Improved compact breathing system design
• Left- or right-side mounting
• COSY with 8" arm and integrated cable management
• Easily removed for cleaning and sterilization

Three drawers allow you to keep items handy and organized.

Fixed and adjustable handles provide easy positioning and maneuvering.

Common rail profiles at the front and rear on both sides of the workplace allow attachment of MR-validated components and accessories.

Central brake with four wheels effectively enables fast and easy interlock or release for safe handling.

Fig. 5.2 Draeger Fabius (Draeger Medical, Inc., Telford, PA) magnetic resonance imaging compatible anesthesia machine. (Courtesy of Draeger.)

personnel are readily available, and to then proceed to the iMRI suite.

◆ Oximetry

Pulse oximeters are very useful for monitoring oxygen saturation in the blood and should be employed in the management of all patients. Conventional pulse oximeters cannot be used during iMRI as they are susceptible to interference from changing magnetic fields or are deactivated by the magnetic field. Nonferrous and fiber-optic oximeters are currently available. The oximeter machine should remain 2 meters away from the MRI scanner to prevent migration. The oximeter probe should be placed on a distal extremity as far from the magnetic field as possible. Some patients have suffered thermal injury to their digits due to looping of the oximeter wire.[14–16] Fortunately, MRI-compatible oximeters are available commercially (**Fig. 5.3**).

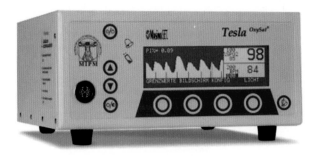

Fig. 5.3 Tesla magnetic resonance imaging compatible oximeter. (Courtesy of Mammendorfer Institut für Physik und Medizin GmbH.)

◆ Electrocardiogram Monitoring

Electrocardiogram (ECG) monitoring is mandatory during MRI and can be problematic. It is not possible to monitor a conventional ECG during MRI due to several issues that can present themselves in an adverse manner. The ECG lead wires that traverse the magnetic field will cause electrical distortion of ECG signals and the MR images. In addition, changing magnetic fields can generate artifacts in the ECG tracing. Spike artifacts that mimic R waves are often produced due to changing magnetic fields. Unfortunately, changes in the ECG waveform are present to some degree even in the filtered systems that are designed for MRI use. Telemetric ECG eliminates the need for wires.[17] Fiber-optic transmission of ECG signals is also possible although seldom used.

When in a magnetic field, blood flow in the aorta produces T and ST wave abnormalities especially when the orientation of the blood within the aorta is 90 degrees to the magnetic field.[18] Reliable ischemia monitoring and interpretation of arrhythmias is difficult.

Electrocardiogram monitoring carries a risk for burns and thermal injuries.[19] The ECG leads should not be coiled into a loop because significant image degradation occurs even with the use of nonferromagnetic wires.[20] Any electrical connection between the equipment and the magnet may produce RF interference. The voltage induced in the wires may lead not only to burns, but also poses an electrical shock hazard to the patient.[21] Positioning the ECG leads near the center of the scanner, avoiding loops of cable, and keeping the electrodes close to each other will help to minimize problems.[22] Plethysmography can be used as a heart rate monitor, but lacks sensitivity and is not useful for ischemia or arrhythmia detection.[23]

◆ Capnography

Positive pressure ventilation is necessary for cases using general anesthesia. Capnography should be used in all cases requiring general anesthesia. Capnography monitoring provides the anesthesiologist with information on breathing frequency, airway patency, anesthesia circuit integrity, and it is also an index of gas exchange. Carbon dioxide measurements are delayed by several seconds because the tubing length from the patient to the analyzer is long. The oxygen in the MRI suite is supplied by a wall outlet extending to the hospital central supply or by aluminum cylinders. It is better to use an aspirating-type CO_2 monitor than a direct-reading type; the latter may cause artifacts because it will sit within the MRI. There is no doubt that there will be a delay in the gas sample readings because the analyzer is located far from the magnet.

◆ Blood Pressure Monitoring

Noninvasive blood pressure monitoring is mandatory and should not pose any problems. Noninvasive blood pressure monitoring can be done successfully provided the connections between the hose and cuff are made of plastic. Such MRI-compatible systems that rely on oscillometric blood pressure monitoring are based on pneumatic techniques and do not interfere with the MR images (**Figs. 5.4** and **5.5**).[24]

Invasive blood pressure monitoring is frequently used in conventional neurosurgical cases and it can also be used during iMRI-guided surgery. Arterial lines are a necessity for most intracranial procedures and nonferrous transducers are readily available and should be used. Sampling arterial blood gases for oxygenation measurement may be prolonged if the laboratory measuring these values is located far from the iMRI suite (**Fig. 5.5**).

◆ Temperature Monitoring

Temperature monitoring should be performed in all patients. Patient body temperature can increase due to heat generated by the magnetic field. Body temperature may also decrease due to the cool MRI environment particularly in children. The MRI suite is kept cool to protect the superconductors. Intermitted temperature monitoring may be employed using liquid crystal thermometers[25] or thermistors. Thermistors may cause skin burns.[26] Internal temperature probes must be withdrawn from the body before scanning to prevent the generation of an electric current that can result in thermal injury.

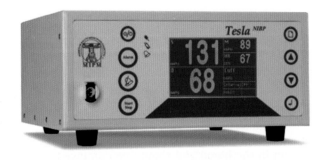

Fig. 5.4 Tesla noninvasive blood pressure monitor. (Courtesy of Mammendorfer Institut für Physik und Medizin GmbH.)

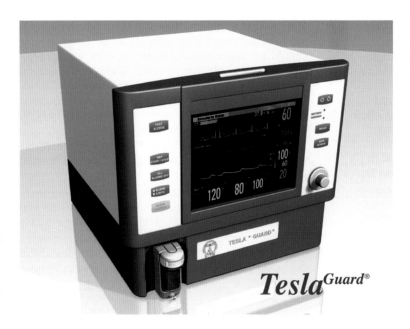

◆ Management of Anesthesia

The anesthetic needs for iMRI are completely different than those necessary for conventional MRI. There are numerous techniques of anesthesia for MRI.[27-29] As mentioned above, it is best to provide general anesthesia to the majority of patients unless there is a contraindication. Sedation with monitored anesthesia care may be employed when there is a need for an awake patient who requires neuromonitoring to avoid disrupting critical neural pathways during the surgery.

Provision of Anesthesia Poses Several Problems

1. Limited access to and visibility of the patient especially when the patient enters the magnet head first
2. The need to avoid ferromagnetic materials
3. Changing magnetic field and RF currents causes interference and/or malfunction of monitoring equipment
4. Monitoring equipment can degrade the MRI image quality

Any object made of metal that is ferromagnetic can be attracted by high magnetic fields. Nonferromagnetic implants are less problematic, but not trouble-free. Intermittent RF used in MRI can cause heat build up in any metal object. Conducting wires can arc under specific conditions such as when they are conducting electrical current.

◆ Induction, Maintenance, and Emergence of Anesthesia

Prior to proceeding with anesthesia, the anesthesiologist must determine where the anesthesia machine, ventilator, and monitoring equipment will be located with respect to the magnetic field. The proper functioning of anesthesia equipment including monitoring devices should be evaluated prior to their clinical use.

The patient is prepared for anesthesia by initiating ECG, pulse oximetry, and blood pressure monitoring. A common approach to the administration of anesthesia is to induce the patient in an adjacent area outside of the magnetic field on the MRI table that will be used during surgery. Commonly used drugs include propofol 1 to 2 mg/kg, fentanyl 1 to 5 μg/kg, and a neuromuscular agent such as vecuronium 0.1 mg/kg. The trachea is intubated and ventilated with an oxygen/air mixture. After induction, additional monitors are utilized that include arterial lines, central venous lines, and urinary catheters. The patient is transported to the MRI suite and the anesthesia is maintained using MRI-compatible equipment and monitors. Should an emergency arise, the patient will have to be removed from the area of high magnetic field strength to enable the use of ferromagnetic equipment to resuscitate the patient.[30]

Anesthesia is maintained by techniques commonly employed in neuroanesthesia. Typically, maintenance anesthesia includes oxygen and nitrous oxide combined with volatile agents in concentrations less than 1 MAC (minimum alveolar concentration). Total intravenous anesthesia can also be used provided the infusion pumps are either MRI-compatible or outside the magnetic field. A common approach is a propofol infusion at doses between 125 to 250 μg/kg per minute along with a fentanyl infusion at 1 to 3 μg/kg per hour. The latter option will necessitate the use of long intravenous tubing. In conventional (nonoperative) MRI, it is not mandatory to have the anesthesia provider in the MRI suite although this is a matter of controversy.[31] However, monitors need to be mirrored and observed and it is necessary to directly view the anesthesia machine.

Infusion pumps are typically used to provide neuroanesthesia. They afford precise titration of medications such as nitroprusside, propofol, and narcotics. One such pump is the

Medfusion 3500 (Medex, Inc., Carlsbad, CA), which can function properly in a magnetic field of up to 150 gauss.

Other unique patient challenges also exist in an MRI environment. In the case of awake craniotomies, all anesthesia considerations apply as they would in a conventional operating room. Additional considerations such as sound protection for the patient are unique to MRI-guided surgery. The use of the contrast material gadolinium, which can cause hypotension, nausea, and vomiting, is specific for MRI.

At the end of the procedure, the patient is taken out of the MRI suite and allowed to emerge from anesthesia. Following emergence, the patient is taken to the postanesthesia care unit or the neurosurgical intensive care unit where they are monitored and receive oxygen. Careful monitoring during patient transfer is mandatory. Nonanesthesia staff can assist with patient transfer by helping to eliminate obstacles during patient transport such as availability of elevators.

Emergencies

Any emergency situation in the MRI suite should be treated with basic life support until the patient can be transported out of the scanner for more definitive treatment.

Quality Assurance

To assure quality, operating room standards should be applied to the MRI suite. In fact, involvement of the anesthesia department in the planning and construction of MRI suites can help to prevent many problems from developing. For example, before selecting an installation site for the MRI-guided surgical suite, a thorough structural survey must be performed because all environmental iron is magnetized. It may be necessary to reroute oxygen, air, and nitrous oxide supply pipes and electrical wiring to or away from the MRI suite.

Compliance with the American Society of Anesthesiology (ASA) recommendation for monitoring is not an easy task. The following recommendations taken from the ASA guidelines for NORA (non-operating room anesthetizing) locations should be followed closely and implemented.[32] These are the minimal guidelines necessary for the administration of anesthesia and the ASA recommends exceeding them based on the judgment of the involved anesthesia personnel.

1. Reliable oxygen source for length of procedure including a full E cylinder backup.
2. Adequate and reliable suction.
3. Adequate and reliable scavenging system for waste anesthetic gases.
4. Self-inflating resuscitation bag capable of delivering positive pressure ventilation with an inspired oxygen fraction (F_iO_2) of 0.90.
5. Complete anesthetic drugs, supplies, and equipment for the planned activity.
6. Adequate monitoring equipment to adhere to standards for basic anesthetic monitoring.

7. Sufficient electrical outlets to support an anesthesia machine and monitoring equipment. The power supply should be ungrounded and isolated by an isolation transformer or electric circuits. Alternatively ground fault circuit interruption should be available if an isolated power supply is not possible. In such a case, a source for an emergency power supply is also needed.
8. There should be adequate space for equipment and personnel and transportation. The patient, anesthesia machine, and monitoring equipment should be well illuminated.
9. An emergency cart with a defibrillator, emergency drugs, and other equipment adequate to provide cardiopulmonary resuscitation should be immediately available.
10. There should be staff to support the anesthesiologist in the event assistance is needed. A means of calling for help should be present.
11. All applicable building and safety codes and facility standards should be obeyed.
12. Appropriate postanesthesia management should be available to recover patients. Transporting patients to the postanesthesia unit may require additional trained staff members in addition to equipment.

References

1. Derrey S, Maltête D, Chastan N, et al. Deep brain stimulation of the subthalamic nucleus in Parkinson's disease: usefulness of intraoperative radiological guidance. The stereoplan. Stereotact Funct Neurosurg 2008;86(6):351–358
2. Senft C, Seifert V, Hermann E, Gasser T. Surgical treatment of cerebral abscess with the use of a mobile ultralow-field MRI. Neurosurg Rev 2009;32(1):77–84, discussion 84–85
3. Kremer P, Tronnier V, Steiner HH, et al. Intraoperative MRI for interventional neurosurgical procedures and tumor resection control in children. Childs Nerv Syst 2006;22(7):674–678
4. Hall WA, Liu H, Martin AJ, Pozza CH, Maxwell RE, Truwit CL. Safety, efficacy, and functionality of high-field strength interventional magnetic resonance imaging for neurosurgery. Neurosurgery 2000;46(3):632–641, discussion 641–642
5. Hall WA, Truwit CL. Intraoperative MR-guided neurosurgery. J Magn Reson Imaging 2008;27(2):368–375
6. American Society of Anesthesiologists. Statement of Nonoperating Room Anesthesizing Location. Available at: http://www.asahq.org/publicationsAndServices/standards/14.pdf.
7. Wichmann W, Von Ammon K, Fink U, Weik T, Yasargil GM. Aneurysm clips made of titanium: magnetic characteristics and artifacts in MR. AJNR Am J Neuroradiol 1997;18(5):939–944
8. Loewy J, Loewy A, Kendall EJ. Reconsideration of pacemakers and MR imaging. Radiographics 2004;24(5):1257–1267, discussion 1267–1268
9. Menon DK, Peden CJ, Hall AS, Sargentoni J, Whitwam JG. Magnetic resonance for the anaesthetist. Part I: Physical principles, applications, safety aspects. Anaesthesia 1992;47(3):240–255
10. Rao CC, McNiece WL, Emhardt J, Krishna G, Westcott R. Modification of an anesthesia machine for use during magnetic resonance imaging. Anesthesiology 1988;68(4):640–641
11. Gooden CK, Dilos B. Anesthesia for magnetic resonance imaging. Int Anesthesiol Clin 2003;41(2):29–37
12. Nixon C, Hirsch NP, Ormerod IE, Johnson G. Nuclear magnetic resonance. Its implications for the anaesthetist. Anaesthesia 1986;41(2):131–137
13. Nixon C. Magnetic resonance imaging. Can Anaesth Soc J 1986;33(3 Pt 1):420
14. Shellock FG, Slimp GL. Severe burn of the finger caused by using a pulse oximeter during MR imaging. AJR Am J Roentgenol 1989;153(5):1105

15. Dempsey MF, Condon B. Thermal injuries associated with MRI. Clin Radiol 2001;56(6):457–465

16. Gooden CK, Dilos B. Anesthesia for magnetic resonance imaging. Int Anesthesiol Clin 2003;41(2):29–37

17. Roth JL, Nugent M, Gray JE, et al. Patient monitoring during magnetic resonance imaging. Anesthesiology 1985;62(1):80–83

18. Peden CJ, Menon DK, Hall AS, Sargentoni J, Whitwam JG. Magnetic resonance for the anaesthetist. Part II: Anaesthesia and monitoring in MR units. Anaesthesia 1992;47(6):508–517

19. Kanal E, Borgstede JP, Barkovich AJ, et al; American College of Radiology. American College of Radiology White Paper on MR Safety. AJR Am J Roentgenol 2002;178(6):1335–1347

20. Peden CJ. Monitoring patients during anaesthesia for radiological procedures. Curr Opin Anaesthesiol 1999;12(4):405–410

21. Patteson SK, Chesney JT. Anesthetic management for magnetic resonance imaging: problems and solutions. Anesth Analg 1992;74(1):121–128

22. Wendt RE III, Rokey R, Vick GW III, Johnston DL. Electrocardiographic gating and monitoring in NMR imaging. Magn Reson Imaging 1988;6(1):89–95

23. Selldén H, de Chateau P, Ekman G, Linder B, Sääf J, Wahlund LO. Circulatory monitoring of children during anaesthesia in low-field magnetic resonance imaging. Acta Anaesthesiol Scand 1990;34(1):41–43

24. Patteson SK, Chesney JT. Anesthetic management for magnetic resonance imaging: problems and solutions. Anesth Analg 1992;74(1):121–128

25. Marsh ML, Sessler DI. Failure of intraoperative liquid crystal temperature monitoring. Anesth Analg 1996;82(5):1102–1104

26. Hall SC, Stevenson GW, Suresh S. Burn associated with temperature monitoring during magnetic resonance imaging. Letter Anesthesiology 1992;76(1):152

27. Patteson SK, Chesney JT. Anesthetic management for magnetic resonance imaging: problems and solutions. Anesth Analg 1992;74(1):121–128

28. Burk NS. Anesthesia for magnetic resonance imaging. Anesthesiol Clin North America 1989;7:707–721

29. Thompson JR, Schneider S, Ashwal S, Holden BS, Hinshaw DB Jr, Hasso AN. The choice of sedation for computed tomography in children: a prospective evaluation. Radiology 1982;143(2):475–479

30. Kanal E, Barkovich AJ, Bell C, et al; ACR Blue Ribbon Panel on MR Safety. ACR guidance document for safe MR practices: 2007. AJR Am J Roentgenol 2007;188(6):1447–1474

31. Kempen PM. Rethinking anesthesia care during MRI. ASA Newsl 2005;69(5):5–6

32. ASA Guidelines for Nonoperating Room Anesthetizing Locations. Park Ridge, IL: American Society of Anesthesiologists; 2001; last amended on 15 October 2003

6

Safety Considerations

Alastair J. Martin

Magnetic resonance imaging (MRI) is an exceptionally powerful and safe imaging modality. In contrast to many of its radiologic counterparts, the modality does not expose the patient or the operator to ionizing radiation and therefore avoids the principle safety concern in x-ray–based imaging systems. The MR environment, however, is quite complex and there are aspects that pose substantial, but largely avoidable, safety hazards. Most notably, MRI systems are always "on" in the sense that safety hazards exist even when the system is inactive. This is in contrast to virtually all other radiologic systems and represents a substantial educational challenge for patients and personnel who work in and around MRI suites.

In this chapter, we address the many facets of MRI safety and pay particular attention to the implications for interventional procedures. Many of the safety concerns related to MRI are heightened in the interventional setting as a result of the additional equipment and personnel that enter the MR environment. Thus particular attention needs to be paid to suite layout and access, personnel training and screening, and equipment safety testing and labeling. The fundamental basis for safety concerns in MRI will initially be reviewed and then followed by a summary of safety protocols that are commonly employed to minimize risk in diagnostic MRI settings. Impending occupational exposure limits for the various magnetic fields that are created in MRI systems will also be introduced and evaluated for the potential impact on interventional MRI approaches. Finally, recommendations for safety protocols in interventional MR systems will be addressed.

◆ Safety Concerns of Magnetic Resonance Systems

MR systems are composed of three major subcomponents: (1) the static magnetic field (B_0), (2) the time-dependent gradient fields (dB/dt), and (3) the radiofrequency (RF) transmission system (B_1). Each of these components produce distinct safety considerations and thus will be considered separately.

Static Magnetic Field (B_0)

The most widely recognized safety concern with MR imaging relates to the presence of a large, invisible, static magnetic field. The static magnetic field of commercially available MR systems is created with either superconducting or permanent magnets. The primary objective of these designs is to create a very strong and homogeneous magnetic field over a modestly sized volume. Secondary criteria, which have become increasingly important, are to maximize system openness and minimize peripheral magnetic fields. The clinical standard for whole-body MRI systems is well established at 1.5 or 3.0 tesla (T), which is achieved with cylindrical bore superconducting magnets. Lower field strength systems featuring enhanced lateral access are also commercially available for clinical use. Higher field strength magnets for research purposes are becoming more prevalent, but are unlikely to be considered for interventional applications. The static magnetic field has several different regions, ranging from magnet isocenter, where there is a very high and homogeneous magnetic field over a relatively small volume, to the magnetic fringe field, where relatively low magnetic fields extend over large areas. An important transitional zone occurs as you near the magnet, as the magnetic field increases rapidly, producing the potential for magnetic attraction of ferrous objects.

Projectile Risk

The area surrounding the physical magnet produces the potential for substantial deflection forces and torques in magnetic objects. The magnitude of deflection forces is directly proportional to the spatial rate of change in magnetic field and the mass and magnetization of the magnetic object. Thus heavier magnetic objects such as ferrous gas cylinders will experience proportionately greater force than objects with less mass or less inherent magnetization. The spatial rate of change in magnetic field is typically greatest near the magnet aperture, where the field strength is rapidly rising toward its eventual peak value. The spatial rate of change is actually enhanced on shielded magnets, which are designed to minimize magnetic fields outside of the magnet bore. Accordingly, magnetic fields are dampened in the periphery of these magnets, but the magnetic attraction near the bore is enhanced. Furthermore, the rate of magnetic field change increases rapidly as you approach the magnet. This creates a circumstance whereby the magnetic force substantially increases as magnetic objects move even slightly closer to the magnet bore and makes it very difficult to hold back an object once it has begun to be attracted toward the magnet.

Unfortunately, projectiles are not uncommon in MRI suites. In the vast majority of cases these projectiles are small objects that are pulled from patients or staff as they approach the magnet. However, larger objects, including gas cylinders,[1] floor waxing machines, and chairs, have been reported, which have resulted in serious injury and death. Protection from these types of accidents requires strict institutional policies and personnel adherence to the established safety and screening protocols.

Internal Ferrous Objects

The large static magnetic field of MRI systems poses a very significant safety hazard to patients with internalized magnetic objects. Metallic implants and foreign bodies will experience the same forces described above and may move if not well seated in tissue. There is particular concern for metallic objects in the eye, which can produce ocular injury when exposed to high magnetic fields.[2] There is further concern for implanted medical devices such as aneurysm clips,[3] which experience deflection and force that may have devastating effects. In general, aneurysm clips made from ferromagnetic materials are contraindicated for MRI, whereas weakly or nonferrous clips are considered safe. Other endovascular devices, including stents, coils, and filters, tend not to be made of strongly ferromagnetic magnetic material and are permitted in MRI scanners. However, it is recommended to wait several weeks after placement of endovascular devices made from weakly ferromagnetic materials to allow for endothelialization and more secure seating of the device. There are many other medical implants that may experience forces when exposed to the static magnetic field of an MRI scanner. An excellent and commonly used reference for determining the safety status of a wide range of implants and devices is maintained by Dr. Frank Shellock and is available online (mrisafety.com) and in book form.[4]

Cryogenic Systems

The majority of MRI systems presently operate with a superconducting magnet producing the static magnetic field. These systems require that the conductive windings that create the static magnetic field be cooled to very low temperatures, which is typically achieved by immersing them in liquid helium. Superconductive windings offer no resistance, so once the appropriate current has been injected into the structure it will maintain at that current level, and corresponding magnetic field, indefinitely. Thus this component of the MR system is "always on" and must always be considered. Superconductive systems, however, also pose another safety risk related to the presence of the cryogenic system. If for some reason the superconductor develops resistance, its temperature can rise very quickly due to the high current levels that run in its windings. This phenomenon is referred to as a "quench" and results in rapid loss of the magnetic field and energy transfer from the coil windings to the cryogenic liquid. The liquid helium is elevated above its boiling point, creating a much larger volume of helium gas that must escape the cryostat. MR systems are designed with vents to permit safe expulsion of helium gas, but if this system fails then the gas will rapidly displace air in the magnet room. The loss of oxygen in the magnet room, coupled with the increased pressure as a result of the rapid expulsion of helium gas, can have tragic consequences. Thus the magnet room should be equipped with outward opening doors and be rapidly evacuated in the event of a magnet quench.

Human Exposure to Magnetic Fields

Humans are continuously exposed to a low-level relatively static magnetic field produced by the molten iron core of the earth. This ubiquitous magnetic field varies between 0.3 to 0.6 gauss over the surface of the earth and poses little concern. Higher, time-varying, magnetic fields are associated with man-made creations such as power lines and substantial study has been made of the potential biologic impact of exposure to these fields. There has been particular concern about a possible correlation between exposure to these electromagnetic fields and cancer, although a causal relationship between the two has never been definitively established.[5] The static magnetic field of an MR imager, however, is quite different. It is static, much like the earth's magnetic field, but has substantially higher field strength. Although human exposure to the magnetic field strengths associated with MR systems is relatively new, there has been substantial study on the biologic effects of these fields. Schenck provides a comprehensive review[6] of the studies that have been done and the associated findings. The impact of static magnetic fields on everything from gene expression to circadian rhythms has been evaluated without demonstration of a clearly pathologic effect from the presence of static magnetic fields of the magnitude used for clinical MRI. However, this remains an important area of study and assumptions about the potential for, or lack of, biologic effects from all forms of magnetic fields should not be made until carefully controlled studies have been performed.

Time Varying Gradient Fields

Spatial localization in MR imaging is achieved via the transient application of magnetic field disturbances. The strength of these magnetic fields is substantially less than the static magnetic field, but they are rapidly activated and deactivated during MR scanning. dB/dt is the ratio between the amount of change in amplitude of the magnetic field (dB) and the time it takes to make that change (dt). This temporal variation in magnetic field induces electric fields and forces that create an assortment of other potential safety concerns.

Nerve Stimulation

The electric field that is created when imaging gradients are activated or deactivated has the potential to produce nerve stimulation. The potential for this stimulation is dependent on both the strength and duration of the induced electric field.[7] Because the strength of the magnetic field produced by gradient coils increases with the distance from the isocenter, peripheral nerve stimulation (PNS) is most commonly experienced. Patients can experience a tingling sensation or twitching once a threshold level has been exceeded. This can progress to become painful with relatively modest increases beyond the stimulation threshold.[8,9] At sufficiently high levels, nerve stimulation could potentially induce epileptic seizures or produce cardiac stimulation. These side effects range from minor discomfort to potentially catastrophic; they place a practical biologic limit on the performance of imaging gradients. Gradient coil design also plays a role in determining if and where nerve stimulation may occur,[10] and designs for high performance gradients that minimize the level of stimulation generating electric fields are being explored.[11]

Acoustic Noise

MR systems emit noise while scanning due to the activation and deactivation of the gradient coil system. Linear perturbations of the static magnetic field are transiently created by running current through gradient coil windings that are built into the scanner bore. Substantial forces in the gradient coil windings are induced when current levels change, making the wires want to twitch. The coil windings cannot move because they are embedded in a solid former, but these forces produce a small vibration in the structure. Because gradient switching occurs in the same frequency range (~ kHz) as human hearing, the vibration is emitted as an audible noise. The amplitude and frequency of the emitted noise is both a function of the MR system and the specific pulse sequence that is being performed, but can be appreciable.

The acoustic noise emitted by an MR system can produce temporary hearing loss or permanent impairment and therefore exposure must be limited. Patients within the magnet bore must wear hearing protection and anyone remaining in the magnet room during scanning must similarly consider ear protection.[12] The necessity for ear protection is a function of the amplitude, frequency, and duration of the acoustic exposure and agencies such as the Occupational Safety and Health Administration (OSHA) in the United States set exposure limits. Fortunately, the level of acoustic noise produced by today's MR systems are adequately mitigated by an assortment of hearing protection devices.

Radiofrequency Transmission

MRI requires that the protons within the bore of the magnet be excited from their equilibrium state. The signals that are used to create MR images reflect the signal emitted by these protons as they subsequently return to their equilibrium state. System excitation is achieved by exposing the subject to energy at the resonant, or Larmor, frequency of protons in the static magnetic field. For commercial MR systems this resonant frequency lies in the radiofrequency (RF) portion of the electromagnetic spectrum (i.e., 64 MHz at 1.5 T). This energy is well below the ionization threshold; therefore, it will not directly damage molecules in the same way ionizing radiation can. The primary concern with RF energy is heating related to absorption of this energy.[13]

Specific Absorption Rate

Although RF energy is not ionizing, the RF power that is transmitted into the patient will produce heat due to resistive loss that occurs within tissue. Standards have been established by the Food and Drug Administration (FDA, Silver Spring, MD) and the International Electrotechnical Commission (IEC, Geneva, Switzerland) that aim to limit specific absorption rates (SAR) in tissues such that no thermal damage will be induced. SAR is a measure of energy deposited per mass of tissue and is commonly measured in watts/kg. Many factors can affect how the body responds to the RF energy that is deposited during MRI scanning. The body attempts to maintain thermoregulatory equilibrium through convection, conduction, radiation, and evaporation, although many underlying health conditions can affect how well a subject responds to a thermal challenge.[14] Accordingly, SAR limitations have been established and are broken down into different operating modes that require variable patient monitoring. In Europe, there are three operating modes of an MRI scanner: level 0 (normal operating mode) where SAR < 1.5 W/kg, level I (firstlevel controlled operating mode) where SAR is between 1.5 to 4.0 W/kg, and level II (second level controlled operating mode) where SAR > 4.0 W/kg. Level I requires additional patient monitoring and level II typically cannot be entered unless as part of an approved research study. The FDA has similar limits that further reflect time averaging of the exposure to protect against heat build-up with long exposures.

RF Burns

SAR restrictions are established to limit heat deposition in tissue, but inherently cannot account for the presence of conductive structures within the bore. In many instances there can be conductors associated with local RF receiver coils, EKG monitoring, and other external objects in close contact with patients. These conductors can channel the RF transmit field and produce substantially elevated focal deposition of RF energy, resulting in what is called an "RF burn." MRI-compatible conductive devices that are within the bore are designed to limit this effect, but care must be taken to avoid the formation of an induction loop when setting up the patient. There have also been reports of RF burns in patients in the absence of defective or poorly positioned conductive equipment.[14,15] These cases tend to be associated with direct contact with RF coil elements or cables, or the formation of effective conductive loops in patients who may be perspiring during the study. Guidelines for avoiding excessive heating have been established[14] and are effective if adhered to.

Implanted Devices

Implanted devices that contain conductors will also interact with the transmitted RF field. These can be substantially more problematic and may preclude patients from undergoing an MR examination. Patients with cardiac pacemakers and implantable cardiac defibrillators (ICDs) are presently contraindicated for MRI, due largely to the potential for device malfunction and focal heating near electrodes. Other devices, such as deep brain stimulator (DBS) electrodes, are permitted to undergo MRI with very specific restrictions on SAR and the type of MR system and transmit RF coil. These restrictions arose following reported adverse heating events with DBS patients undergoing MRI,[16] but may be overly restrictive.[17] Indeed, reports of patients with pacemakers and ICDs who undergo MRI are increasing – provided additional precautions are taken.[18,19] Safety of internalized conductive devices remains a very active research area and improved MRI compatibility of many of these devices can be anticipated in the near future.

◆ ACR MRI Safe Practice Guidelines

The potential safety concerns in an MRI suite must be countered with processes and protocols that avoid or minimize the potential for adverse events. The American College of Radiology (ACR) formed a Blue Ribbon Panel on MR Safety to provide guidance and standards for safe MRI examinations. These guidelines were initially published in 2002[20] and are regularly revised[21] to keep up with this dynamic field. The most recent installment was published in 2007[22] and addresses the many facets of MRI safety, from static magnet fields to MRI contrast agents. This living document is an excellent resource and should be referred to when establishing institutional MR safety policies. It should be noted, however, that this reference primarily applies to conventional clinical MRI systems, and therefore does not specifically consider niche applications such as interventional MRI.[23]

MR Zones

A key aspect of the ACR standard is the concept of different zones in facilities with MRI scanners. Zone I is defined as freely accessible and having negligible MRI-related safety concerns. Zones II to IV have increasing safety concerns and therefore require progressively greater access restrictions and screening of equipment and personnel. Zone II is the region just outside zones III and IV where patients or staff must be greeted and screened to establish whether further access is appropriate. At this level, there remain insignificant MR risks, but access control must begin in earnest prior to entry into zones with more substantial risks. Zone III is the region in which free access by staff or equipment could result in serious injury or death. This transition zone must be constantly supervised by trained MR personnel and secured against unauthorized entry. It typically encompasses the region outside any doors that access the actual magnet room and may contain regions where the magnetic field exceeds 5 mG, which should be appropriately marked. Zone IV is the magnet room itself, which should only ever be accessed by trained personnel, screened hospital staff, and patients, and equipment that is established to be MRI safe.

This zone approach requires appropriately designed MRI suites with access controls that are enforced and adhered to by staff. Further, protocols should be established for handling patients who experience cardiac or respiratory arrest in high-risk MR zones. The primary aim of this protocol should be to provide the patient with the necessary acute life support while transferring them out of the area of magnetic risk. The magnet room itself should specifically be secured immediately after extracting the patient to avoid entry when code responders descend on the MRI suite.

Patient and Personnel Screening

An integral part to the ACR guidelines is the screening process: this relies heavily on MR personnel, who must be appropriately trained. Recommendations on screening are also available in a recent publication by Shellock and Spinazzi.[24] Personnel training may be aimed at assuring the safety of the staff themselves (referred to as level 1 MR personnel), or may be more extensive (level 2 MR personnel). Level 2 trained personnel will assume responsibility for evaluating the safety of non-MR personnel and should have a broad understanding of the MR environment and how it may interact with humans, devices, and equipment. All non-MR personnel need to be screened prior to entering a zone III area and this screening should be largely the same for staff and patients. An up-to-date screening form must be obtained or be on file for anyone entering a zone III area and examples of these forms are available.[14,22,24] MR screening personnel should verbally confirm key aspects of the screening form and not rely solely on responses provided on the form. Key questions include whether they have had prior MR studies or surgical procedures, and whether they have a pacemaker or any other foreign object in their body.

Due to a variable sensitivity and lack of specificity, conventional metal detectors are not recommended at MR gateways. Ferromagnetic detection systems are now available and can be considered as an adjunct to the screening performed by level 2 MR personnel. Once non-MR personnel enter a zone III or IV area they must be continuously monitored or in communication with trained MR personnel.

Device and Equipment Screening

All equipment that is to enter zone IV must be previously certified to be MRI compatible and, where possible, labeled accordingly. Any non-MR compatible equipment within zone III should be labeled as such and have physical restraints to prevent accidental introduction into zone IV. For equipment where this is impractical, the device must be continually under the supervision of level 2 MR personnel while within zone III. Examples of non-MR safe equipment that may exist in zone III include chairs, carts, and pumps. A strong handheld magnet can be used to test for ferromagnetic materials, but should not be relied upon for establishing MR safety. It is also important to be aware of whether the equipment's MR certification of safety is established for the specific MR system (i.e., is it safe up to 3 T?).

Patients who present with potential contraindications for MR imaging must undergo additional screening prior to entry into the MR environment. If, for example, the patient reports that they have an aneurysm clip, then the particular type of clip must be established along with the surgical date. Similarly, if there is the possibility of metallic objects in the eye, then x-ray–based imaging must be performed to establish whether the patient is appropriate for MR study. If the patient has an implanted device that has special MR restrictions, such as a deep brain stimulator, then these requirements must be identified and adhered to.

◆ Occupational Health and Safety

MR safety policies have by and large been focused on the patient within the bore of the magnet. This patient typically stands to benefit from the MR procedure and will only be exposed to the MR environment relatively briefly. Staff that work within an MRI suite, however, are routinely exposed to the MR environment even if they never enter the magnet bore. Thus there has been considerable interest in possible biologic effects that could be attributable to exposure to this environment. Should a causal relationship between exposure to a particular aspect of the MR environment and some measurable health effect be demonstrated, then steps can be taken to limit this exposure and monitor for the effect. This is routinely done for staff operating equipment that emits ionizing radiation, as their exposure is monitored with a dosimeter and strict limits are placed on annual and lifetime exposure levels. Creating a similar paradigm in the MR environment is very challenging. Minimization of the potential for projectiles and the use of ear protection where appropriate are relatively straightforward examples of safety requirements that also directly affect staff. However,

potential biologic effects from the electromagnetic fields (EMF) of MR systems have not been definitively established; therefore, it is not clear what safety measures are necessary.

The European Union (EU), however, in 2004 proposed a Physical Agents Directive that introduced occupational exposure limits for EMFs.[25] This directive would require by law that all member states of the EU abide by their exposure limits. Exposure limits of particular concern to interventional MRI,[26] and clinical[27] and research[28] MRI in general, include a proposed static magnetic field "action value" of 0.2 T and limits to time-variable magnetic fields comparable to that produced by the gradients of MR systems. RF exposure, which is largely localized within the magnet bore, was much less likely to be problematic. The static magnetic field action value requires that employers take steps to assure that an exposure limit is not exceeded. However, the directive presently has not established this exposure limit, so the implications of this aspect remain uncertain. The proposed limits to the time varying magnetic field, however, are potentially much more problematic. Unlike RF exposure, gradient strength can be quite high near magnet openings and any procedure that involves the interventionalist reaching into the magnet (**Fig. 6.1**) during scanning will almost certainly substantially exceed the proposed exposure limit. This aspect of the directive remains very controversial and Hill et al[26] discuss the scientific background that went into developing the exposure limit. They conclude that the scientific basis for the proposed exposure level is incomplete and inconclusive and may be unnecessarily conservative in the 1 kHz range, where imaging gradients typically operate.

The controversy and implications on patient care have delayed implementation of the proposed EU directive from 2008, until 2012. This delay does not change the potential impact of the directive, but does allow an opportunity to review the logic of the guidelines and perform scientific evaluations that might provide better insight into appropriate occupational limits for MR workers. The aim of the legislation is to protect workers from potential risks: this must be a priority regardless of whether a country is within the EU. The question remains whether the standards are appropriate and logical, or whether they are unnecessarily restrictive. Hill et al note that a consequence of the proposed EU directive would be to allow an interventionalist to stand near a computed tomography (CT) scanner during operation, but not an MR system.[26] The implication would be that the interventionalist is safer being exposed to ionizing radiation than the time varying magnetic fields produced by the gradient system of an MRI scanner. This flies in the face of conventional radiologic practices and must be addressed prior to mandating safety policies. An amendment to the EU directive is expected in 2009, with adoption of this policy anticipated to be enacted in all EU countries by 2012. The final language in this directive may play a key role in determining if and how interventional MRI will be practiced in the future. It is anticipated that the FDA in the United States will closely follow this legislation and consider similar standards. Thus it is crucial that a policy that provides sufficient occupational safety, without becoming unnecessarily restrictive, be enacted.

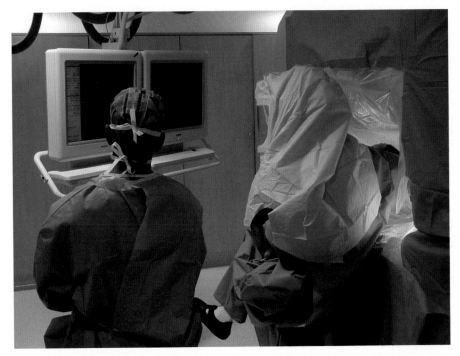

Fig. 6.1 This photograph shows a neuro-surgeon reaching into the bore of a sterilely draped magnetic resonance imaging (MRI) scanner to manipulate a device. Real-time MRI scanning is performed during these manipulations and presented to the surgeon on radiofrequency-shielded (RF-shielded) examination room monitors. This concept is central to many interventional MRI procedures, but exposes the surgeon to time varying magnetic fields that substantially exceed the limits in the proposed European Union directive.

◆ Safety Protocols for the Interventional MRI Suite

The interventional MRI suite poses a particular challenge for establishing and maintaining MR safe practices. Each installation must design their site and establish procedures that place a strong emphasis on MR safety. They must further actively educate and train staff who will be involved in interventional MR procedures and continually refresh and emphasize the importance of adhering to established safety protocols. Hushek et al have published safety protocol recommendations specific to interventional MR practices,[29] which provides a good overview of the special issues that must be addressed.

Interventional MRI Suite Planning

Establishing a functional and defensible suite layout is key to safely and effectively performing MR-guided interventional procedures. Each interventional MRI suite is unique and may have to balance MR system requirements, space limitations, radiological and interventional system use, and variable applications. However, the ACR concept of different MR zones must be carefully considered when developing suite layout. The zone concept must be adapted to the special needs of an interventional MRI system, where additional equipment and personnel will need to access zones III and IV. Access restrictions must be carefully thought through to avoid unnecessary limitations on surgical staff movement while maintaining the integrity of established safety protocols. Appropriate line of sight or video surveillance must be integrated to permit constant monitoring of the MR environment by level 2 trained MR personnel. Consideration must further be made for anesthetic

induction, transportation of anesthetized patients, scrub sinks, and room and staff sterility. If appropriate, room ventilation and air filtration must be established to meet operating room requirements. Demarcation of the spatial extent of the magnetic fringe field (5 G or 30 G), either through physical walls, floor markings, or ceiling mounted devices, is utilized in virtually all interventional MRI installations and serves as reminder of the unique environment.

Figure 6.2 shows an example of a hypothetical interventional MRI suite that serves as both a radiologic and interventional MRI suite. The various zones in this installation are identified and include two separate paths into the magnet room. Access restrictions are implemented between zones II and III (yellow doors) and between zones III and IV (red doors). The latter will by default be locked and only one pathway into the scanner will be active at any given time. Access between zones must be under the supervision and control of level 2 MR personnel. For conventional radiologic procedures, magnet room access would be via the scan control room, where the MR technologist would greet the patient and review screening. Interventional magnetic resonance imaging procedures, which typically require access for anesthesia and sterile personnel, would be provided an alternate route that requires the staff to be trained as level 1 MR personnel. The suite further permits direct viewing of the magnet room from both zone III areas and features floor demarcation of the magnet's 30 G line.

Staff Training

All staff that are involved with interventional MRI procedures and may be required to enter zones III or IV should be trained to level 1 MR personnel and undergo regular

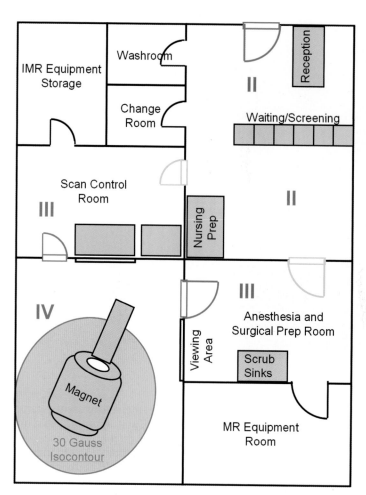

Fig. 6.2 A floor plan for a hypothetical interventional magnetic resonance imaging (MRI) suite is presented. The suite utilizes the American College of Radiology (ACR) concept of zones and creates secure access requirements before moving from zone II to zone III (*yellow doors*) and from zone III to zone IV (*red doors*). Two access routes to the magnet room are provided, with only one access path permitted at any given time. Conventional radiologic patients would access the magnet room via the scan control room and be accompanied by an MR technologist. During interventional MRI procedures, access via the anesthesia/surgical prep area would be made available to level 1 trained MR personnel. Windows into the magnet room are provided from both zone III areas and the 30 G line is demarcated on the magnet room floor. A local storage area for dedicated interventional MRI equipment is further provided to minimize the potential for loss of this equipment or exchange for non-MR compatible versions.

training updates. It is important that these staff be aware of MR safety requirements as typically there will be insufficient level 2 MR personnel to continuously track all aspects of interventional MRI procedures. The larger number of staff that is associated with interventional MRI procedures, however, creates its own safety risk as there exists the potential for untrained staff to pass through conventional screening. A relatively common method for minimizing this risk is to have uniquely colored surgical scrubs that are dedicated to the interventional MRI suite. This scrub would ideally lack pockets to prevent the accidental introduction of loose ferrous objects. This concept has two principle advantages: (1) staff who transiently appear from other departments are easily identified, and (2) the requirement to change into a specific scrub reinforces to staff the unique environment that they are entering and hopefully emphasizes the need for heightened safety awareness. Level 2 MR personnel must further work with anesthesia personnel to assure that patients entering the room under general anesthesia have been properly screened and prepared.

Patient Screening and Preparation

Patients scheduled to undergo an interventional MRI procedure must initially undergo conventional screening to assure that they are not contraindicated for MRI. This should be performed as an integral part of surgical preparation and a level 2 MR staff member must interview the patient prior to anesthetic induction. The patient is then permitted to enter the anesthesia preparation area to be induced. MRI screening must continue at this point to assure that the anesthetized patient is appropriately prepared to enter the MR system. Specific attention must be paid to the presence, and conformation, of any conductive leads that are attached to the patient. If incorrectly placed, these leads could lead to RF burns that will not be felt and reported by the anesthetized patient. All unnecessary or unsafe conductors must be removed and the remaining leads run linearly from the patient, parallel to B_0, and as far from the bore walls as possible. Insulation should further be provided between these wires and the patient to minimize the potential for thermal injury. Finally, the MR technologist should assure that ear protection is in place prior to MRI scanning.

Equipment Certification

Interventional equipment that is specifically designed for use in an MR environment is increasingly becoming available. MR-compatible versions may suffer some functional limitations and cost substantially more than their traditional counterparts, but should be utilized whenever possible. In instances where compatibility is yet to be established or unknown, then certification by an experienced MR physicist or engineer can be considered. This certification should follow the methods established by the American Society for Testing and Materials (ASTM, www.astm.org). They maintain standards for evaluating MR-induced displacement forces (ASTM F2052–06), torque (ASTM F2213–06), and RF induced heating (ASTM F2182–02). They also have developed marking standards for indicating the conditions that are acceptable for devices in an MR environment (ASTM F2503–08). In situations where non-MRI compatible, or unverified, equipment must be brought to the MRI suite (zones III or IV), then they should be constantly monitored and, whenever possible, physically tethered to avoid the possibility of entering an MR unsafe region.

◆ Summary

MRI guidance of interventional procedures affords a host of potential benefits. The MR environment, however, is complex and poses challenges for staff and equipment. Although MRI does not require ionizing radiation, there are safety hazards associated with the strong static magnetic field, incident RF energy, gradient fields, and cryogenic system. Staff must be thoroughly trained in MR safety and patients and staff carefully screened prior to entering the MR environment. Vigilant adherence to predefined MR safety practices, such as those established by the ACR, provides the greatest likelihood of avoiding MR accidents. Interventional MRI introduces a very novel work environment and occupational health and safety standards remain controversial. Efforts are ongoing to institute exposure limits and guidelines that appropriately protect interventional MRI staff without being unnecessarily restrictive. Ultimately, safety in an interventional MRI setting can only be achieved by appropriate facility design, in-depth and regularly updated personnel training, and careful screening of patients, staff, and equipment that enter the MRI suite.

References

1. Chaljub G, Kramer LA, Johnson RF III, Johnson RF Jr, Singh H, Crow WN. Projectile cylinder accidents resulting from the presence of ferromagnetic nitrous oxide or oxygen tanks in the MR suite. AJR Am J Roentgenol 2001;177(1):27–30
2. Kelly WM, Paglen PG, Pearson JA, San Diego AG, Soloman MA. Ferromagnetism of intraocular foreign body causes unilateral blindness after MR study. AJNR Am J Neuroradiol 1986;7(2):243–245
3. Klucznik RP, Carrier DA, Pyka R, Haid RW. Placement of a ferromagnetic intracerebral aneurysm clip in a magnetic field with a fatal outcome. Radiology 1993;187(3):855–856
4. Shellock FG. Reference Manual for Magnetic Resonance Safety, Implants, and Devices: 2008 Edition. Los Angeles: Biomedical Research Publishing Group; 2008
5. Moulder JE. Power-frequency fields and cancer. Crit Rev Biomed Eng 1998;26(1-2):1–116
6. Schenck JF. Safety of strong, static magnetic fields. J Magn Reson Imaging 2000;12(1):2–19
7. Irnich W, Schmitt F. Magnetostimulation in MRI. Magn Reson Med 1995;33(5):619–623
8. Ham CL, Engels JM, van de Wiel GT, Machielsen A. Peripheral nerve stimulation during MRI: effects of high gradient amplitudes and switching rates. J Magn Reson Imaging 1997;7(5):933–937
9. Schaefer DJ, Bourland JD, Nyenhuis JA. Review of patient safety in time-varying gradient fields. J Magn Reson Imaging 2000;12(1):20–29
10. Zhang B, Yen YF, Chronik BA, McKinnon GC, Schaefer DJ, Rutt BK. Peripheral nerve stimulation properties of head and body gradient coils of various sizes. Magn Reson Med 2003;50(1):50–58
11. Mansfield P, Haywood B. Controlled E-field gradient coils for MRI. Phys Med Biol 2008;53(7):1811–1827
12. Moelker A, Maas RA, Lethimonnier F, Pattynama PM. Interventional MR imaging at 1.5 T: quantification of sound exposure. Radiology 2002;224(3):889–895
13. Shellock FG. Radiofrequency energy-induced heating during MR procedures: a review. J Magn Reson Imaging 2000;12(1):30–36
14. Shellock FG, Crues JV. MR procedures: biologic effects, safety, and patient care. Radiology 2004;232(3):635–652
15. Knopp MV, Essig M, Debus J, Zabel HJ, van Kaick G. Unusual burns of the lower extremities caused by a closed conducting loop in a patient at MR imaging. Radiology 1996;200(2):572–575
16. Henderson JM, Tkach J, Phillips M, Baker K, Shellock FG, Rezai AR. Permanent neurological deficit related to magnetic resonance imaging in a patient with implanted deep brain stimulation electrodes for Parkinson's disease: case report. Neurosurgery 2005;57(5):E1063, discussion E1063
17. Larson PS, Richardson RM, Starr PA, Martin AJ. Magnetic resonance imaging of implanted deep brain stimulators: experience in a large series. Stereotact Funct Neurosurg 2008;86(2):92–100
18. Nazarian S, Roguin A, Zviman MM, et al. Clinical utility and safety of a protocol for noncardiac and cardiac magnetic resonance imaging of patients with permanent pacemakers and implantable-cardioverter defibrillators at 1.5 tesla. Circulation 2006;114(12):1277–1284
19. Sommer T, Naehle CP, Yang A, et al. Strategy for safe performance of extrathoracic magnetic resonance imaging at 1.5 tesla in the presence of cardiac pacemakers in non-pacemaker-dependent patients: a prospective study with 115 examinations. Circulation 2006;114(12):1285–1292
20. Kanal E, Borgstede JP, Barkovich AJ, et al; American College of Radiology. American College of Radiology White Paper on MR Safety. AJR Am J Roentgenol 2002;178(6):1335–1347
21. Kanal E, Borgstede JP, Barkovich AJ, et al; American College of Radiology. American College of Radiology White Paper on MR Safety: 2004 update and revisions. AJR Am J Roentgenol 2004;182(5):1111–1114
22. Kanal E, Barkovich AJ, Bell C, et al; ACR Blue Ribbon Panel on MR Safety. ACR guidance document for safe MR practices: 2007. AJR Am J Roentgenol 2007;188(6):1447–1474
23. Shellock FG, Crues JV III. MR Safety and the American College of Radiology White Paper. AJR Am J Roentgenol 2002;178(6):1349–1352
24. Shellock FG, Spinazzi A. MRI safety update 2008: part 2, screening patients for MRI. AJR Am J Roentgenol 2008;191(4):1140–1149
25. Commission-of-the-European-Union. European Union Physical Agents (Electromagnetic Fields) Directive 2004/40/EC. Brussels: European Parliament;2004
26. Hill DL, McLeish K, Keevil SF. Impact of electromagnetic field exposure limits in Europe: is the future of interventional MRI safe? Acad Radiol 2005;12(9):1135–1142
27. Moore EA, Scurr ED. British Association of MR Radiographers (BAMRR) safety survey 2005: potential impact of European Union (EU) Physical Agents Directive (PAD) on electromagnetic fields (EMF). J Magn Reson Imaging 2007;26(5):1303–1307
28. Perrin NM, Morris CJ. A survey of the potential impact of the European Union Physical Agents Directive (EU PAD) on electromagnetic fields (EMF) on MRI research practice in the United Kingdom. J Magn Reson Imaging 2008;28(2):486–492
29. Hushek SG, Russell L, Moser RF, Hoerter NM, Moriarty TM, Shields CB. Safety protocols for interventional MRI. Acad Radiol 2005;12(9):1143–1148

II

Minimally Invasive Cranial Applications

7

Low-Field Brain Biopsy

John Koivukangas and Sanna Yrjänä

Low-field MRI scanners are well suited for brain biopsies because of the short distance from the edge of the magnet to the isocenter and the relatively minor susceptibility artifacts. High-field imaging data obtained routinely in the course of diagnostic imaging preoperatively can be fused to low-field intraoperative images if needed. There are only a few patient series published on brain biopsies performed using low-field imagers. Tronnier et al[1] reported on a series of 60 patients biopsied using a 0.2 tesla (T) imager as early as 1999. However, most of the publications on experiences at low-field strength contain relatively few biopsy cases. Lewin et al[2] included only three biopsies in a series of 130 operations using a 0.2 T scanner. Kanner et al[3] had 15 biopsy cases in their series of 70 neurosurgical procedures performed using the 0.12 T imaging system. Using the 0.12 T scanner, Schulder et al[4] reported only three biopsies out of 93 operations. Indeed, for some of the pioneering centers, the goal of application of intraoperative magnetic resonance imaging (iMRI) has been to improve tumor resection results, with no biopsies being performed.[5]

The low number of brain biopsies may reflect treatment practices preferring tumor resection over biopsy in many centers using low-field MRI. Although in some centers a "watch and wait" approach favors diagnostic biopsy over more risky tumor resection, the tendency in other centers prefers removing as much tumor as possible while obtaining a histologic diagnosis. Advocates of the latter approach stress delaying future neurologic compromise due to the mass effect of the growing tumor as well as the delay of the malignant transformation of low-grade tumors and reduction of tumor burden for adjuvant therapy of high-grade tumors. Some studies indicate that biopsy may cause morbidity comparable to that of resection, which speaks for the latter approach.[6]

This chapter is based on our experience in Oulu, Finland: (1) since 1996 with one of the first iMRI concepts in the world[7] – the application of a new commercially successful Finnish low-field MRI scanner (at the time, Picker Nordstar Oy, Vantaa, Finland, but later acquired by Philips Healthcare,

Andover, MA), (2) pioneering experience since 1981 with real-time intraoperative ultrasound imaging (iUS),[8] and (3) since 1990 with neuronavigation.[9,10]

Most of the low-field systems originally offered by vendors, with the notable exception of the 0.15 T scanner (PoleStar-N20, Medtronic Navigation, Louisville, CO), have since been replaced by high-field ones. However, the lessons learned in all of the early centers need to be brought over to the newer systems. One of the important aspects of the Oulu experience has been the feasibility of formally sharing the scanner with other specialties, including radiology, pediatric surgery, and ear, nose and throat surgery. Another important aspect has been the realization that iMRI, and other intraoperative technology, is complicated: the full realization of its potential will continue to require dedicated technical and scientific collaboration at leading development centers.

◆ The Oulu Low-Field iMRI Concept and Experiences

The Low-Field iMRI Suite

The Oulu low-field iMRI concept was based on a single room concept featuring a commercially successful low-field scanner that could be turned off and on again within minutes (**Fig. 7.1**). This scanner was originally developed over a 20-year period at Picker-Nordstar Oy, Vantaa, Finland (acquired by Philips). The patient was operated on in the scanner or more commonly adjacent to it. When operating outside of the scanner, the magnetic field could be turned off, and all regular instruments and devices could be used next to the scanner. The ramp-up time for the scanner was 6 minutes. Together with the vendor, we developed the entire suite, including an optical neuronavigator system complete with custom-made visualization software. Because it was an early concept, all aspects of the operating room had to be modified for the new concept of having an MRI scanner in the

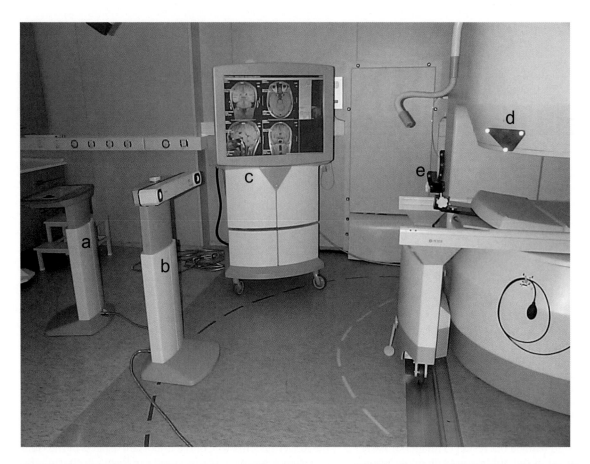

Fig. 7.1 The Oulu single-room intraoperative magnetic resonance imaging (iMRI) suite. **(A)** In-room MRI scanner control panel. **(B)** Polaris optical neuronavigator camera. **(C)** Large movable image display. **(D)** Philips Panorama 0.23 T scanner (Philips Healthcare, Andover, MA) with fiducials. **(E)** Head holder (fiducials not attached) connected by custom made fixation to anti-Trendelenburg elevatable couch adapter.

operating room. Also, the idea of sharing the room with other specialties, and especially with outpatient radiologic imaging was a departure from the usual neurosurgical suite setting.[11]

Preoperative Workup

It is important for the neurosurgeon to meticulously plan each procedure. The patient also needs to be well informed as to the purpose and nature of the procedure. For over 10 years, we have routinely informed our patients about iMRI procedures using preoperative neuronavigation either in the patient examination room on the ward or in the actual iMRI suite.

The patient education session facilitates preoperative workup, in which the patient has recently been imaged; these images are used with a neuronavigator to not only plan the operation hands on, but to show the patient and significant others what the operation will actually look like. Because our clinic was one of the early developers of neuronavigation, several of these expensive and sensitive systems were available. For biopsies, patients were routinely imaged with MRI on the day before surgery, with fiduciary markers (i.e., fiducials) or other markings. We simply took one of our neuronavigators into the patient examination room, fixed the patient's head with a ring cushion, and performed a navigation exercise, including

registration of the device to the skin fiducials on the patient's head. At first, we were apprehensive about whether or not the patient was interested in following the procedure on the navigation display. As it seemed to lessen anxiety, and certainly served to inform the patient about the upcoming surgery, it soon became a routine part of workup of all of our iMRI patients. Since 2002, the patient education session has been performed on the day before surgery in conjunction with the preoperative MRI study in the actual iMRI scanner.[12]

Biopsy Documentation

The patient information and planning session forms the first part of the overall documentation of the iMRI procedure using the Onesys Navigator software program to be reported elsewhere (**Fig. 7.2**). This is a novel graphical user interface, integrated to the electronic medical record. It allows us to condense all of the essential information and images related to any procedure onto one single workspace with links to the pertinent images on various hospital databases, including the Picture Archiving and Communication System (PACS). On this unique workspace the preoperative, intraoperative, and postoperative information can be collected for later quick retrieval. The workspace also serves prospective

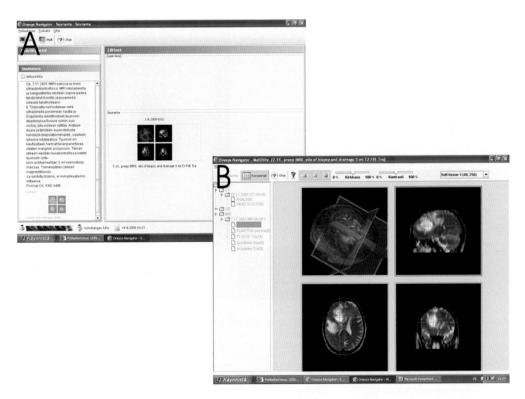

Fig. 7.2 The Onesys Navigator workspace. **(A)** Basic layout with pertinent patient information on left including clinical notes before, during, and after biopsy and later throughout management process; on the right, a link icon to the essential magnetic resonance imaging (MRI) dataset used for biopsy. **(B)** By clicking the icon, a three-dimensional interactive view of the dataset with orthogonal slices through the intended biopsy site of a 65-year-old man with a large right frontal lobe glioblastoma multiforme.

follow-up studies, with scientific information being an integral part of the Hospital Information System (HIS) and not standalone documentation.

Biopsy Technique

Our iMRI concept allowed many kinds of biopsy techniques. We were able to perform biopsies by needle, forceps, and endoscope. Depending on radiologic appearance and site of the tumor, patient characteristics, and consideration of the operating neurosurgeon, the biopsy was performed either on-line or off-line.

On-line biopsy means that the biopsy is performed between the magnet poles, in the imaging space thus enabling near real-time MRI. After determination of the target and the trajectory from the surface of the head, the biopsy needle can be followed with quick images taken along the axis of the instrument (**Fig. 7.3**). These images serve to check the passage of the needle, the actual site of

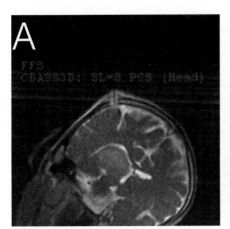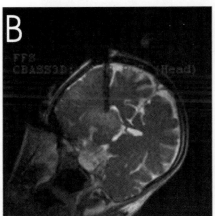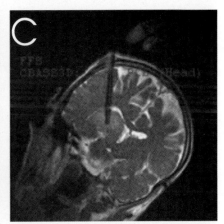

Fig. 7.3 On-line views of biopsy needle passing **(A)** through the burr hole, **(B)** to the superficial part of tumor, **(C)** to deep into the tumor in a 61-year-old man with right thalamic glioblastoma multiforme.

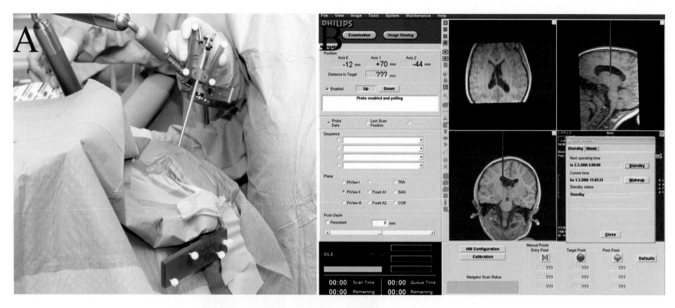

Fig. 7.4 The patient is an 8-year-old girl with right thalamic pilocytic astrocytoma. **(A)** A rigid endoscope is passed using the optical navigator toward a thalamic tumor. When the endoscope is in the lateral ventricle, the biopsy forceps can be passed into the tumor under direct visualization to avoid choroid plexus and blood vessels. **(B)** Green line shows the path of the endoscope.

the biopsy, and any early results of the removal of tissue, including hemorrhage. We used a side-cutting MRI-compatible needle. The on-line system was also used extensively by radiologists for abdominal and spinal procedures, but imposed some physical limitations to its use in brain biopsies. For example, it was not possible to pass the needle vertically due to the scanner gap height of 44 centimeters.

Off-line biopsy means that the patient is moved out of the scanner, and the needle is optically navigated along the planned trajectory.[13] This is analogous to doing the biopsy procedure in a regular operating room with a neuronavigator or stereotactic system, based on preoperative imaging.

In the iMRI suite, however, it is possible to immediately check the site of biopsy to confirm the accuracy of the intended procedure and to rule out any early complications. Off-line biopsy method also enables iMRI-guided placement of an endoscope in cases where biopsy is performed through the cerebral ventricles and direct vision of the procedure is required (**Fig. 7.4**).

In the Oulu concept, the role of multimodality imaging—intraoperative ultrasound—has long been crucial. Off-line biopsy allows for the use of iUS to help choose the site of biopsy and especially the intended trajectory. iUS allows real-time assessment of major vascular structures using color Doppler (**Fig. 7.5**). It also gives supplementary information on

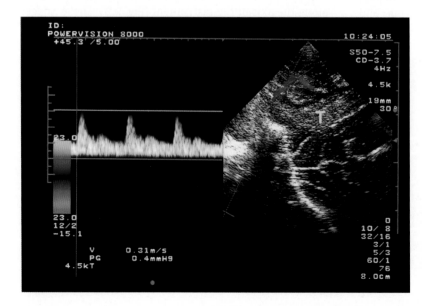

Fig. 7.5 One of the advantages of intraoperative ultrasound imaging used in conjunction with intraoperative magnetic resonance imaging is real-time visualization of especially major arteries along the intended biopsy path to tumor (T) using color Doppler (PowerVision 8000, Toshiba, Tokyo, Japan). The patient is a 35-year-old man with left frontotemporal astrocytoma WHO grade III.

calcifications and cystic septae. The trajectory of the planned iMRI biopsy can be aligned with the plane of the ultrasound image by using a neuronavigator, and the passage of the needle can be followed in real time with the ultrasound scanner. Here, too, the result of the removal of the biopsy tissue can be controlled with MR images. The drawback of US is that the ultrasound probe requires an opening in the bone, in which case we simply used a burr hole opening, which admitted the probe instead of a small twist drill hole that would suffice for passage of a biopsy needle.

The off-line biopsy method was also chosen in cases where the neurosurgeon elected to perform an open biopsy procedure using a small craniotomy and approach to the tumor under the operating microscope. A special instrument set for navigated cortical (sulcus or fissure) dissection to better access the tumor was used. This allowed for direct visualization of the lesion, for larger and more representative biopsy tissue samples, and for drainage of necrotic or cystic tumor components. Such biopsy technique may be of crucial importance in heterogeneous subcortical tumors to assure correct grading of glioma.[14] Open biopsy may also be chosen for safety reasons in cases where risk for hemorrhage is increased.

Biopsy instrumentation consisted of several alternatives. In on-line biopsies the nonferrous metallic NeuroGate (Daum Medical, Schwerin, Germany) was used early in the program (**Fig. 7.6A**). It consisted of a 20 mm diameter base that was twisted into a burr hole, and a ball and ring construct that could be aimed from the burr hole to the target and then fixed to allow accurate passage of the biopsy needle. The Navigus (Medtronic Navigation, Inc., Louisville, CO) was also tested (**Fig. 7.6B**). This device facilitates prospective stereotaxy and is widely used for iMRI procedures.[15] It does not require a separate navigational system. We usually used the nonferrous metal 150 mm side-cutting biopsy needle NeuroCut (Daum Medical, Schwerin, Germany), which can be used with the above guidance systems as well as with neuronavigator or ultrasound guidance. In open biopsy, we use a small biopsy forceps.

◆ Lessons

All of the image-guided technology, including the neuronavigator and visualization system was custom-made for this scanner. Visualization was extremely simple and was based on the tool-coordinate system developed in the early 1990s for our navigator at that time.[10] It also enabled us to match the iMR images with the real-time US images.[16] The development of the Oulu concept was done in a project with continual development of technique on site by a dedicated group of physicians, engineers, and physicists. We were concerned about adequately informing our iMRI biopsy patients, so a navigated "rehearsal" of the procedure in conjunction with preoperative imaging became part of our overall patient consent routine. Collection of pertinent textual information and images into a single workspace facilitated quick retrieval and review of biopsy cases for both clinical follow-up and for scientific review of our work.

The Oulu low-field iMRI concept and experience taught us that it is possible to share iMRI facilities, purportedly at any field strength, not only with other surgical specialties, but also with radiologists doing both interventional procedures and even routine diagnostic imaging of hospital outpatients. We were very concerned about infections because a system quite this versatile was rare in the world at the time. In over 200 iMRI cases, our rate of infections was less than 3%, and no infections occurred in the biopsy procedures.

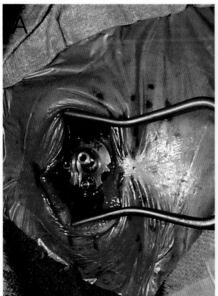
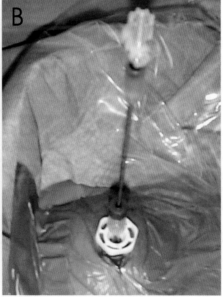

Fig. 7.6 Two burr hole biopsy needle guides. **(A)** The metallic NeuroGate (Daum Medical, Schwerin, Germany) with ball joint that could be adjusted for angle and then held in place by a metal ring plate. **(B)** The Navigus System (Medtronic Navigation, Inc., Louisville, CO) designed for prospective stereotaxy, allows guidance without other navigation systems based on target, pivot, and alignment stem points.

Obviously, biopsy is reserved for those cases in which the lesion cannot be adequately removed, for example, because of its location, extent, multiplicity, suspected histology, patient's age, and medical condition. In our experience, one of the contributions of iMRI and other image-guided technique is that the proportion of biopsies compared with resections has actually decreased as safer and more effective tumor removal has been achieved.

Current understanding of patient management is based on an accurate and comprehensive understanding of the histology of the lesion. Although with various genetic probes our management of patients will become increasingly individualized, we still divide tumors with respect to the histologic appearance of the tissue (based on World Health organization [WHO] grading criteria). Thus it is important that the tissue samples be representative of the true nature of the tumor. Representative biopsy sampling is paramount in the case of the gliomas, in which the diagnosis is based on the histologically most malignant part of the tumor. Accurate histologic diagnosis leads to better assessment of prognosis and serves to guide the overall management of the patient. Thus histologic diagnosis is required by oncologists for determination of the optimal treatment regime.

Preoperative workup with a high-field MRI scanner will generate images based on the various imaging sequences, tractography and spectroscopy. Functional MRI (fMRI) can help to avoid biopsy sites and trajectories that may impair speech and motor areas, for example. iUS can provide supplementary real-time information about the lesion as well as manipulation of the surgical area. Color Doppler can show important vascular structures including the arteries of the Sylvian fissure or veins surrounding the tumor. Computer tomography (CT) can be used to improve the spatial accuracy of the MR images, which can suffer from magnetic field inhomogeneity. Finally, on-line iMRI shows the position of the biopsy needle as it is passed through the brain toward the tumor.

The question of the high cost of iMRI technology can be solved by multitasking; many centers have elected to acquire this technology on a cost-sharing basis. On the basis of our experiences, a formal division of MRI scanning time, adjusted according to need, requires close collaboration with the radiology department. New models can be developed, including sharing the facilities with the neurovascular interventionists, who may wish to check for complications associated with placement of coils and stents, and with radiation oncologists who need MRI time for better three-dimensional planning of cancer treatment. Indeed, the iMRI unit can also be shared with neurosurgeons doing radiosurgery.

Acknowledgments Although most of the procedures were performed by JK, the inclusion of some example cases done by other staff neurosurgeons is greatly appreciated.

Disclosures The authors have no financial interests in the low-field iMRI system which was a major public project funded by the vendor, TEKES (the Finnish Funding Agency for Technology and Innovation), the Department of Labor, Finland, and Oulu University Hospital. The Onesys Navigator software for managing clinical information in huge health care databases has been developed by and is available from Onesys Oy/Inc (www.onesysmedical.com), in which one author (JK) has a financial interest.

References

1. Tronnier VM, Staubert A, Wirtz R, Knauth M, Bonsanto M, Kunze S. MRI-guided brain biopsies using a 0.2 Tesla open magnet. Minim Invasive Neurosurg 1999;42(3):118–122
2. Lewin JS, Nour SG, Meyers ML, et al. Intraoperative MRI with a rotating, tiltable surgical table: a time use study and clinical results in 122 patients. AJR Am J Roentgenol 2007;189(5):1096–1103
3. Kanner AA, Vogelbaum MA, Mayberg MR, Weisenberger JP, Barnett GH. Intracranial navigation by using low-field intraoperative magnetic resonance imaging: preliminary experience. J Neurosurg 2002;97(5):1115–1124
4. Schulder M, Sernas TJ, Carmel PW. Cranial surgery and navigation with a compact intraoperative MRI system. Acta Neurochir Suppl (Wien) 2003;85:79–86
5. Nimsky C, Ganslandt O, Buchfelder M, Fahlbusch R. Glioma surgery evaluated by intraoperative low-field magnetic resonance imaging. Acta Neurochir Suppl (Wien) 2003;85:55–63
6. McGirt MJ, Woodworth GF, Coon AL, et al. Independent predictors of morbidity after image-guided stereotactic brain biopsy: a risk assessment of 270 cases. J Neurosurg 2005;102(5):897–901
7. Yrjänä SK, Katisko JP, Ojala RO, Tervonen O, Schiffbauer H, Koivukangas J. Versatile intraoperative MRI in neurosurgery and radiology. Acta Neurochir 2002;144(3):271–278, discussion 278
8. Koivukangas J. Ultrasound imaging in operative neurosurgery: an experimental and clinical study with special reference to ultrasound holographic B (UHB) imaging. Acta Universitatis Ouluensis Series D 115. Oulu, Finland: University of Oulu Printing Center; Doctoral thesis, 1984
9. Koivukangas J, Louhisalmi Y, Alakuijala J, Oikarinen J. Ultrasound-controlled neuronavigator-guided brain surgery. J Neurosurg 1993;79(1):36–42
10. Koivukangas J, Louhisalmi Y, Alakuijala J, Oikarinen J. Neuronavigator-guided cerebral biopsy. Acta Neurochir Suppl (Wien) 1993;58:71–74
11. Yrjänä S. Implementation of 0.23 T magnetic resonance scanner to perioperative imaging in neurosurgery. Acta Universitatis Ouluensis Series D 860. Oulu, Finland: Oulu University Press; Doctoral thesis, 2005. Available at: http://herkules.oulu.fi/isbn9514279271/isbn9514279271.pdf. Accessed August 18, 2009
12. Koivukangas J, Katisko J, Yrjänä S, Tuominen J, Schiffbauer H, Ilkko E. Successful neurosurgical 0.23T intraoperative MRI in a shared facility. Proceedings of the 12th European Congress of Neurosurgery (EANS). Bologna, Italy: Monduzzi Editore Medimond; 2003:439–444
13. Vahala E, Ylihautala M, Tuominen J, et al. Registration in interventional procedures with optical navigator. J Magn Reson Imaging 2001;13(1):93–98
14. McGirt MJ, Villavicencio AT, Bulsara KR, Friedman AH. MRI-guided stereotactic biopsy in the diagnosis of glioma: comparison of biopsy and surgical resection specimen. Surg Neurol 2003;59(4):277–281, discussion 281–282
15. Hall WA, Liu H, Truwit CL. Navigus trajectory guide. Neurosurgery 2000;46(2):502–504
16. Katisko JP, Koivukangas JP. Optically neuronavigated ultrasonography in an intraoperative magnetic resonance imaging environment. Neurosurgery 2007; 60(4, Suppl 2)373–380, discussion 380–381

8

High-Field Brain Biopsy

Walter A. Hall and Charles L. Truwit

Brain biopsy allows neurosurgeons to access areas of the brain safely and accurately to determine the nature of an ongoing intracranial process. With the introduction of stereotaxis, the surgeon could now translate a three-dimensional (3D) database into the coordinate system of a rigid head frame and direct a biopsy needle to an area of interest during which the biopsy needle could be stabilized to prevent inadvertent displacement. Initially, biopsies were performed using computed tomography (CT) guidance; however, this imaging modality was rapidly replaced by magnetic resonance imaging (MRI) because of its ability to demonstrate the brain in multiple projections and its exquisite soft tissue discrimination and anatomic detail. Neuronavigational systems became popular in the 1990s and replaced frame-based stereotaxis for the performance of neurobiopsy. All of the above-mentioned biopsy techniques require the acquisition of preoperative images either several days or immediately before the surgical procedure is planned when the cranium is closed. Once the surgical procedure begins, the penetration of the skull and the incising of the dura will result in the subsequent loss of cerebrospinal fluid (CSF). This egress of CSF is unavoidable, but can lead to the displacement of the target tissue due to the shifting of the brain. Brain shift is one of the leading reasons for non-diagnostic brain biopsies. The degree to which the target tissue has moved cannot be easily determined during surgery and can necessitate that the tissue be examined by frozen section analysis by a pathologist to determine whether the procedure will lead to an accurate diagnosis of the underlying central nervous system (CNS) disorder.

The only current surgical technique that will allow the neurosurgeon to compensate for the displacement of the brain that occurs during surgery is intraoperative MRI- (iMRI-) guided brain biopsy.[1–5] During this procedure, the imaging is acquired in near-real time so that the advancement of the biopsy needle through the brain can be monitored by the surgeon until the target has been encountered. iMRI-guidance was used more than a decade ago to perform

a brain biopsy with the first procedures using a 0.5 tesla (T) interventional MRI system.[6,7] In 1997, we performed the first successful 1.5 T high-field brain biopsy using a closed short-bore iMRI system (Philips Healthcare, Andover, MA). In performing the first high-field brain biopsies there was no way to direct the biopsy needle toward the target or to stabilize the needle once the target had been reached. For these reasons, the biopsies were performed under general anesthesia to avoid the potential for displacement of the needle during the procedure. The ability to direct and stabilize the biopsy needle was achieved in 1999 when we combined the use of a disposable skull-mounted trajectory guide with the 1.5 T short-bore iMRI system.[2,8] Lesions located in the supratentorial compartment and the posterior fossa can be safely sampled using iMRI-guidance and this trajectory guide. Even brainstem lesions can be accessed using iMRI-guidance because a needle trajectory that begins with a coronal entry point can be chosen that avoids the ventricular system.

◆ Preoperative Preparation

All patients receive intravenous (IV) antibiotics (cefazolin 1 g IV) and corticosteroids (dexamethasone 10 mg IV) before beginning the procedure. The neurosurgeon has previously reviewed all of the patient's MRI studies to determine which imaging sequences will best demonstrate the lesion that is to be biopsied and in which scan orientations it will be best to image the biopsy needle as it passes through the brain. Low-grade brain tumors and demyelinating disease are best demonstrated on T2-weighted (T2W) orthogonal half-Fourier acquisition single-shot turbo spin-echo (HASTE) or turbo fluid-attenuated inversion-recovery (FLAIR) images. Secondary metastatic brain tumors or primary high-grade glial tumors are associated with blood–brain barrier breakdown and are best visualized on T1-weighted (T1W) images after the administration of gadolinium. Administration of the contrast agent is usually reserved until the time when the trajectory guide is being used for targeting to prevent the diffusion of the contrast material out into areas where the blood–brain barrier has broken down, which may not represent the true focus of confluent tumor tissue. Superficial and cerebellar lesions are usually imaged in the coronal and axial planes because the needle is generally passed the shortest distance from the surface of the brain to the target. Brainstem and deep central supratentorial lesions are usually reached by passing the biopsy needle through the frontal lobe while the imaging is obtained in the coronal and sagittal planes.

Anesthesia

Brain biopsies can be performed under local or general anesthesia. We prefer to perform our MRI-guided brain biopsies under general anesthesia for several reasons. Because of the length of time that is required to perform an MRI-guided brain biopsy due to the necessity to obtain intraoperative imaging, it can be difficult for patients to remain calm and immobile for the entire procedure. The biopsy procedure can last from 1 to 3 hours depending on the complexity of the surgery. Many lesions are located in areas in the brain where it is difficult for a patient to maintain the head in the proper orientation for prolonged periods. If the procedure was performed under local anesthesia and the patient received IV sedation, it is possible that the patient may startle with the initiation of the scanning because of the loud noise that is associated with some of the MRI sequences. Abruptly displacing the head with the biopsy needle within the brain could lead to neurologic injury – or worse – because the head must be located at the center of the magnet during imaging, which is at least an arm's length away from the flared openings of the MRI scanner.

Positioning

Once under general anesthesia the patient is brought from the main operating room to the iMRI suite where transfer is made from the transport cart to the padded MRI-compatible surgical table. The vast majority of brain biopsies are performed with the patient in the supine position. Even occipital and cerebellar biopsies can be performed in a supine patient by turning the head to the side and taping the ipsilateral forehead down onto the side of the surgical table to prevent inadvertent posterior rotation of the head. A shoulder roll is placed if the head is to be turned. If the lesion is in the posterior fossa, then the head is placed on folded towels instead of on a foam rubber donut because the edge of the donut can interfere with the passage of the biopsy needle; the donut will compress due to the weight of the patient's head. One of the circular radiofrequency (RF) coils is placed underneath the head on either the towels or the donut in a plastic bag to prevent soiling of the coil (**Fig. 8.1**). The second coil is then wrapped in gauze and sandwiched between two sterile plastic sheets. The plastic in the center of the coil is then excised before the coil is stapled to the

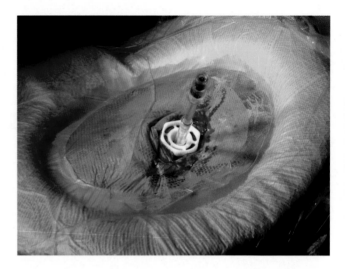

Fig. 8.1 Brain biopsy is performed through one of the radiofrequency surface coils with the second coil placed under the head of the patient in a phased array. The alignment stem has been placed in the guide tube for alignment and the white plastic locking nut is used to secure the guide tube in place after an accurate trajectory to the target has been achieved. (Courtesy of Walter A. Hall and Charles L. Truwit.)

sterile drapes surrounding the surgical field. After the second RF coil is stapled to the surgical drapes in a location that is opposite to the first coil, an Ioban drape (3M Medical Products, Minneapolis, MN) is placed over the entire surgical field to establish and maintain a sterile environment. Positioning the RF coils in this way will allow the entire biopsy to be performed through one coil, which will enhance visualization of the target site during the biopsy by improving the signal-to-noise ratio and affording the high resolution imaging. To date, we have not needed to place any patient in the prone position to perform a cerebellar biopsy.

◆ Procedure

The disposable Navigus trajectory guide[8] that we use for brain biopsies is commercially available and manufactured by Medtronic Navigation, Inc., Louisville, CO (**Fig. 8.2**). The guide has two bases that can be attached to the skull either in a burr hole or to allow for a twist drill craniostomy. We prefer the base that rests in a burr hole because it allows for the visualization of the cortical surface and any blood vessels that may lie underneath the dura mater once it has been incised. In penetrating the skull with a twist drill it is possible to injure a superficial cortical vessel resulting in a subarachnoid hemorrhage. There is also another version of the trajectory guide base that is angled allowing for a more oblique angle to be attained thereby allowing for the sampling of inferior anterior frontal lesions where the skin incision is placed behind the hairline (**Fig. 8.3**).

After general anesthesia is administered, an MRI-visible button with a single adhesive side is placed on the head where it is anticipated that the burr hole will be drilled. For

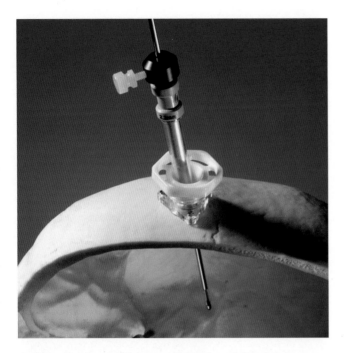

Fig. 8.2 The disposable Navigus trajectory guide (Medtronic Navigation, Inc., Louisville, CO) attached to the skull with the brain biopsy needle locked in place to prevent inadvertent migration. The base, guide tube, reduction cannula, biopsy needle, and plastic collar brake are visible. (Courtesy of Medtronic Navigation, Inc., Louisville, CO. Used with permission.)

lesions located directly below the cortical surface, it is particularly important to localize the site for penetrating the skull. Inaccurate localization can result in the surgeon (1) being unable to sample a lesion because the obliquity of the angle needed to direct the biopsy needle to the target, or

(2) removing additional cranial bone to just expose the lesion. The hair is not shaved, but is parted along the line of the incision before the skin is prepped with an iodine-based scrub, alcohol, and DuraPrep (3M Medical Products, Minneapolis, MN). Local anesthesia containing epinephrine is used to infiltrate the skin and the incision is made that is just long enough to allow for the trajectory guide base to be secured in the burr hole. A cranial perforator is used to make the burr hole. In areas of the skull where the bone is particularly thin such as in the temporal region, the cranial opening may need to be enlarged with a Kerrison rongeur to accept the burr hole design trajectory guide base. The dura mater is cauterized and then opened in a cruciate fashion and the trajectory guide base is secured in place with three self-taping titanium screws using a disposable screwdriver that is included in the kit. Once the base is in place, a single diameter guide tube is snapped into the base and secured in place with a plastic locking nut that will prevent the inadvertent redirection of the guide tube during the procedure. An alignment stem is next inserted into the guide tube to begin the targeting process. Visualization of the alignment stem can be difficult on MRI and is entirely dependent on the fluid with which the stem is filled. For enhancing lesions a mixture of saline and gadolinium is necessary to optimize visualization of the stem on T1W scan sequences. For nonenhancing lesions that are best demonstrated on T2W MRI, saline alone is used to fill the stem for recognition. After insertion of the alignment stem into the guide tube, the trajectory is determined in two planes that will best allow for access of the target lesion using prospective stereotaxis.

Up to this point, if the biopsy has been performed outside the 5 gauss line in the non-MRI–compatible section of the surgical suite, the surgical drapes that hang below the edge of the surgical table are then cut off to enable the surgical table to dock properly with the gantry of the MRI scanner,

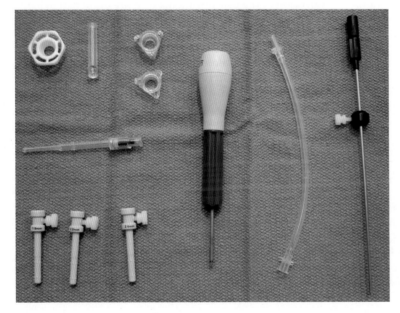

Fig. 8.3 The various components of the brain biopsy trajectory guide kit (locking nut, guide tube, straight base, angled base, alignment stem, three different diameter reduction cannulas, and screwdriver) and the titanium biopsy needle with the plastic collar brake (right) and its flexible aspiration tubing. (Courtesy of Walter A. Hall and Charles L. Truwit.)

which will allow the patient to be transported through the scanner to the opposite end of the room where the targeting and the biopsy are performed. At the far end of the magnet, the alignment stem is manipulated using prospective stereotaxis to determine a safe and accurate trajectory to pass the biopsy needle into the lesion that is being sampled.

Prospective Stereotaxis

Prospective stereotaxis represents a unique way to determine the path of the biopsy needle to the target of interest using a trajectory guide.[2,5,9] Determining a safe and successful surgical path with prospective stereotaxis starts at the biopsy site and moves away from the brain toward the distal end of the alignment stem. Once the location of the biopsy has been chosen (target point), there are two additional points that need to be selected to allow for alignment of the trajectory guide with the target. The location of the second point is at the tip of the alignment stem and is known as the pivot point. The desired location of a cross section of the alignment stem above the scalp out in space represents the third point. The intersection of two orthogonal MRI scan planes will define the desired location of the alignment stem. By rapidly updating the MRI scans in these two plane orientations, the alignment stem is shifted until all three points are colinear, which will ensure that the biopsy needle will encounter the target once it is passed through the trajectory guide.

After the alignment stem is filled with a solution that will allow it to be visualized on the chosen MRI sequences, it is inserted into the guide tube to perform prospective stereotaxis.[2,5,9] The guide tube has a ball joint that allows it to be freely rotated in space such that all three points can be aligned in less than 5 minutes (**Fig. 8.4**). Once the three points are aligned, MRI along the entire length of the alignment stem occurs to verify that the trajectory guide is pointing directly at the target and that the biopsy needle will encounter the target after passing through the brain. If the surgical path is considered appropriate and accurate, the locking nut is tightened to prevent redirection or displacement of the trajectory guide tube.

Upon completion of the prospective stereotaxis, the alignment stem should be pointing directly at the target in two orthogonal projections as confirmed on MRI. The alignment stem is removed from the guide tube, which is secured in place by tightening the locking nut prior to passing the biopsy needle. A reduction cannula is inserted into the guide tube, which allows the biopsy needle to be locked at a specific depth to prevent migration to either more superficial or deeper levels. The MRI-compatible disposable titanium biopsy needle (Ad-Tech Medical Instrument Corp., Racine, WI) is passed gradually through the brain in a stepwise fashion toward the target in near-real time during which time periodic snapshot MRI updates are obtained (**Figs. 8.5** and **8.6**). The biopsy needle that we use is 15 cm in length and allows for any location within the intracranial compartment to be successfully accessed.

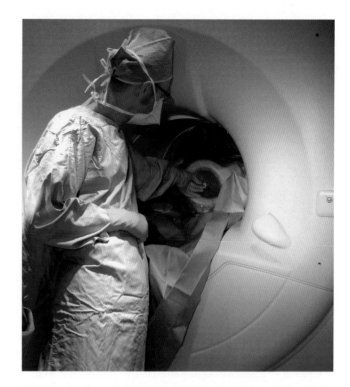

Fig. 8.4 Because of a ball joint, the alignment stem can be rotated freely in space to orient the stem toward the target point in less than 5 minutes using prospective stereotaxis. The shore-bore nature of the magnet allows the neurosurgeon to easily manipulate the alignment stem with having to move the patient out of the scanner. (Courtesy of Walter A. Hall and Charles L. Truwit.)

For the majority of lesions to be biopsied, HASTE imaging is used to determine the surgical trajectory because of the rapid scanning acquisition time. If the target lesion that is to be biopsied is best seen on contrast-enhanced images then the intravenous contrast is administered immediately before the biopsy needle is passed to prevent the inadvertent diffusion of the contrast media into the brain parenchyma surrounding the target. Upon reaching the target, the reduction cannula is tightened around the biopsy needle to prevent displacement and imaging is performed in two orthogonal planes along the entire length of the needle. The imaging demonstrates the location of the end of the needle from where the tissue samples will be taken and confirms the overall accuracy of the procedure. In performing the biopsy, a 10 mL syringe filled with sterile saline is utilized to gently aspirate the tissue sample into the open 1-cm-long side aperture of the needle (**Fig. 8.7**). The biopsy needle is connected to the aspiration syringe by flexible tubing to limit the manipulation of the outer cannula of the biopsy needle during tissue sampling and to assure that the position of the needle remains constant during the procedure. After the tissue is aspirated into the biopsy needle, the inner cannula that contains the sample is withdrawn from the outer cannula and the specimen is flushed onto a piece of nonadherent Telfa dressing (Tyco Healthcare Group, Albertville, AL). To assure that an accurate sample of the target tissue is obtained and to avoid sampling error, multiple

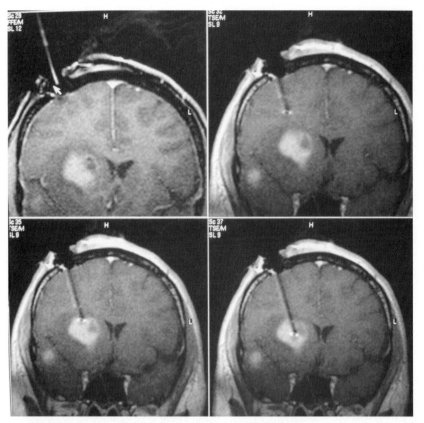

Fig. 8.5 Brain biopsy of a right frontal mass on oblique coronal T1-weighted contrast-enhanced magnetic resonance images. The alignment stem (*arrow*) is seen directed toward the target in the upper left panel. The remaining three images demonstrate the progression of the biopsy needle being advanced through the brain in a step-wise fashion in near-real time to the target point. (Courtesy of Walter A. Hall and Charles L. Truwit.)

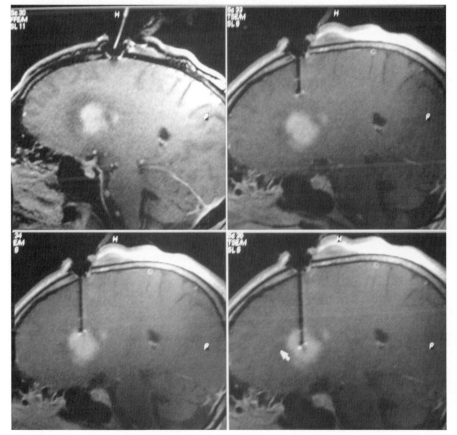

Fig. 8.6 Brain biopsy of a right frontal mass on oblique sagittal T1-weighted contrast-enhanced magnetic resonance images. The alignment stem is seen directed toward the target in the upper left panel. The other three images show the biopsy needle being advanced through the brain in a step-wise fashion in near-real time to the target point. (Courtesy of Walter A. Hall and Charles L. Truwit.)

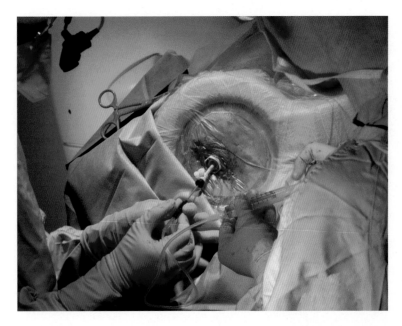

Fig. 8.7 Brain biopsy being performed entirely within the magnetic field using all magnetic resonance imaging-compatible instrumentation. A 10-cc syringe filled with saline is used to gently aspirate the tissue being sampled into the biopsy needle through a 1-cm-long side port. Flexible plastic tubing connected to the end of the biopsy needle limits the amount of manipulation of the outer cannula of the biopsy needle, assuring that the position of the biopsy needle does not change. (Courtesy of Walter A. Hall and Charles L. Truwit.)

specimens are taken at different depths and from different locations for frozen section and permanent pathologic analysis. It is still our practice to confirm the presence of pathologic tissue in the specimen before leaving the operating room to assure that a definitive diagnosis will be obtained from the procedure.

While the frozen section is being performed by the pathologist, the biopsy needle is removed from the target and the sample site is evaluated for the presence of intraoperative hemorrhage using three distinct MRI sequences that allow for the detection of hyperacute blood (**Fig. 8.8**). Because hyperacute blood, before the conversion of intracellular oxyhemoglobin to deoxyhemoglobin, can be difficult to detect on MRI, it is necessary to combine HASTE, gradient echo (GE)-T2*, and turbo FLAIR scan sequences to accurately identify intraoperative hemorrhage.[7] The presence of a sig-

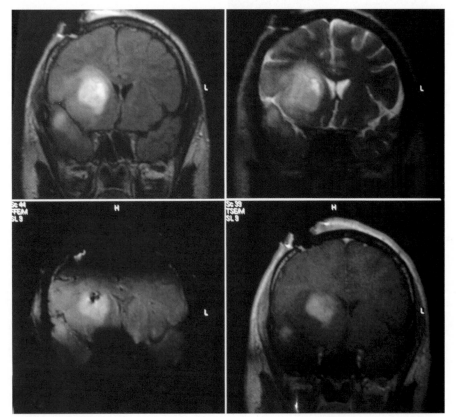

Fig. 8.8 Because the presence of hyperacute blood can be difficult to detect on magnetic resonance imaging (MRI), a combination of turbo fluid-attenuated inversion-recovery (FLAIR; upper left), half-Fourier acquisition single-shot turbo spin-echo (HASTE; upper right), and gradient echo-T2* (lower left) sequences are necessary to accurately exclude the presence of intraoperative hemorrhage. The black area on the gradient echo-T2* scan in the enhancing target lesion represents air and not hemorrhage because it is not present on the turbo FLAIR and HASTE scans. A T1-weighted contrast-enhanced oblique coronal MRI scan is present in the lower right panel. (Courtesy of Walter A. Hall and Charles L. Truwit.)

nal void on all three sequences is representative of hemorrhage whereas if the signal is absent only on the GE-T2* images it is indicative of the presence of air. The biopsy needle comes with a disposable plastic collar brake that can be used to mark the depth of the needle and to prevent the advancement of the needle past the target tissue. Before withdrawing the biopsy needle to perform the MRI that detects the presence of intraoperative hemorrhage, the collar brake is tightened onto the needle to mark the depth from where the samples were taken. In the event that the pathologist is unable to identify pathologic tissue on the frozen section specimens that will lead to an accurate diagnosis on the analysis of the permanent sections, the needle can be immediately repositioned within the target without the need for retargeting the lesion.

If diagnostic tissue is confirmed by frozen section, the patient is moved out of the MRI scanner to the area outside the 5 gauss line for closure. The base of the trajectory guide is disengaged from the skull by unscrewing the self-tapping titanium screws and the wound is irrigated with an antibiotic solution. To restore the outer contour of the skull, a titanium burr hole cover (OsteoMed, Dallas, TX) is attached to the skull using two 4 mm self-tapping titanium screws. The galea of the scalp is closed with inverted interrupted absorbable sutures and the skin is closed with a continuous running absorbable stitch.

ChloraPrep antibacterial skin preparation (Enturia, Inc., formerly Medi-Flex, Inc., Leawood, KS) is applied to the incision to prevent infection and a Primapore dressing (Smith & Nephew, Hull, England) is placed over the wound for 48 hours. Patients are instructed to keep the wound dry for 3 days after which it can become wet and come into contact with soap or shampoo. The patient is then transported from the surgical table to a gurney before being transported to the recovery room for extubation. Patients are usually observed overnight and discharged the following morning, although on occasion a patient has been sent home on the same day of surgery at their own request provided they have been observed for several hours after surgery.

Spectroscopy-Guided Biopsy

To enhance the diagnostic yield of brain biopsy, magnetic resonance spectroscopy (MRS) was combined with the use of the trajectory guide.[10-14] Two MRS techniques were used during brain biopsy to identify an appropriate location for tissue sampling: single voxel spectroscopy (SVS) and turbo spectroscopic imaging (TSI). Single voxel spectroscopy ($1.5 \text{ cm}^3 \times 1.5 \text{ cm}^3 \times 1.5 \text{ cm}^3$ voxel, 1-Hz spectral resolution, echo time (TE)/repetition time (TR) = 136/2000 millisecond, 4.5-minute acquisition time) was performed on the area of interest and compared with the comparable control location in the contralateral hemisphere of the brain. Turbo spectroscopic imaging (32×32 mm grid of

spectra in a single plane, $0.66 \text{ cm}^3 \times 0.66 \text{ cm}^3 \times 2.0 \text{ cm}^3$ spatial resolution, 4.4-Hz spectral resolution, TE/TR 272/2000 millisecond, turbo factor = 3, 11-minute acquisition time) was obtained on a single axial brain slice to measure the metabolites phosphocholine, creatine, N-acetyl aspartate (NAA), and lactate/lipid. Those regions where phosphocholine is elevated on SVS or TSI are felt to represent areas of rapid membrane turnover with increased cellular density that should correlate with the presence of tumor tissue. These areas of elevated phosphocholine are generally chosen for targeting if a neoplasm is suspected to be present. Areas of normal brain tissue will demonstrate elevated NAA, a neuronal marker. There is generally more spectral contamination seen with TSI than with SVS due to the lower spatial resolution of TSI compared with SVS. Quantitative spectral analysis of TSI data are limited by its low spectral resolution. After performing an MRS-guided brain biopsy, the standard three imaging sequences determined to demonstrate the presence of intraoperative blood are performed in the axial plane to determine whether there has been a hemorrhage at the time of the brain biopsy.

References

1. Hall WA, Martin AJ, Liu H, Nussbaum ES, Maxwell RE, Truwit CL. Brain biopsy using high-field strength interventional magnetic resonance imaging. Neurosurgery 1999;44(4):807–813, discussion 813–814

2. Hall WA, Liu H, Martin AJ, Maxwell RE, Truwit CL. Brain biopsy sampling by using prospective stereotaxis and a trajectory guide. J Neurosurg 2001;94(1):67–71

3. Hall WA, Liu H, Martin AJ, Pozza CH, Maxwell RE, Truwit CL. Safety, efficacy, and functionality of high-field strength interventional magnetic resonance imaging for neurosurgery. Neurosurgery 2000;46(3):632–641, discussion 641–642

4. Hall WA, Liu H, Martin AJ, Truwit CL. Minimally invasive procedures. Interventional MR image-guided neurobiopsy. Neuroimaging Clin N Am 2001;11(4):705–713

5. Martin AJ, Hall WA, Roark C, Starr PA, Larson PS, Truwit CL. Minimally invasive precision brain access using prospective stereotaxy and a trajectory guide. J Magn Reson Imaging 2008;27(4):737–743

6. Hall WA, Truwit CL. Intraoperative MR imaging. Magn Reson Imaging Clin N Am 2005;13(3):533–543

7. Hall WA, Truwit CL. Intraoperative MR-guided neurosurgery. J Magn Reson Imaging 2008;27(2):368–375

8. Hall WA, Liu H, Truwit CL. Navigus trajectory guide. Neurosurgery 2000;46(2):502–504

9. Liu H, Hall WA, Truwit CL. Neuronavigation in interventional MR imaging. Prospective stereotaxy. Neuroimaging Clin N Am 2001;11(4): 695–704

10. Martin AJ, Liu H, Hall WA, Truwit CL. Preliminary assessment of turbo spectroscopic imaging for targeting in brain biopsy. AJNR Am J Neuroradiol 2001;22(5):959–968

11. Liu H, Hall WA, Martin AJ, Truwit CL. An efficient chemical shift imaging scheme for magnetic resonance-guided neurosurgery. J Magn Reson Imaging 2001;14(1):1–7

12. Hall WA, Martin AJ, Liu H, Truwit CL. Improving diagnostic yield in brain biopsy: coupling spectroscopic targeting with real-time needle placement. J Magn Reson Imaging 2001;13(1):12–15

13. Hall WA, Liu H, Truwit CL. MR spectroscopy-guided biopsy of intracranial neoplasms. Tech Neurosurg 2002;7:291–298

14. Hall WA, Truwit CL. 1.5 T: spectroscopy-supported brain biopsy. Neurosurg Clin N Am 2005;16(1):165–172, vii

9

MRI-Guided Catheter Placement

Gregory T. Sherr and Cornelius H. Lam

Intraoperative magnetic resonance imaging (iMRI) allows neurosurgeons to interactively perform surgery using MRI guidance. This relatively new technology provides exceptional visualization of intracranial anatomy and pathology. Its availability and use are quickly becoming a standard for comprehensive care hospitals and practices in the United States, Europe, and beyond. To embrace this technology, some of neurosurgery's most difficult problems are being given renewed attention with an eye toward an iMRI solution. For example, traditionally one of the great challenges in neurosurgery has been to accurately cannulate the tiny ventricular system of a child with a shunt catheter. Likewise, deep cystic lesions next to critical parts of the brain in both the adult and pediatric populations are often equally difficult to cannulate and divert.

In recent years, more refined techniques for placing these catheters have been evolving as the rate of technology development accelerates. Important milestones along the way have included the development of modern flexible plastic catheters, ultrasound/endoscopic assistance, and now iMRI guidance. Real-time or near-real-time image-guided catheter placement across the frontal, parietal, and occipital lobes has become an important new technique in complex cases. Another advantage is that, unlike other neuronavigation techniques such as computer-guided stereotaxy, iMRI allows the neurosurgeon to adjust for the brain shift that occurs once the cranium is open.[1] With the advent of iMRI, catheter placement into dangerous locations such as the 4th ventricle or posterior fossa cysts near the brainstem have become a safer possibility.

◆ Milestones Leading to iMRI Shunting Techniques

Alternate shunting techniques that have helped to lay the foundation for iMRI procedures include ultrasound- (US-) guided catheter placement in premature neonates, endoscopic third ventriculostomies, and image-guided shunting of complex multiloculated hydrocephalus or cystic lesions. In adults, the frontal horns are often large enough to allow blind cannulation of the lateral ventricle using anatomic landmarks only. The smaller the patient or lesion/ventricle though, the more difficult the target can be to access. The frontal approach is often preferable because it is familiar to most neurosurgeons. Likewise, in children the alternative occipital approach is a good second choice that takes advantage of common accessible landmarks and wide central access to the ventricular system. Both approaches are safe and in experienced hands can be performed accurately, but with varying skull geometries, ventricular shapes, and congenital anomalies, the approach can be very difficult. These customary methods could be improved upon so that placement of the catheter could be done in a single pass sparing the brain from repeated trauma. Clearly, the same concern extends to both adult and pediatric patients with complicated clinical scenarios.

US techniques presaged the advent of modern MRI-guided practices. The first formal published description of US-assisted shunt catheter placement was by Shkolnik in 1981. In that paper, the author succinctly described the advantages of using image guidance. Most importantly, he described a new and reliable method of assuring that the final placement of the shunt tip was in an optimal site in the lateral ventricle.[2] However, perhaps the greater gain with US was that the neurosurgeon could finely adjust the trajectory of the catheter in real time. Before then, there was no way to know with any immediate confidence that both the path through the brain and the final location were correct. In retrospect, US guidance seems crude compared with the detailed anatomy seen on MRI. Yet, in retrospect, the anatomic knowledge gained with US was leaps and bounds ahead of the blind passage technique.[3–5] The ultrasound therefore laid the groundwork for iMRI in terms of guidance for catheter placement. If insertion of the catheter is undertaken in a patient with relatively normal anatomy, fine discrimination of cerebral structures may not be important. US would likely be a good choice and confer some speed and accessibility advantages for an experienced surgeon in that case.[6,7] However, like other advances in technology, MRI and MR-guided surgeries improve on the prior ultrasound techniques with very fine detailed imagery which is especially important in cases with distorted, abnormal or small/pediatric anatomy.

Similarly, with advances and miniaturization in optics, endoscopic techniques have also helped create the groundwork for MRI-guided surgery. In addition to the evolution of surgical techniques and instruments, there was a parallel improvement of diagnostic techniques. Both processes of development influenced each other. Modern diagnostic imaging is able to provide us with almost all the individual anatomic and pathologic or anatomic details of a specific patient and is able to show us the individual anatomic windows. With the knowledge of these details, it is possible to target and to treat an individual lesion through a relatively small (keyhole) approach.[8,9] The problems of adopting a miniature incision are narrow viewing angles, reduction of light intensity in the operating field, and the necessity for almost coaxial control of the microinstruments. The rigid endoscope with its rounded wide view lens, powerful light source, and relatively small diameter made directed, exploratory microsurgery possible. Procedures at the skull base or deep in the brain such as a third ventriculostomy could be done with the aid of real-time feedback and continuous trajectory adjustment based on up to the moment data.

iMRI developed from, and alongside these precursor techniques represents a natural next step in the attempt to embrace new technology, decrease morbidity, and to refine the accuracy of our surgeries. The first MRI-guided surgical suites came on-line in the mid-1990s; since then the technology has matured to much higher magnet strength and better designs of both MRI-compatible surgical instruments and the suites themselves. Tumor surgeons were the first to embrace this leap in technology. One group found that 41% of their glioma resections (grades 1–4) were extended after imaging, increasing the percentage of gross total resections from 27 to 40%.[10] Next, deep brain stimulator surgery with its high demand for precision targeting of deep seated nuclei was adapted and augmented by the push toward iMRI. At the same time, cannulation of complex cystic lesions and difficult shunt placement procedures were being attempted. This was aided in part by the development of tools and scanning protocols designed to facilitate brain lesion needle biopsy.

Early iMRI-guided brain biopsies were performed freehand in the same way that early computed tomography- (CT-) guided brain biopsies were accomplished. Initially, there was no way to direct the brain biopsy needle toward the target or to stabilize the needle after the region of interest had been reached. The need for needle stabilization devices soon became apparent and they were rapidly designed and developed. Early work on a disposable trajectory guide (Navigus, Medtronic Navigation, Inc., Louisville, CO) was undertaken at our facility. This was done in combination with a unique targeting technique known as prospective stereotaxy to perform brain biopsy in near-real time using a 1.5 T

iMRI system.[1] Certainly, if this new method could work for needle biopsy, it could just as easily help place a drainage catheter.

◆ Clinical Experience

At the University of Minnesota, we have performed over 1000 intraoperative MRI cases in the decade since coming on-line in 1996. The different neurosurgeons within the department found a wide variety of uses and applications for MRI-guidance. Deep brain stimulator lead placement, tumor removal/biopsy, and catheter placement in anatomically difficult patients are some of the typical indications. There are in fact two different surgical MRI suites at two different hospitals in our academic program in Minneapolis. One is a 1.5 tesla system and the second has a 3.0 tesla magnet. The higher resolution or speed in acquisition can be helpful in working close to vital and sensitive structures such as the medulla oblongata where millimeters of accuracy count.

The drive to use iMRI in pediatric and adult oncology cases has been strong. More often, it is the pediatric cases that present the kind of technical challenge where interventional MRI can be the greatest help. In an early paper covering cases from 1997 to 2000, nine posterior fossa intraoperative magnet cases out of 11 were pediatric. The mean age was 6.4 years and the median age 7. Seven midline craniotomies were performed, of which three were reoperations. Two were burr hole placements, one for cyst aspiration with P32 instillation, and the other for tumor biopsy.[11,12] In each case, iMRI was chosen as the superior option for the complexity of the case in the setting of such diminutive anatomy.

Nimsky et al indicate that among the iMRI pediatric cases at their institution, it was the monitoring of catheter placement and consecutive cyst alterations that proved the most beneficial application of the technology. In many of their catheter placement cases, intraoperative imaging resulted in a modification of the surgical strategy. It served as an intraoperative quality control that helped them to monitor the effects of the ongoing surgery (e.g., the extent of a resection or depth of a catheter), in comparison with the treatment plan. They state that besides its application in brain tumors, iMRI has also proven to be particularly helpful in children undergoing complicated catheter placements for cyst drainage, as well as in pituitary and epilepsy surgery.[13]

An example of how to best use the iMRI for catheter placement is a case where there was an expanding cystic lesion adjacent to a sensitive, vital structure. A 4-year-old child with cerebral palsy was brought in to the emergency department with recurrent and worsening hydrocephalus despite an existing traditional frontal ventriculoperitoneal shunt. From birth, the boy had had a complex cystic lesion that was incorporated into his ventricular system. Recently, the lesion had begun expanding the 4th ventricle (**Fig. 9.1**). This had worsened over a period of months and with it a gradual neurologic decline. iMRI was used on two different occasions in attempts to place a catheter that

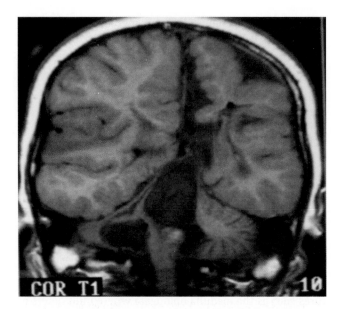

Fig. 9.1 Presenting lesion in a 4-year-old boy with cerebral palsy and frontal ventriculoperitoneal shunt failure now with an expanding 4th ventricular cyst lesion.

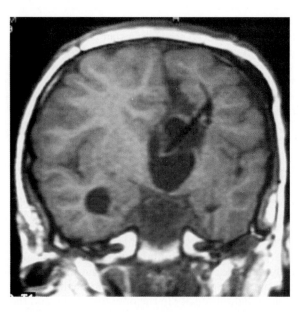

Fig. 9.2 Initial intraoperative magnetic resonance imaging shunt placement, but 4th ventricular cystic lesion continued to expand.

adequately controlled and drained the expanding cystic lesion. First, a left-sided frontal approach was used to place a 3rd ventricular/cyst catheter in the hope that the cysts and ventricular system were in continuity and the entire system could be decompressed from above (**Fig. 9.2**).

Follow-up CT scans showed this was only partially successful and a more definitive procedure would have to be attempted from below to fully decompress the 4th ventricle. The patient returned to the operating room a few days later. This time a suboccipital approach was undertaken and the

catheter was meticulously placed within the 4th ventricle cystic lesion along the plane of the brainstem with good results (**Figs. 9.3** and **9.4**). Catheter placement required two passes because the first trajectory caused the catheter tip to lie against the anterior wall of the ventricle. This was seen immediately and corrected with a subsequent pass using more frequent updates of MRI scanning as the catheter was slowly advanced into better position. This would likely not have been recognized intraoperatively using other imaging techniques and the implications of not correcting it immediately

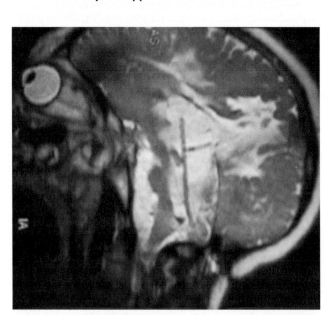

Fig. 9.3 Intraoperative magnetic resonance imaging scan during placement of a new catheter into the 4th ventricular cystic lesion, with excellent midline alignment.

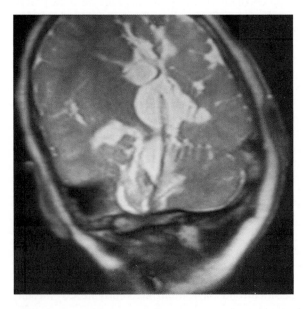

Fig. 9.4 Intraoperative coronal magnetic resonance imaging showing the complex trajectory required for proper and effective catheter placement.

would have been critical. Any catheter migration or even irritation of the brainstem could have been devastating. Such quality control and precise localization is a truly unique advantage of iMRI-guided procedures.

Another unique shunting procedure that was accomplished in the 1.5 tesla intraoperative MRI (iMRI) suite was not cerebral, but rather a case of an expanding cervicothoracic syrinx that was treated with placement of a syringosubarachnoid shunt (**Fig. 9.5**). Here the basic procedure was the same with some adjustments in patient position and surgical technique. This adult patient required careful prone positioning with minimal chest rolls and padding to allow passage into the scanner. Preoperative scans were completed to precisely localize the incision over the syrinx. A sterile MRI-opaque fiducial was left in place as a marker. Then, the floating table top with the patient in place was brought out of the magnetic field and over onto the surgical pedestal outside the 5 gauss line. There, a standard laminectomy was accomplished using the familiar ferrous spinal instruments. Further intraoperative scans were then obtained to minimally open the dura, place the syringosubarachnoid catheter to the proper depth within the syrinx, and then close the case (**Fig. 9.5**). Immediate collapse of the syrinx was documented when the postoperative scan was completed to ensure no bleeding or other complication had occurred. Incidentally, this patient did require a reoperation when the syringosubarachnoid shunt migrated into the syrinx 3 months after initial placement. Surgery was repeated in the iMRI suite in the same manner as before with lasting success.

Pseudotumor cerebri also represents a unique problem for traditional shunting techniques. An obese 22-year-old woman underwent several optic nerve sheath fenestrations for worsening vision difficulties and painful frontal headaches, but was reluctant to have a shunt placed. She knew that her ventricles were the typical "slit like" ones that make catheter placement in this population so difficult (**Fig. 9.6**). Finally, her headaches became so intractable that she agreed to have the procedure done. After careful consideration of the alternatives, an iMRI-guided right frontal approach was chosen. Here, another advantage of well-defined, anatomically precise image guidance is evident. The exact depth and trajectory of the catheter is crucial in her case. The treating neurosurgeon has to think beforehand about the best possible way of maximizing the cannulation of her ventricle. Given the small target, it would be quite possible that only one set of drainage holes on the catheter's lateral surface will fit in these tiny ventricles. Continued patency is always a problem in such a case and any way to increase the effectiveness or number of functioning holes should be considered. One idea would be to use a more lateral angle of attack outside the usual landmarks and rely on iMRI navigation to help place more of the catheter tip within the ventricle. In this case, a slightly more lateral burr hole was made and widened to accommodate a reservoir. The catheter was carefully and slowly advanced with subtle

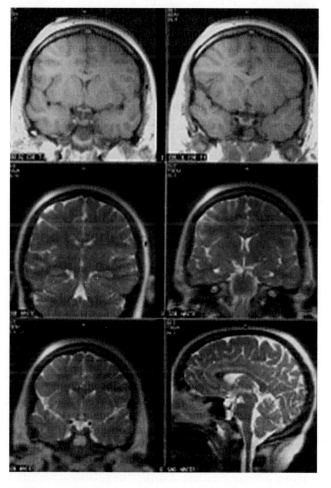

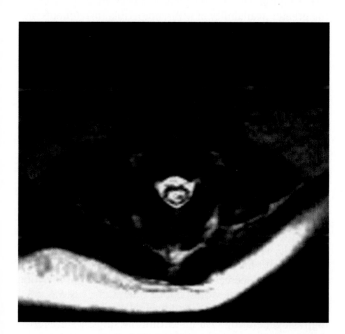

Fig. 9.5 Intraoperative magnetic resonance imaging-placed syringosubarachnoid shunt placement via laminectomy. The catheter can be clearly seen within the syrinx.

Fig. 9.6 Small slit-like ventricles that are present in pseudotumor cerebri.

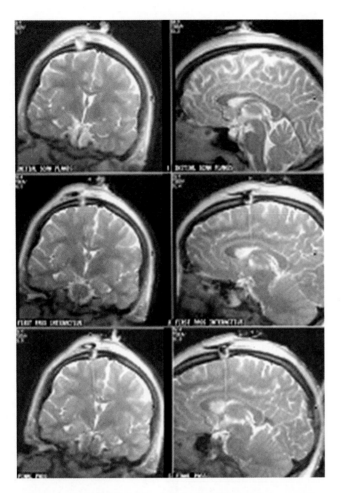

Fig. 9.7 Placement of a catheter in the lateral ventricle in a pseudo-tumor cerebri patient.

adjustments in trajectory over several scans to guide it into place (**Fig. 9.7**). Ultimately, the placement of the shunt was successful in relieving her severe headaches.

Another example of the effective use of iMRI catheter placement occurred in a 43-year-old man with a recurrent craniopharyngioma. This lesion had been resected twice before; once by craniotomy and once transsphenoidally. Yet again, he developed a bitemporal visual field deficit from compression of the optic chiasm by this suprasellar cystic lesion. Aspiration of the cyst with placement of an Ommaya reservoir into the cyst under MRI-guidance was effected.

◆ Methodology

Much of the methodology that we have developed is tailored to the type of MRI suites we have helped to design and install through a research partnership with industry. Given that our two operative scanners are set up very differently and serve different patient populations, we often adjust our surgical plan depending on which hospital and iMRI suite we are utilizing. However, many basic features

are the same. Each MRI suite is kept at positive pressure relative to surrounding rooms. The room is also equipped with numerous radiofrequency- (RF-) shielded power outlets and gas lines for suction, air, oxygen, and nitrous oxide. MRI-compatible anesthesia and patient monitoring equipment are incorporated into the suite.[14] The 1.5 Tesla suite (Intera I/T; Philips Healthcare, Andover, MA) is principally arranged so that the surgical bed can be moved outside the 5 gauss line for an unencumbered procedure using many ferromagnetic instruments. Once a scan is needed, the reverse process occurs where the MRI/surgical bed simply reconnects to the floating table top leading into the scanner. Anesthesia sits on the opposite/far side of the surgery suite with extended tubing connections that allow the transfer to occur without having to change hoses or lines. MRI scans are obtained first as a baseline prior to the catheter insertion then one or more times mid-case and again postoperatively to check for any bleeding and to document the catheter's final position.

The 3.0 tesla suite (Intera, Philips Medical Systems) is perhaps better suited for catheter placement than the 1.5 T intraoperational system in that it has a higher spatial resolution and also allows for more focused cerebral procedures on the opposite side of the magnet. The patient's body remains inside the scanner at all times, but they are positioned such that their head is accessible at the opposite side of the scanner, where it can be draped and prepped in a sterile fashion for catheter insertion (**Fig. 9.8**). This system was designed for minimally invasive cranial procedures to be performed entirely at the back end of the scanner. Although this limits patient positioning to a minor degree, the rapid acquisition of high-field images offers significant improvement in patient flow and throughput, particularly with respect to sterile surgical draping. This advance has also been made possible by the greater availability of MRI-compatible instruments and equipment.[1]

In general, the patient's head is placed in the surgical position with two-phased array RF coils positioned adjacent to the head in a sensitivity encoding (SENSE) pair. One coil is usually placed underneath the patient's head on a foam rubber donut and the other coil is placed opposite to the first. One coil is wrapped in gauze and then sandwiched between two sterile plastic adhesive drapes. This coil is then stapled to sterile surgical towels placed around the surgical site. A clear plastic sterile drape with an Ioban center and an irrigation collection bag (3M, Minneapolis, MN) is applied to the surgical field and the adhesive back side is attached to the back of the scanner in such a manner as to allow sterile patient transport to the isocenter of the scanner.[1]

Sterility is of the utmost concern especially when introducing shunt hardware that will reside in the patient permanently. Any increase in wound complications or infection rates from iMRI use would not be tolerated. This was not a small consideration in that additional machinery and moving/heat generating systems within the surgery suite introduce many new variables. Therefore, in designing these two suites, details regarding draping and wound protection were carefully considered. Imaging can be performed

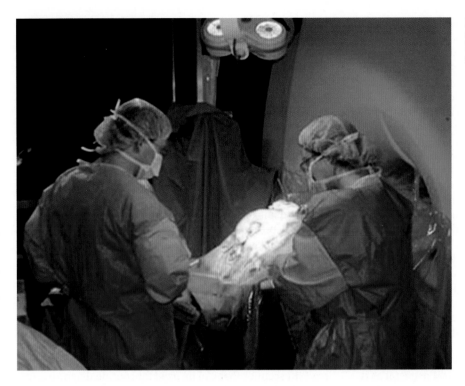

Fig. 9.8 Typical head location for surgery outside the magnet while the torso and body remain inside the scanner during catheter-placement surgeries.

during the surgery while taking careful precautions to maintain sterility. Again, the room is kept at a positive pressure and air recirculation occurs ~27 times per hour. Surgical instruments are removed from the operative field and the wound is covered with a sterile towel during scans. The specialized sterile surgical plastic draping that is meant to fit over the aperture of the MRI also protects the surgeons from accidently contaminating themselves by touching the walls of the scanner.

Head position is also very important in shunt placement surgery. Most surgeons prefer to have the head midline to best gauge the surgical landmarks. This may pose a problem for some patients or for some types of cases. The iMRI allows alternative head positioning and facilitates difficult catheter placement by giving the surgeon a view of the surrounding anatomy in three different planes that helps with anatomic orientation irrespective of the position of the head. Patients with torticollis or those requiring unique trajectories into the brain due to pathologic anatomy are better accommodated once the head is stabilized.

The actual guidance of a catheter through the brain may be done in a variety of ways. The traditional freehand approach is the simplest and quickest surgical method. Rapid scan acquisition time is important to facilitate three-dimensional image-guidance for the surgeon. In a closed-bore cylindrical iMRI, the patient and the surgeon would have to be partially in the magnet during the procedure and stabilization of the catheter or biopsy needle could be difficult. Aside from the awkwardness experienced by the surgeon that is associated with reaching into the magnet, the risk of contamination of the sterile surgical field may increase. On the other hand, tactile feedback during the catheter insertion could be very

helpful and freehand passage provides immediate information in terms of cyst wall firmness and compliance. Alternately, a guidance device may be employed that is fixed either to the head holder or in a burr hole in the skull.

The aforementioned Navigus trajectory guide is a low-profile disposable device that stabilizes and holds a plastic catheter gently without distortion. The small size is critical as the catheter may be long and encroach upon the walls of the MRI scanner if positioning of the head is not done carefully preoperatively. Our experience indicates that catheter placement is possible with the Navigus with millimeter accuracy. In either technique, a steel stylet may not be used, but many different catheter introducers are available that are made of plastic or titanium. Both materials provide excellent visualization of the catheter on MRI. Many catheters are now open on one end to accommodate endoscopic insertion. The stylet should be marked in terms of depth to ensure that the catheter remains in the proper position during repeat imaging and upon redirection toward the target. If an endoscope is used, insertion and visualization is performed outside the 5 gauss line due to the current incompatibility of this type of instrumentation with MRI. Finally, temporary fixation of the catheter after placement cannot be overemphasized, as movement of the patient in the midst of surgery is unavoidable. Careful partial closure of the scalp, fixation to the scalp, or partial insertion of the catheter into the soft tissue should prevent migration of a well-placed catheter during the movement of the patient either for abdominal placement of the distal tubing or for any other surgical or anesthetic manipulation that is necessary outside the magnetic field.

In the case of the boy with the growing cystic lesion (**Fig. 9.1**), access to the 4th ventricle was accomplished by keeping him supine, but turning the head a full 90 degrees away from the surgeon. His head and neck were also flexed forward. To accomplish this, a customized Malcolm-Rand carbon fiber headholder was applied before the operation. The child's head was then turned and flexed into the required operative position and secured to the floating table top.[7] A suboccipital incision was made in the midline and the dissection was carried down to the posterior ring of C1 thereby allowing further exposure of the foramen magnum from above. This opening was widened using Kerrison rongeurs. The shunt was then placed using repeat scanning to follow the path of the catheter superiorly. From the surgeon's point of view, however, this would seem more like a lateral trajectory given that the patient's head was completely turned to the side. This approach to the posterior fossa would probably not be attempted using other methods of shunt placement but with the help of the iMRI, the task was accomplished easily.

Subsequent scans are performed by the MRI technologist at a mobile scan console in the surgical work space. The patient is simply reintroduced into the 3.0 T scanner by sliding the table top on which they are secured a distance of one meter rather than realigning the surgical pedestal as is necessary in the 1.5 T suite. Anesthesia is also much closer to the patient affording better oversight and control of the airway. The basic process is the same in that iterative scans are done to track changes in the catheter position as it is advanced into position.

Before and after the procedure is completed, hemorrhage scans are performed and compared. These images consist of a baseline and postoperative turbo FLAIR (fluid-attenuated inversion recovery), ultrafast T2-weighted half-Fourier acquisition single-shot turbo spin echo (HASTE), and T2*-weighted gradient echo scans. These particular sequences are exceptionally sensitive for detecting the presence of hemorrhage. This imaging review provides an additional level of safety and precision to the surgical procedures performed.[15,16]

◆ Discussion

These difficult example cases show the power of iMRI surgery to make an otherwise difficult or possibly dangerous catheterization procedure less ominous. Although there are other methods to cannulate a fluid collection in the central nervous system, none gives the dynamic and high-resolution near-immediate feedback of an iMRI. Clearly, this technology is under development. Nonetheless, it has already been updated and refined over a decade of practical use, principally in an academic setting. This technology is now becoming both a functional tool and a vibrant frontier in neurosurgery. We do not yet know the full extent of the possible adaptations or uses of iMRI let alone what additional advances are possible. Thus far, we can say that iMRI appears safe and in many cases may become the gold standard for precision-guided neurosurgical cases. Certainly, intracerebral catheter

placement is one of those clinical scenarios. Other issues that must be considered when deciding on whether to perform MRI-guided shunt placement include cost, ease of use, and the need for increased personnel. On the other hand, the potential for someday incorporating the full capabilities of MRI technology while benefitting from its superior navigating ability makes a strong argument for incorporating this instrumentation into one's practice if available.

All iMRI systems provide basic T1- and T2-weighted imaging capabilities, but only with field strengths of 1.5 T or higher can some perform high-resolution MR spectroscopy (MRS), MR venography (MRV), MR angiography (MRA), brain activation studies, chemical shift imaging, and diffusion-weighted imaging. Identifying vascular structures by MRA or MRV may prevent their injury during surgery. Demonstrating elevated phosphocholine within a tumor may improve the diagnostic yield of brain biopsy. Mapping out neurologic function may influence the surgical approach to a cyst or tumor.[1] These techniques are already applicable to other aspects of neurosurgery and could also be used in catheter placement.

An iMRI can be both an economic boon and a drain on the facility that adopts its use. On the one hand, it is a unique technology that the public would likely be impressed with and might thereby help attract patients. It is also a functioning MRI scanner that can be used for routine diagnostic imaging by the radiology department when it is not being used for surgical cases. On the other hand, acquisition of an iMRI system is associated with considerable expense, and its utilization can increase the length of time for an operative procedure and its overall cost. Despite these additional expenses, iMRI can lead to a potential overall cost reduction in the treatment of certain patients if long-term cure can be achieved, repeat catheter placement and shunt failures can be avoided, or procedure-related morbidity can be reduced. Often, a partnership between anesthesia, radiology, and neurosurgery that share both the costs and benefits will make the effort successful.

As surgeons, we greatly appreciate the capability of monitoring the progress of our surgery (catheter advancement, tumor resection, biopsy, cyst drainage, aneurysm clipping, etc.). MRI scanning allows us to objectively monitor our progress while also verifying the global status of the brain. In the case of an intraoperative complication such as intracerebral hemorrhage, diffuse cerebral edema, hydrocephalus, etc., we can better control the collateral damage and adjust our surgical plan almost immediately instead of waiting for the postoperative discovery of a clinical decline. Auxiliary adjuncts of iMRI such as diffusion-weighted MRI, MRA, and MRV could clearly demonstrate vascular complications such as ischemia. iMRI does not only reflect surgical anatomy, it also gives information about the functional integrity and dynamic changes in the brain during the course of surgery as well.[17]

Trauma neurosurgeons are very familiar with the problem of acute distortions of anatomy complicating ventriculostomy landmarks. Any significant hemorrhage, skull fracture, or internal injury causing edema will force an adjustment in surgical technique. This is especially true after a craniotomy has been performed. Often, once the skull has been breached, the anatomy changes dramatically. The brain is not a firm organ and the parenchyma, cerebrospinal fluid (CSF) and blood vessels are prone to shift during neurosurgical procedures, rendering preoperative MR images invalid. Brain shift of up to 1 cm occurs in almost all neurosurgical cranial procedures due to CSF loss, brain edema, and iatrogenic physiologic changes. This ever-changing spatial organization of the brain structures during surgery necessitates the use of intraoperative near-real-time MRI modalities. Of all advances in the imaging field, MRI appears to be the most important new modality both in terms of diagnosis and intraoperative guidance that has developed over the last two decades.[17] With catheter insertion, fluid drainage is the primary endpoint. Collapse of a cyst or ventricle by default will affect brain location.

Catheter placement can also be a combined modality procedure. Many authors report using both iMRI and frameless stereotaxy in the same case to help plan, execute, and verify their catheter placement. In a recent paper by Albayak et al, they state that this combination greatly helps to augment the neurosurgeon's surgical accuracy and keenness considerably by providing him or her with the unique opportunity to delineate the normal anatomy and the lesion much more precisely, and to monitor the planned progress of the surgical case in a near-real-time fashion.[17]

As we look forward, there are many advancements that have been discussed in the neurosurgical literature that would make this type of surgery and technology even better and perhaps more practical than currently existing modalities. Could there be a way to obtain continuous MR imaging during a procedure in much the way US guidance shows the real-time progress of shunt placement? Would integration of the different views be possible such that an intraoperative dynamic three-dimensional model could be generated? Could functional, diffusion, perfusion, and electrophysiologic data be overlaid on the basic MRI sequences creating a kind of up to the moment virtual reality image of the brain during the case? Catheter placement in anatomically complex patients remains one of the best uses of iMRI technology. Whether the region of interest is pathologically too small for conventional methods or perhaps too near to vital structures, finely detailed iMRI is the most precise way to cannulate the target. Nonetheless, using this technology can add cost, time, and complexity to a given procedure. Therefore, until iMRI becomes more routine, individual patient and case selection are of paramount importance to ensure success. The advantages of this technology are better visualization, planning, and execution of the surgery. The imaging can account for unseen changes such as brain shift after craniotomy and add a safeguard in that any intraoperative complication should

be seen quickly affording an immediate opportunity for an equally rapid corrective countermeasure. Certainly in cases of complex, loculated cysts or pseudotumor cerebri, it has demonstrable advantages over other methods of catheter placement. Nonetheless, the theoretically proposed and partially proven beneficial effects of iMRI on various neurosurgical procedures need to be validated by larger surgical series and in randomized prospective trials.

References

1. Hall WA, Truwit CL. Intraoperative MR-guided neurosurgery. J Magn Reson Imaging 2008;27(2):368–375 Review
2. Shkolnik A, McLone DG. Intraoperative real-time ultrasonic guidance of ventricular shunt placement in infants. Radiology 1981;141(2):515–517
3. Whitehead WE, Jea A, Vachhrajani S, Kulkarni AV, Drake JM. Accurate placement of cerebrospinal fluid shunt ventricular catheters with real-time ultrasound guidance in older children without patent fontanelles. J Neurosurg 2007; 107(5, Suppl)406–410
4. Babcock DS, Barr LL, Crone KR. Intraoperative uses of ultrasound in the pediatric neurosurgical patient. Pediatr Neurosurg 1992;18(2):84–91
5. Merritt CRB. Physics of ultrasound. In: Rumack CM, Wilson SR, Charboneau JW, eds. Diagnostic Ultrasound. 2nd ed. St. Louis: Mosby-Year Book; 1998:3–35
6. Rubin JM, Chandler WF. Intraoperative sonography of the brain. In: Rumack CM, Wilson SR, Charboneau JW, eds. Diagnostic Ultrasound. 2nd ed. St. Louis: Mosby-Year Book, 1998: 631–652
7. Ruge JR, Dauser RC, Storrs BB. Posterior fossa cysts: supratentorial shunt placement with ultrasound guidance. Childs Nerv Syst 1991; 7(3):165–168
8. Hopf NJ, Perneczky A. Endoscopic neurosurgery and endoscope-assisted microneurosurgery for the treatment of intracranial cysts. Neurosurgery 1998;43(6):1330–1336, discussion 1336–1337
9. Kestle JR, Drake JM, Cochrane DD, et al; Endoscopic Shunt Insertion Trial participants. Lack of benefit of endoscopic ventriculoperitoneal shunt insertion: a multicenter randomized trial. J Neurosurg 2003; 98(2):284–290
10. Nimsky C, Ganslandt O, Gralla J, Buchfelder M, Fahlbusch R. Intraoperative low-field magnetic resonance imaging in pediatric neurosurgery. Pediatr Neurosurg 2003;38(2):83–89
11. Lam CH, Hall WA, Truwit CL, Liu H. Intra-operative MRI-guided approaches to the pediatric posterior fossa tumors. Pediatr Neurosurg 2001;34(6):295–300
12. Lam CH, Horrigan M, Lovick DS. The Seldinger technique for insertion of difficult to place ventricular catheters. Pediatr Neurosurg 2003;38(2):90–93
13. Nimsky C, Ganslandt O, Gralla J, Buchfelder M, Fahlbusch R. Intraoperative low-field magnetic resonance imaging in pediatric neurosurgery. Pediatr Neurosurg 2003;38(2):83–89
14. Hall WA, Martin AJ, Liu H, et al. High-field strength interventional magnetic resonance imaging for pediatric neurosurgery. Pediatr Neurosurg 1998;29(5):253–259
15. Hall WA, Galicich W, Bergman T, Truwit CL. 3-Tesla intraoperative MR imaging for neurosurgery. J Neurooncol 2006;77(3):297–303
16. Fenchel S, Boll DT, Lewin JS. Intraoperative MR imaging. Magn Reson Imaging Clin N Am 2003;11(3):431–447 Review
17. Albayrak B, Samdani AF, Black PM. Intra-operative magnetic resonance imaging in neurosurgery. Acta Neurochir (Wien) 2004;146(6):543–556, discussion 557 Review

10

Implantation of Deep Brain Stimulator Electrodes Using Interventional MRI

Philip A. Starr, Alastair J. Martin, and Paul S. Larson

In this chapter we describe our technical approach to interventional magnetic resonance imaging (iMRI) guided deep brain stimulator (DBS) electrode placement, based on 53 DBS lead insertions into the subthalamic nucleus (STN) in patients with Parkinson's disease. The conceptual foundation for the interventional MRI approach to STN-DBS derives from prior experience of our group and others with the standard technique: frame-based stereotaxy with microelectrode guidance. The criteria for successful STN lead placement have been physiologic (region in which microelectrode recording detected STN cells including cells with movement-related responses), or clinical (lead placements that resulted in successful reduction in parkinsonian symptoms). During the past 10 years, many groups have performed post hoc correlation of lead location by postoperative MRI with single unit physiology,[1–4] thresholds for stimulation-induced adverse events,[5–7] and clinical success.[6,8–15] These studies have shown that the STN can be visualized on MRI by its T2 hypointensity, and that the dorsolateral region of the MRI-defined STN reliably contains movement-related cells. Brain coordinates predicting clinical success have been elucidated.[6,8–15] This experience provided a conceptual justification for the use of imaging criteria alone to define and confirm accuracy of target placement.

◆ Description of Procedure

The technique evolved as an extension of the prior work of Hall and Truwit in high-field MRI-guided brain biopsy,[16,17] described in earlier chapters. The prior biopsy work utilized a smaller "joystick" aiming device (Medtronic Navigus, Medtronic Navigation, Inc., Louisville, CO), whereas the present work employed a skull-mounted device (Medtronic NexFrame, Medtronic, Inc., Minneapolis, MN) that utilizes a "rotate/translate" mechanism, providing finer control at the expense of a less-intuitive aiming paradigm.

Our approach uses a standard configuration (closed bore) 1.5 T MRI that is located in a radiology suite rather than an "intraoperative" MRI specifically configured for neurosurgery. Key features of this approach are as follows. (1) Planning, insertion, and MRI confirmation of DBS lead placement are integrated into a single procedure while the patient is on the MRI gantry. (2) The platform for inserting the DBS lead is a burr hole mounted trajectory guide rather than a traditional stereotactic frame and arc system. (3) Target coordinates are defined with respect to the MRI isocenter rather than with respect to a separate stereotactic space using fiducial markers. (4) Patients are under general anesthesia in the supine position and no microelectrode recordings (MER) or test stimulation are performed. (5) Target images are acquired after burr hole creation and intracranial air entry, reducing the potential for errors associated with "brain shift" that can occur with conventional techniques in between image acquisition and probe insertion.

Specialized devices and MRI-compatible equipment used are listed in **Table 10.1**, and MRI protocols in **Table 10.2**.

Patient Preparation and Positioning

Patients were allowed to take their usual morning dose of antiparkinsonian medications. After premedication with midazolam and fentanyl, general anesthesia was induced with propofol in a room adjacent to the MRI suite. Anesthesia was maintained with sevoflurane and intermittent fentanyl and vecuronium boluses. Ventilation was adjusted to maintain end-tidal CO_2 between 35 and 40 mm Hg. After placement of an intraarterial catheter into the wrist, patients' heads were placed into a carbon fiber headholder designed to mount directly to the MRI gantry. The frontal

Table 10.1 Equipment Utilized for Magnetic Resonance Imaging- (MRI-) Guided Deep Brain Stimulation (DBS)

Item	Manufacturer	Description
Philips Intera 1.5 T Intraoperative MRI	Philips Healthcare, Andover, MA	Bore dimensions: length 157 cm, diameter 60 cm. Used for routine diagnostic imaging, as well as interventional procedures
Malcolm Rand Headset	Integra Life Sciences (Plainsboro, NJ)	MRI-compatible carbon-fiber headholder
Stimloc cranial base and cap	Medtronic, Inc. (Minneapolis, MN)	For long-term cranial fixation of permanent electrodes. This device is currently being used at University of California-San Francisco for most DBS lead implants.
NexFrame trajectory guide and alignment stem	Medtronic, Inc.	Disposable skull-mounted aiming device
NexFrame peel-away introducer	Medtronic, Inc.	A standard peel-away introducer design intended to be used in conjunction with the NexFrame family of trajectory guides to deliver devices into the brain
Ceramic stylet for NexFrame peel-away introducer	Medtronic, Inc.	A nonmetallic rigid stylet that fits the inner diameter of the peel away introducer, for use in inserting the introducer into the brain
Model 3389 28 cm DBS electrode	Medtronic, Inc.	One of a family of DBS electrodes currently used for DBS implantation procedures. The length (28 cm) is shorter than that used in standard frame-based procedures.
Titanium stylet for DBS electrode	Medtronic, Inc.	Custom MRI-compatible stylet associated with relatively low MR artifact
Gas-powered MRI compatible cranial drill	Anspach, Inc. (Palm Beach Gardens, FL)	The nitrogen tank used to power the drill is not MRI-compatible and is kept outside of the MRI room.
Titanium surgical instruments	KMedic Instruments (Kenosha, WI)	Set includes Adson forceps, Metzenbaum scissors, Mayo scissors, 3 mm Kerrison rongeur, Penfield dissectors, DeBakey forceps, hemostats, needle holder

area was shaved using clippers. An array of four flexible surface coils positioned at the sides, top, back, and front of the head, was used for MR signal reception (**Fig. 10.1**).

Trajectory Planning for Burr Hole Location

Patients were then moved into the bore of the MRI. An MRI-compatible anesthesia machine was used. A landmark was established on the frontal scalp near the presumed coronal suture and advanced to magnet isocenter. A gadolinium-enhanced volumetric gradient echo MRI was obtained (scan parameters in **Table 10.2**, protocol 1) parallel to the line between the anterior commissure and posterior commissure (AC-PC line). On the MRI console, approximate anatomic targets were selected bilaterally at a point 12 mm lateral, 3 mm posterior, and 4 mm inferior to the midcommissural point. (This target was used only for trajectory planning; final anatomic target selection was performed in a subsequent step described below.) Single-slice obliqued parasagittal reformatted images were reconstructed that passed through the approximate targets, but avoided the lateral ventricle. A trajectory that avoided sulci and cortical veins was then selected on the oblique image (**Fig. 10.2**). At

the point where the trajectory crossed the scalp, a rapidly updating "MRI fluoroscopy" sequence (**Table 10.2**, protocol 2, described further below) was prescribed with its center at the intended entry. The surgeon reached into the bore of the magnet and manually placed an MRI visible pointer at the intended entry. The entry point was marked on the scalp with a pen, the patient moved to the back of the bore, and the skull marked percutaneously by injecting methylene blue through a 22-gauge needle at the scalp entry site.

Initial Exposure and Mounting of Trajectory Guide

The frontal area was prepped and draped with an MRI bore drape designed to keep the surgical field sterile yet tolerate head movement between the center and back of the bore (a distance of ~1 m) (**Fig. 10.3A**). A pressurized nitrogen tank, electrical power sources for bipolar cautery, one headlight, and one floor light were placed outside the MRI room with the regulator hose and electrical cords directed through the waveguide. Monopolar cautery was not used. After making coronally oriented incisions, 14 mm frontal burr holes were drilled with an MRI compatible cranial drill. The base rings for the Stimloc (Medtronic, Inc., Minneapolis, MN) lead

Table 10.2 Magnetic Resonance Imaging (MRI) Pulse Sequences for Intraoperative MRI-Guided Deep Brain Stimulation (DBS)

Protocol Type and Purpose

	1. Volumetric gadolinium-enhanced (3D T1-weighted gradient echo)	2. MR "fluoroscopy" sequence	3. High-resolution axial T2-FSE	4. Volumetric T2-FSE	5. Low-resolution T2-FSE	6. High-resolution T2-FSE	7. Intermediate-resolution T2-FSE	8. High-resolution volumetric (3D T1-weighted gradient echo)
Purpose	Trajectory planning	Marking of scalp entry point, and alignment of the fluid-filled stem	Identification of STN target point, and confirmation of stylet position	Identification of the alignment stem pivot points	Confirmation of trajectory of alignment stem	Confirmation of trajectory of stylet during brain entry	Confirmation of lead depth	Postplacement lead location measurements
Acquisition plane	Axial	Oblique axial	Axial	Coronal and sagittal	Oblique coronal and sagittal	Oblique coronal and sagittal	Axial	Axial
Slice thickness (mm)	2.0	1.2	2.0	1.0	2.0	1	1.0	1.5
Field of view (mm)	260 × 207	128 × 104	260 × 222	256 × 256	250 × 188	256 × 216	256 × 192	260 × 222
Number of slices	75	1	21	9	3	11	15	120
TR (repetition time)	20	5.5	3000	2000	2000	2000	3000	20
TE (echo time)	2.9	2.8	90	100	103	96	90	3.2
Matrix size	176 ×114	128 × 103	384 × 224	256 × 256	256 × 192	256 × 172	256 × 192	192 × 152
Flip angle	30	60	90	90	90	90	90	30
NEX (# excitations)	1	1	6	1	1	1	1	1
Echo train length	N/A	N/A	16	54	24	56	42	N/A
Bandwidth (kHz)	54	75	40	182	115	160	88	50
SAR (Watts/kg)	0.3	0.9	1.0	0.8	1.2	1	0.5	0.3
Scan time (minutes: seconds)	4:09	5 frames per second*	8:42	1:28	0:18	1:22	4:06	8:54

Abbreviations: N/A, not applicable; 3D, three dimensional; T2-FSE, T2-weighted fast spin echo; STN, subthalamic nucleus; SAR, specific absorption rate.

*Each scan duration is 600 milliseconds, but they are "stacked" so as to present at 5 frames/second.

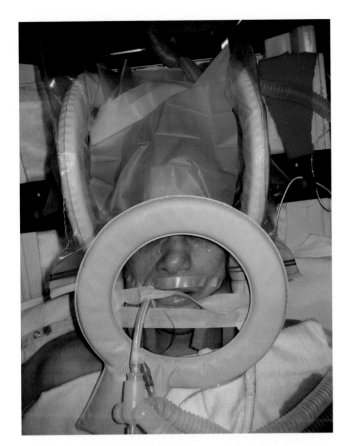

Fig. 10.1 Position of the head in an magnetic resonance imaging-compatible headholder, showing placement of radiofrequency surface coils. The connection between the endotracheal tube and ventilator is led through the center of the anterior coil. The posterior coil, placed under the headholder, is hidden under a towel. The side headholder pins pass through the centers of the side coils.

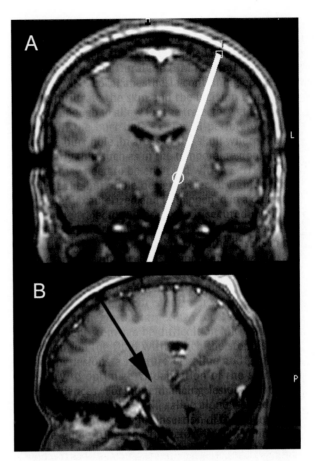

Fig. 10.2 Method of trajectory planning on magnetic resonance imaging (MRI) console by using reformatted oblique slices passing through the target, angled to exclude the lateral ventricle (protocol 1, **Table 10.2**). **(A)** First step: on a coronal plane passing through the target, an oblique sagittal plane is defined (white line) that avoids the lateral ventricle. **(B)** Second step: the oblique sagittal plane selected in **(A)** is constructed on the MRI console, and a safe trajectory to the target (*black arrow*) is planned.

anchoring device and the NexFrame DBA (deep brain access; Medtronic) trajectory guides were mounted over the burr holes. The dura mater was opened bilaterally and the leptomeninges coagulated. The trajectory guide alignment stems were filled with sterile saline and mounted into the trajectory guide (**Fig. 10.3B**).

Target Definition and Aiming of Alignment Stem

Patients were moved to reposition the head at magnet isocenter. Table movement was then disabled and no further patient movement was allowed until the leads were inserted and placement confirmed by imaging. A high-resolution T2-weighted (T2W) axial MRI was performed with 2 mm slice thickness, aligned such that one slice passed 4 mm inferior to the commissures (protocol 3, **Table 10.2**). The brain target was selected on this image (**Fig. 10.4**). The intended target was generally very close to the "default" coordinates of 12 mm lateral, 3 mm posterior, and 4 mm inferior to the midcommissural point. However, small adjustments in the default coordinates were made based on direct visualization of the borders of

STN and red nucleus (RN), so as to place the target within dorsolateral STN at least 2 mm from medial, lateral, and posterior borders. Axial and coronal volumetric T2W MRI scans were performed through the pivot points of the alignment stems (protocol 4, **Table 10.2**) (**Fig. 10.5**). The XYZ coordinates of target and pivot, with respect to the MRI isocenter, were determined by placing a "region of interest" cursor over the desired location. The final XYZ of the pivot was a synthesis of the values on coronal and sagittal views.

For the first side to be implanted, the XYZ coordinates of target and pivot were used to prescribe the MR fluoroscopy sequence (**Table 10.2**, protocol 2). The target and pivot points define a line and the MRI scan is prescribed such that it is perpendicular to and centered on this trajectory at a location 9 to 10 cm superior to the burr hole. The surgeon donned a sterile hood to maintain the sterile field and reached into the bore of the magnet to manually align the stem to the target line, while viewing the MR fluoroscopy image on an in-room monitor. When the desired alignment

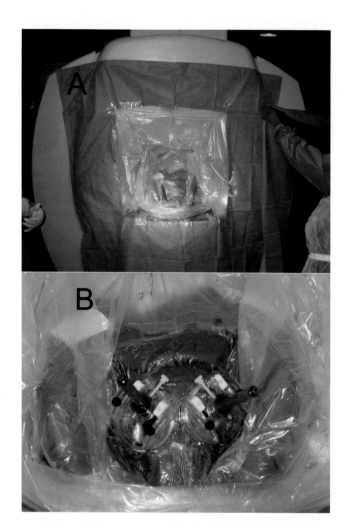

Fig. 10.3 Surgical draping and trajectory guides. **(A)** Patient's head at the back of the magnetic resonance imager bore, showing placement of the sterile drape. **(B)** Close-up view of trajectory guides with alignment stems.

was achieved, the NexFrame was locked into place. Rapid, low-resolution oblique coronal and sagittal images (protocol 5, **Table 10.2**) were obtained along the orientation of the stem, and the final anticipated target reconstructed graphically (**Fig. 10.6**). Occasionally, the oblique scans predicted a trajectory not perfectly aligned with the intended target. In these cases a new alignment scan was prescribed with its center slightly modified and a new manual alignment performed by the surgeon. The distance from the target to the relevant level of the trajectory guide (the step-off between thick and thin sections of the alignment stem) was measured on the oblique images to allow calculation of the position of the depth stop in the subsequent step. This distance was increased by 4.5 mm so that the sheath and stylet would slightly overshoot the target.

Insertion of Guidance Sheath and Lead

The alignment stem was replaced with a five-channel multilumen insert, and a ceramic stylet within a plastic peel-away sheath was placed into the center lumen. A depth stop

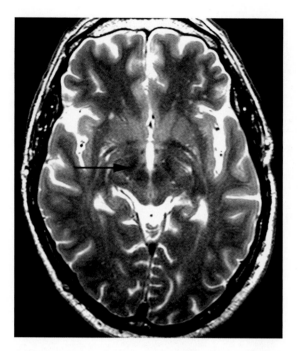

Fig. 10.4 Magnetic resonance imaging (MRI) used to define the target in dorsolateral subthalamic nucleus (*black arrow* points to right subthalamic nucleus) (protocol 3, **Table 10.2**).

was placed on the stylet at the appropriate length as described above. The stylet/sheath assembly was advanced into the brain in two to three stepwise movements, monitored via in-plane MRI, using oblique sagittal and coronal T2W sequences (protocol 6, **Table 10.2**). The alignment and insertion procedure were then repeated for the contralateral side. A high-resolution axial T2W image was obtained through the target area to assess sheath/stylet position at the target (protocol 3, **Table 10.2**) (**Fig. 10.7**).

If the placement of the peel-away sheath/stylet assembly was found to be inappropriate for either side (defined as distance between intended and actual stylet position of greater than 2 mm in the axial plane 4 mm below the commissures) a side channel of the NexFrame multilumen insert (MLI) was considered to provide a parallel track with an offset of 3 mm in a direction perpendicular to the lead trajectory. If an offset of 3 mm could not provide an appropriate placement, the sheath/stylet were removed, alignment indicator replaced, and the NexFrame trajectory readjusted by repeating the alignment scans.

Two 28-cm DBS leads (Medtronic model 3389–28), were prepared by replacing their standard wire stylet with custom made nonferrous titanium wire stylets supplied by Medtronic, Inc., so as to allow imaging of the lead with their wire stylets in place, without excessive artifact. On one side, the ceramic stylet within the peel-away sheaths was removed and a "bridge" snapped over the MLI. The bridge provided a space between itself and the MLI for the sides of the peel-away sheath, and contained a lead-holding screw. A depth stop was placed on the lead 42.5 mm higher than the depth stop on the ceramic stylet (to account for the extra height of the bridge and lead holder) and the lead was advanced through the sheath to target. Lead insertion was repeated on

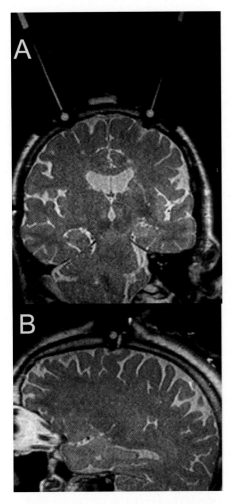

Fig. 10.5 Magnetic resonance imaging (MRI) used to define the coordinates of the pivot points for the trajectory guides, prior to aligning the alignment stem (protocol 4, **Table 10.2**). **(A)** Coronal image (with alignment stems nearly in-plane). **(B)** Sagittal image (alignment stem is out of plane on this image, so only the pivot point is seen).

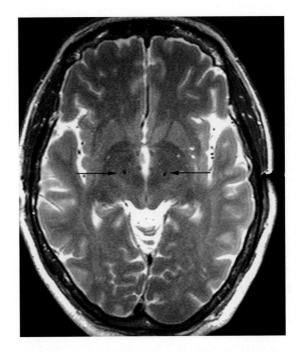

Fig. 10.7 Axial T2-weighted magnetic resonance image at 4 mm below the commissures, showing sheath/ ceramic stylet assembly at target (indicated by *black arrows*) (protocol 3, **Table 10.2**).

the contralateral side. An axial T2W MR image was used to confirm lead depth (protocol 7, **Table 10.2**).

Closure, Final Imaging, and Implantable Pulse Generator (IPG) Placement

Patients were moved to position the head at the back of the bore for easier surgical access. The peel-away sheaths were removed and the DBS leads anchored to the skull with Stim-loc clips. The titanium wire stylets were removed from the

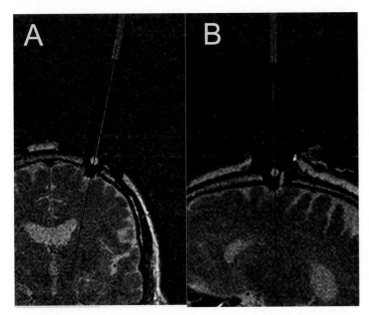

Fig. 10.6 Rapid acquisition **(A)** oblique coronal and **(B)** oblique sagital images passing through the target and pivot point, after the trajectory guide has been aligned (protocol 5, **Table 10.2**). The thin black lines show the predicted trajectory of the deep brain stimulator lead.

leads, and the Stimloc cranial caps set in place. The NexFrame trajectory guides were removed and the scalp closed with sutures. The mean surgical time (from initial scalp incision to scalp closure) for simultaneous bilateral implants was 225 ±30 minutes, and for unilateral implantation was 217 ± 62 minutes.

Patients were moved back to isocenter for a final high-resolution volumetric T1W MRI (protocol 8, **Table 10.1**), to be used for measurement of lead tip location and trajectory. Patients were awakened, recovered in the postanesthesia care unit, monitored overnight in a stepdown unit, and discharged the day after lead implantation. Lead extenders and dual-channel pulse generator (Medtronic Kinetra) were placed 1 to 2 weeks later in the standard operating room.

◆ Brain Penetrations and Placement Accuracy Using the Interventional MRI Approach

In 46 implants (87%) only a single brain penetration with the peel-away guidance sheath was necessary to place the lead at the final location. In four implants (8%), the first placement of the stylet/sheath, at target depth, was considered inaccurate based on a >2 mm radial error (measured in the plane 4 mm below the commissures). In these cases, the sheath/stylet were withdrawn completely and replaced either through a parallel port of the multilumen insert (three cases), or by replacing the alignment stem into the NexFrame and performing a new target alignment (one case). In another three implants, the sheath/stylet was advanced only partially into the brain on the first pass, and removed because the projected sheath/stylet trajectory, based on oblique sagittal and coronal images in the plane of the sheath/stylet, appeared to predict a >2 mm distance between intended and desired target. In these three cases, the sheath/stylet was removed, the alignment stem replaced, a new target alignment was performed with the alignment stem and the sheath/stylet advanced a second time. The total number of instrument passes into the brain for the 53 DBS lead implants was 60. The maximum number of passes per lead was three. In each procedure, we measured the radial error, defined as the scalar distance between the location of the intended target and actual location of the ceramic stylet, in the axial plane 4 mm inferior to the commissures, on high-resolution axial T2W images. The mean (± SD) radial error for the initial pass of the peel-away sheath/ceramic stylet assembly was 1.18 ±0.65 mm.

◆ Complications

There were no MRI visible hemorrhages (either symptomatic or asymptomatic) in the 53 STN implantations. Two hardware infections occurred early in the series, both at the frontal incision (implants #7 and #11), requiring removal of all implanted hardware. One of these was accompanied by cerebritis, requiring a prolonged stay in the intensive care unit, with eventual full recovery. Of note, both of these occurred prior to the availability of an MRI-compatible cranial drill. At that time, the procedure required performing the initial exposure and burr hole in the room adjacent to the MRI suite, followed by a move into the MRI bore with partial redraping of the field (described in reference 18). Since the introduction of an MRI-compatible drill and performance of all parts of the implant in the MRI room with a single draping procedure (beginning with implant #12), no further infections associated with the interventional MRI procedure have occurred.

In one patient, both leads were found to be inadequately placed, based on failure to achieve expected clinical results following multiple programming attempts. In retrospect, this patient had unusual STN anatomy (medially located STNs), a variant that was not fully appreciated on the targeting MRI, such that the intended target in the interventional MRI procedure did not reflect actual STN position. Expected clinical benefit was achieved following surgical replacement of the lead to a more medial location (10 mm from the midline), using the traditional stereotactic method.

In a historical comparison group of 76 STN-DBS electrodes implanted using traditional frame-based stereotaxy and MRI,[6] there were two hemorrhages (one symptomatic and one asymptomatic), no hardware infections, and one suboptimally placed lead that required surgical repositioning.

◆ Future Development of MRI-Guided DBS

A long-range goal of the MRI approach to DBS implantation is to utilize the method with speed and simplicity within any diagnostic MRI scanner, without special modification for surgery. As currently realized, however, there are several cumbersome aspects. (1) Reaching into the bore of the magnet for manual steering is awkward, especially for those with limited reach. This could be addressed with a mechanical remote control. (2) There is some loss of image quality with surface coils compared with rigid "birdcage" coils. (3) The current trajectory guide is not optimized to deal with targeting errors, due to limited side channel availability and inability to interpolate smaller distances between center and side channels. (4) The MRI console does not have easy turnkey software to perform this procedure, and requires an operator with detailed technical knowledge of the software provided by the console manufacturer. Moreover, the accuracy of many steps in the procedure relies on the operator's ability to accurately identify the geometric center of the pivot point and fluid stem. (5) At this time, the technique requires in-room visualization by the surgeon of the MR fluoroscopy images used to manually perform the stem alignment. Expensive manufacturer-installed in-room monitors could be replaced by a simpler monitor projector set-up, as has been described for MRI-guided cardiac interventions.[19]

◆ Summary

We have developed a technical approach to placement of deep brain stimulators that adapts the procedure to a standard-configuration 1.5 T diagnostic MRI scanner in a radiology suite. The technique uses near-real-time MRI, in conjunction with a skull-mounted aiming device, as the sole method of guiding DBS electrodes to the STN and confirming localization. Preoperative imaging, device implantation, and postimplantation MRI are integrated into a single procedure performed under general anesthesia, providing real-time, high-resolution MRI confirmation of electrode position. The method is conceptually simpler than the current standard technique for DBS placement, as it eliminates the stereotactic frame, the subsequent requirement for registration of the brain in stereotactic space, physiologic testing, and the need for patient cooperation. With further technical refinement, the MRI method should improve the accuracy, safety, and speed of DBS electrode placement.

References

1. Abosch A, Hutchison WD, Saint-Cyr JA, Dostrovsky JO, Lozano AM. Movement-related neurons of the subthalamic nucleus in patients with Parkinson disease. J Neurosurg 2002;97(5):1167–1172

2. Theodosopoulos PV, Marks WJ Jr, Christine C, Starr PA. Locations of movement-related cells in the human subthalamic nucleus in Parkinson's disease. Mov Disord 2003;18(7):791–798

3. Rodriguez-Oroz MC, Rodriguez M, Guridi J, et al. The subthalamic nucleus in Parkinson's disease: somatotopic organization and physiological characteristics. Brain 2001;124(Pt 9):1777–1790

4. Romanelli P, Heit G, Hill BC, Kraus A, Hastie T, Bronte-Stewart HM. Microelectrode recording revealing a somatotopic body map in the subthalamic nucleus in humans with Parkinson disease. J Neurosurg 2004;100(4):611–618

5. Ashby P, Kim YJ, Kumar R, Lang AE, Lozano AM. Neurophysiological effects of stimulation through electrodes in the human subthalamic nucleus. Brain 1999;122(Pt 10):1919–1931

6. Starr PA, Christine CW, Theodosopoulos PV, et al. Implantation of deep brain stimulators into the subthalamic nucleus: technical approach and magnetic resonance imaging-verified lead locations. J Neurosurg 2002;97(2):370–387

7. Shields DC, Gorgulho A, Behnke E, Malkasian D, DeSalles AA. Contralateral conjugate eye deviation during deep brain stimulation of the subthalamic nucleus. J Neurosurg 2007;107(1):37–42

8. Okun MS, Tagliati M, Pourfar M, et al. Management of referred deep brain stimulation failures: a retrospective analysis from 2 movement disorders centers. Arch Neurol 2005;62(8):1250–1255

9. Anheim M, Batir A, Fraix V, et al. Improvement in Parkinson disease by subthalamic nucleus stimulation based on electrode placement: effects of reimplantation. Arch Neurol 2008;65(5):612–616

10. Plaha P, Ben-Shlomo Y, Patel NK, Gill SS. Stimulation of the caudal zona incerta is superior to stimulation of the subthalamic nucleus in improving contralateral parkinsonism. Brain 2006;129(Pt 7):1732–1747

11. Saint-Cyr JA, Hoque T, Pereira LCM, et al. Localization of clinically effective stimulating electrodes in the human subthalamic nucleus on magnetic resonance imaging. J Neurosurg 2002;97(5):1152–1166

12. Lanotte MM, Rizzone M, Bergamasco B, Faccani G, Melcarne A, Lopiano L. Deep brain stimulation of the subthalamic nucleus: anatomical, neurophysiological, and outcome correlations with the effects of stimulation. J Neurol Neurosurg Psychiatry 2002;72(1):53–58

13. Zonenshayn M, Sterio D, Kelly PJ, Rezai AR, Beric A. Location of the active contact within the subthalamic nucleus (STN) in the treatment of idiopathic Parkinson's disease. Surg Neurol 2004;62(3):216–225, discussion 225–226

14. Godinho F, Thobois S, Magnin M, et al. Subthalamic nucleus stimulation in Parkinson's disease: anatomical and electrophysiological localization of active contacts. J Neurol 2006;253(10):1347–1355

15. McClelland S III, Ford B, Senatus PB, et al. Subthalamic stimulation for Parkinson disease: determination of electrode location necessary for clinical efficacy. Neurosurg Focus 2005;19(5):E12

16. Hall WA, Liu H, Martin AJ, Maxwell RE, Truwit CL. Brain biopsy sampling by using prospective stereotaxis and a trajectory guide. J Neurosurg 2001;94(1):67–71

17. Hall WA, Martin AJ, Liu H, Nussbaum ES, Maxwell RE, Truwit CL. Brain biopsy using high-field strength interventional magnetic resonance imaging. Neurosurgery 1999;44(4):807–813, discussion 813–814

18. Martin AJ, Larson PS, Ostrem JL, et al. Placement of deep brain stimulator electrodes using real-time high-field interventional magnetic resonance imaging. Magn Reson Med 2005;54(5):1107–1114

19. Guttman MA, Ozturk C, Raval AN, et al. Interventional cardiovascular procedures guided by real-time MR imaging: an interactive interface using multiple slices, adaptive projection modes and live 3D renderings. J Magn Reson Imaging 2007;26(6):1429–1435

III

Intracranial Tumor Resection

11

Utilization of Low-Field Intraoperative MRI in Glioma Surgery–An Overview

Volker Seifert and Christian Senft

Cytoreductive surgery has been the first step in the treatment of glial tumors for decades. Even though malignant, high-grade gliomas might be distinguished macroscopically from healthy brain parenchyma more easily than low-grade gliomas in the majority of cases, intraoperative visualization of tumor remnants frequently remains difficult. Even in dedicated neurosurgical centers, these difficulties account for tumor tissue visible on early postoperative magnetic resonance imaging (MRI) scans in a number of patients.[1,2]

It is a well-recognized, distinct feature of gliomas to diffusely infiltrate brain tissue, rendering them impossible to be completely resected biologically or histopathologically. However, radiographically complete resections of gliomas are not simply the neurosurgeon's goal: in recent years, several well-conceived and well-conducted studies have indicated that the extent of resection is one of the most important prognostic factors for patients with both high-grade and low-grade gliomas.[2–6]

To provide the neurosurgeon with information about the extent of resection intraoperatively, different techniques and modalities have been developed and assessed. MRI is the gold standard for the diagnostic and follow-up imaging of gliomas, and intraoperative MRI (iMRI) provides optimal image quality in a familiar way. Although there is ongoing interest in other modalities such as ultrasound or computed tomography (CT), both have significant drawbacks concerning image quality or radiation exposure. Consequently, the intraoperative resection control for tumors of glial origin represents the main indication for the use of iMRI.[7]

Several different iMRI systems have been developed and are available today. These systems can be categorized by the magnet's field strength, by the magnet's configuration, and by the way in which the patient is brought to the scanner or the scanner to the patient. In this chapter, we will review the experiences that others and we have had using low-field iMRI systems in glioma surgery.

◆ Prevailing Low-Field iMRI Systems

Peter Black from the Brigham and Women's Hospital in Boston and General Electric Co. (General Electric Medical Systems, Waukesha, WI) pioneered iMRI with the development of the first iMRI scanner to be used in the neurosurgical operating room (OR) in the 1990s. For technical reasons, this device was equipped with two vertical superconductive magnets employing a magnetic field strength of 0.5 tesla. It required major modifications of OR infrastructure to meet the demands for low radiofrequency (RF) interference as well as the adaptation of surgical tools, instruments, microscopes, and so on, which all needed to be MRI-compatible. There was a 60 cm vertical gap between the magnets, in between which the patient's head was placed. The surgeon also stood between the two magnets. Due to the shape and appearance of the system, the Signa SP was nicknamed the "double-donut" system.[8,9] The main drawbacks of this system was the constrained working area of the surgeon, who has to stand in between the magnets, and the patient positioning restrictions (**Fig. 11.1**).

Simultaneously, Siemens Corporation (SiemensAG, Erlangen, Germany) developed a C-shaped resistive MRI scanner with a static magnetic field with a strength of 0.2 tesla (Magnetom Open). In contrast to the Signa SP, which marked the center of the operating theater, the Magnetom Open was set up at one end of the OR, separated from the surgical area by RF shielding, thus allowing for the use of standard instrumentation during surgery. The patient had to be transferred to the magnet, which featured a 240-degree opening, allowing for safe placement of the anesthetized patient's head into the scanner's field of view.[10,11] However, image acquisition necessitated transferring the patient from the operating site to the scanner, which was time-consuming.

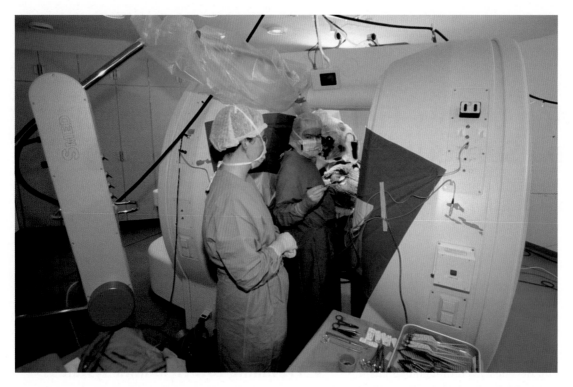

Fig. 11.1 Example of surgery with the GE Signa SP (0.5 tesla; General Electric Medical Systems, Waukesha, WI). The surgeon stands in between the magnets; surgery is performed within the magnetic field using special instruments.

Although the AIRIS II MRI scanner (Hitachi Medical Corp., Tokyo, Japan), employing a magnetic field strength of 0.3 tesla, was developed primarily as a conventional diagnostic tool, it was also employed as an iMRI scanner.[12,13] It is an open MRI unit with two horizontally oriented magnets with a vertical opening of 17 inches. Surgeries can be performed either in the adjacent OR, or with the patient positioned on the scanner's table.

The PoleStar (Medtronic Navigation, Inc., Louisville, CO) is one of the most frequently used low-field systems today with a static magnetic field strength of 0.12 (Model N-10) or 0.15 (Model N-20) tesla. It was developed to overcome the necessity of using special, MRI-compatible instruments and surgical devices, demanded for by other iMRI systems, while avoiding cumbersome patient transfer to the scanner. The PoleStar was designed as a mobile MRI unit with two vertical magnets spaced 25 or 27 cm apart, respectively. During surgery, conventional instruments can be used while the magnet is parked underneath the operating table (**Fig. 11.2**). The scanner is moved upward for intraoperative image aquisition.[14,15]

◆ Safety Considerations

In other groups' as well as our experience, there are no specific safety concerns in using low-field iMRI, and there are no risks on top of those related to cranial surgery in a conventional OR setting.[10,12,16–18] There are no reports of

patients being harmed by the use of low-field iMRI itself despite large numbers of patients being treated.[19,20] On the contrary, iMRI even allows for the intraoperative detection of complications, such as hematomas.[21,22] Further, low-field iMRI is not limited to adult patients only. Several groups have successfully performed surgeries with the help of iMRI in series of pediatric patients with comparable results to adult patients without complications pertaining to MRI.[23,24]

◆ Image Quality in Low-Field MRI

Although there is a variety of different magnet designs, field strengths, and investigational concepts, there are many similarities in the information obtained to guide and monitor neurosurgical procedures. All of the above-mentioned systems have been successfully used to monitor craniotomy and extent of resection in patients with gliomas.[12,14,18,21,25–30]

However, each has its own set of advantages and disadvantages, and as iMRI still evolves, no single system has gained universal use. Image quality in MRI is directly linked to the field strength of the magnet and to the homogeneity and stability of the static and gradient magnetic fields. Undoubtedly, high-field, 1.5 or even 3 tesla systems offer an excellent image quality that cannot be reached by low-field systems. They are, however, very expensive, and are yet limited to a small number of centers worldwide.

In iMRI in general, there is a constant trade-off between signal-to-noise ratio, access to the patient, and usable field of

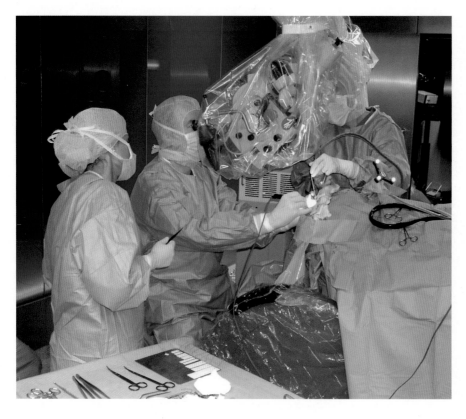

view. The optimal design of a magnet with regard to homogeneity would be a complete sphere without opening, which is obviously impossible in both conventional "closed" and intraoperative "open" MRI systems.[31] To overcome this problem and to achieve an acceptable signal-to-noise ratio in low-field open MRI systems, longer acquisition times are necessary. Although weaker magnets are usually less expensive and can allow near-real-time imaging, they suffer from poorer image resolution. High-field systems on the other hand are more expensive and permit only interruptive scanning.

From an image-quality point of view, cylindrical superconductive systems bear significant advantages relative to static magnetic field strength and homogeneity.[32] In the Signa SP scanner, the central segment of a cylindrical system was taken out, allowing for direct access to the patient in the scanner at the expense of a decreased field strength at the imaging isocenter compared with 1.5 tesla. Nonetheless, image quality is still almost comparable to high-field imaging and sufficient for the delineation of both contrast-enhancing and noncontrast-enhancing lesions such as high- and low-grade gliomas.[21]

In contrast to this system, the PoleStar MRI system offers more convenience for the surgeon with a larger working space, yet its field strength is even lower, and the magnet's field of view is considerably smaller, requiring accurate patient positioning and rendering a slightly lower signal-to-noise ratio. Still, the PoleStar provides good quality visualization of contrast-enhancing tumors and fair quality for nonenhancing lesions (**Figs. 11.3** and **11.4**).[16,33] In our experience, the image quality in high-grade gliomas is comparable in both systems, but image quality in low-grade gliomas is to some extent better when using the Signa SP.[30]

Contrast-enhancing gliomas are displayed best on T1-weighted imaging with application of contrast agent; usually higher doses of contrast agent are recommended for optimal lesion to white matter contrast.[34] Several groups have experienced difficulties with visualizing the tumor margins on regular T2-weighted imaging in nonenhancing tumors with different low-field MRI units; fluid-attenuated inversion recovery (FLAIR) sequences were found to be superior in these cases.[9,16,35]

◆ Indications for iMRI

The introduction of image-guided frameless neuronavigation was an important step toward an enhanced visualization of the surgical field. However, although helpful in planning the initial surgical approach, the method of neuronavigation is of limited use during or at the end of tumor resection because of intraoperative anatomical alterations called "brain-shift," caused by surgical retraction, cerebrospinal fluid (CSF) loss, edema, and tumor removal itself (**Fig. 11.5**).[36] As a result, neuronavigation that is based solely on preoperative imaging data is not reliable in terms of determining residual tumor tissue intraoperatively.

Bergsneider et al compared tumor resection with the aid of frameless neuronavigation with low-field strength iMRI without neuronavigation in a small series of patients and found a higher percentage of tumor volume resected in the iMRI group, again indicating the superiority of iMRI versus neuronavigation alone.[37] Moreover, iMRI bears the advantage of enabling the surgeon to update anatomic

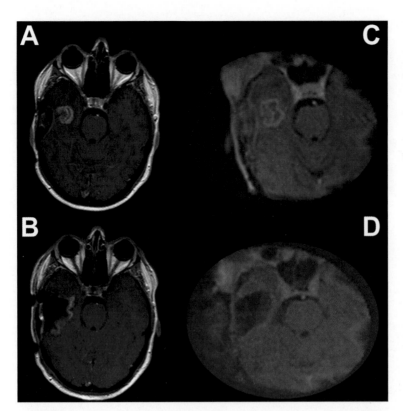

Fig. 11.3 Comparison of diagnostic contrast-enhanced 1.5 tesla T1-weighted magnetic resonance imaging acquired **(A)** preoperatively and **(B)** postoperatively with intraoperative low-field imaging at 0.15 tesla **(C)** before and **(D)** after complete tumor resection in a patient with a recurrent glioblastoma; the hyperintense rim inside the resection cavity corresponds to hemostatic material.

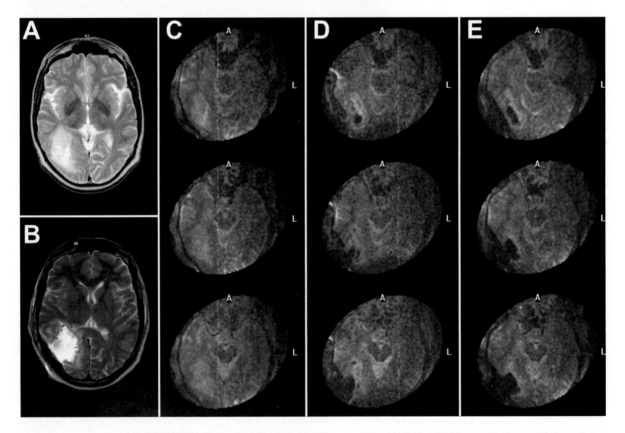

Fig. 11.4 Comparison of T2-weighted magnetic resonance imaging acquired **(A)** preoperatively and **(B)** postoperatively at 1.5 tesla with intraoperative low-field imaging at 0.15 tesla **(C)** before and **(D,E)** during continued tumor resection in a patient with a right-sided WHO grade II-astrocytoma of the dorsal right temporal lobe.

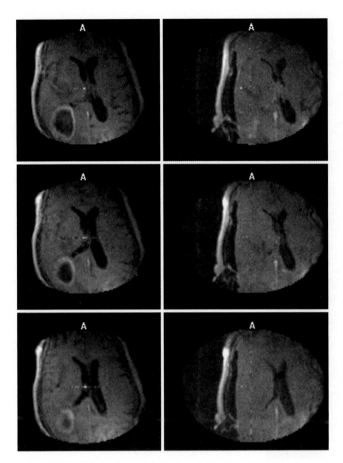

Fig. 11.5 Comparison of intraoperatively acquired 0.15 tesla magnetic resonance images (T1-weighted, contrast-enhanced sequences) before (left column) and after tumor resection (right column). In addition to complete removal of contrast-enhancing tumor tissue (histology: anaplastic astrocytoma), a marked brain shift can be recognized.

data intraoperatively; hence it is possible to update the neuronavigation intraoperatively to precisely locate and target remaining tumor tissue.[16,18]

To update neuroanatomic information intraoperatively, intraoperative imaging techniques such as MRI or ultrasound are mandatory. In this respect, however, ultrasonographic imaging is not only more difficult to interpret, but might also impose severe limitations with regard to reliability of findings, even for experienced surgeons.[38–40] Consequently, intraoperative imaging in glioma surgery is the domain of MRI, allowing even for the incorporation of preoperatively acquired high-resolution datasets (**Fig. 11.6**).

◆ Influence of iMRI on the Course of Surgery

Although iMRI has evolved as a new technology in neurosurgery from the 1990s, first reports dealing with iMRI systems focused primarily on the feasibility of their use. Until today, more than 800 glioma patients have reportedly undergone surgical resection with the aid of any low-field-strength iMRI. With the increasing experience of applying these methods in the neurosurgical routine and the knowledge of their safety, the influence of iMRI on the surgical routine and clinical benefit of the patients has become more important.

In both, high- and low-grade glioma cases, all investigators who reported on the influence of intraoperative low-field MRI on the course of surgery stated that intraoperative scanning had revealed residual tumor tissue in a significant number of cases. The percentage of patients with an extended resection after depiction of residual tumor tissue on intraoperative images is reported to range between 14 to 75% (**Table 11.1; Fig. 11.7**).[11,12,16,18–20,41] Correspondingly, in high-grade glioma cases the respective figures are 10 to 71% (**Table 11.2**).[11,12,16,18,19,27,42,43] Consequently, the rates of complete resection have thus increased by greater than 20%.[17] It is clear that low-field iMRI has had a major influence on the course of surgery in a large number of patients.

◆ Influence of iMRI on Patient Outcome

In studies addressing postoperative morbidity, complication rates range from 5 to 18% postoperatively in all but one series,[12,16,21,25,35,43–45] where an early complication rate of 53% in a group of 13 patients was observed.[37] Permanent deficits occurred in less than 10% of the patients, which is comparable to the complication rates in conventional glioma surgery. In our own series of patients, an extended resection after iMRI scans had revealed residual tumor did not correlate with postoperative morbidity.[16] To prevent patient injury and neurologic deterioration due to overly aggressive resection, the use of iMRI can also be combined with intraoperative monitoring techniques, such as motor or sensory evoked potentials during surgery, even when applied in the fringe field.[46] After careful patient selection, gliomas can undergo maximum resection with acceptable risks for the patients.

Yet, only few studies have aimed to evaluate the influence of low-field iMRI on the clinical course of glioma patients. As mentioned earlier, most studies have thus far focused on the feasibility, safety, and influence on the course of surgery in the application of iMRI in glioma surgery. In a large series of low-grade glioma patients, Claus et al found a trend toward prolonged survival of patients who had undergone total versus subtotal resection in an iMRI-environment.[6] Similar findings were reported by Trantakis et al in patients with high-grade gliomas.[47] Using two different low-field systems, Wirtz et al and Schneider et al independently reported statistically significant prolonged survival times for high-grade glioma patients who had undergone total versus subtotal tumor resection with the aid of iMRI.[19,43] These results add to the growing evidence that extent of resection translates into prolonged survival in glioma patients.[5] However, theses studies did not compare patients treated under iMRI-guidance with a control group of patients. Hirschberg et al performed a matched group-analysis in a series of glioblastoma patients undergoing

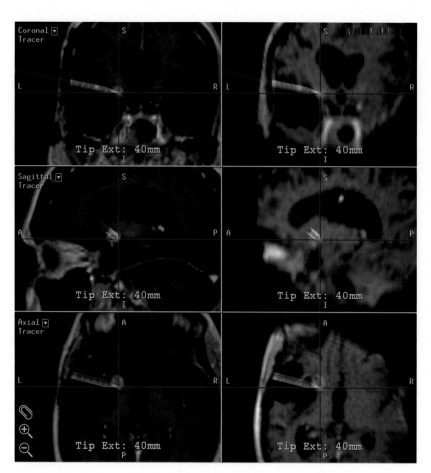

Fig. 11.6 Screenshot image showing an example of combining preoperative 1.5 tesla magnetic resonance-datasets (MR datasets) (left column) with intraoperative 0.15 tesla MR datasets (right column) for neuronavigation in a patient with a recurrent WHO grade III astrocytoma (note: intraoperative images were acquired axially only – sagittal and coronal planes are reconstructed from axial plane).

Table 11.1 Studies Reporting the Use of Low-Field Intraoperative MRI in Low-Grade Gliomas with a Minimum of 10 Patients

Author	Year	System Used	No. of Patients	Increased Resection Due to Intraoperative Imaging
Black et al	1999	Signa SP (General Electric Medical Systems, Waukesha, WI)	29	n.r.
Seifert et al	1999	Signa SP	13	n.r.
Wirtz et al	2000	Magnetom Open (Siemens AG, Erlangen, Germany)	29	45%
Zimmermann et al	2000	Signa SP	16	n.r.
Bohinski et al	2001	AIRIS II (Hitachi Medical Corp., Tokyo, Japan)	10	40%
Zimmermann et al	2001	Signa SP	11	n.r.
Buchfelder et al	2002	Magnetom Open	11	14%
Nimsky et al	2002	Magnetom Open	47	38%
Nimsky et al	2003	Magnetom Open	52	40%
Schulder et al	2003	PoleStar N-10 (Medtronic Navigation, Inc., Louisville, CO)	12	n.r.
Claus et al	2005	Signa SP	156	n.r.
Nimsky et al	2005	Magnetom Open	61	29%
Senft et al	2008	PoleStar N-20	21*	47%

Abbreviations: n.r., not reported; *nonenhancing gliomas.

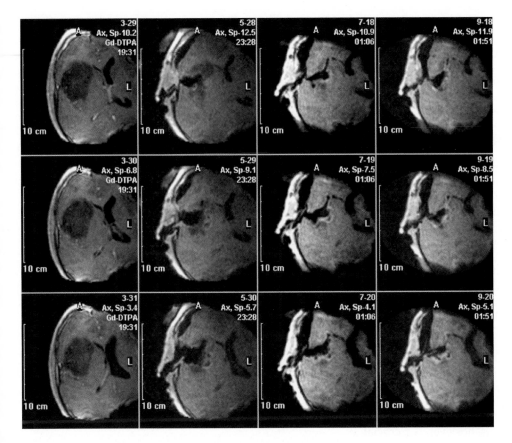

Fig. 11.7 Screenshot image showing continued tumor resection after intraoperative imaging at 0.15 tesla in a patient with a right insular WHO grade II astrocytoma (left column: tumor delineation before tumor resection; middle columns: during continued tumor resection; right column: final scans after tumor resection). A brain shift is also visible.

Table 11.2 Studies Reporting the Use of Low-Field Intraoperative MRI in High-Grade Gliomas with a Minimum of 10 Patients

Author	Year	System Used	No. of Patients	Increased Resection Due to Intraoperative Imaging
Tronnier et al	1997	Magnetom Open (Siemens AG, Erlangen, Germany)	10	n.r.
Black et al	1999	Signa SP (General Electric Medical Systems, Waukesha, WI)	19	n.r.
Knauth et al	1999	Magnetom Open	41	41%
Seifert et al	1999	Signa SP	12	n.r.
Wirtz et al	2000	Magnetom Open	68	63%
Zimmermann et al	2000	Signa SP	16	n.r.
Bohinski et al	2001	AIRIS II (Hitachi Medical Corp., Tokyo, Japan)	30	56%
Zimmermann et al	2001	Signa SP	14	n.r.
Nimsky et al	2002	Magnetom Open	48	10%
Trantakis et al	2003	Signa SP	68	n.r.
Nimsky et al	2003	Magnetom Open	54	13%
Schulder et al	2003	PoleStar N-10 (Medtronic Navigation, Inc., Louisville, CO)	25	n.r.
Bergsneider et al	2005	Magnetom Open	10	n.r.
Hirschberg et al	2005	Signa SP	32	52%
Schneider et al	2005	Signa SP	31	71%
Senft et al	2008	PoleStar N-20	42*	28%

Abbreviations: n.r., not reported; *contrast-enhancing gliomas.

low-field iMRI-guided surgery and found a trend in favor of iMRI, but no statistically significant differences in overall survival between the groups.[42] Therefore, the true benefit of iMRI has not yet been proven, in contrast to other means of intraoperative resection control, such as the administration of fluorescent porphyrins.[3,4]

◆ Comparison with High-Field Systems

Even though the superiority of high-field iMRI systems over low-field iMRI systems seems obvious in terms of image resolution and quality, only a few reports have specifically addressed this issue. Although Nimsky et al[20] described a clearly better image quality and a smoother workflow with a high-field system, the rates of extended resection were comparable between the low- and high-field system. Bergsneider et al[37] found no difference in the extent of resection when comparing a low-field versus a high-field iMRI. High-field systems may offer faster acquisition times and allow for a greater variety of imaging sequences; however, low-field systems, too, can provide the surgeon with reliable information about the extent of resection. In our own experience, this is definitely true at least for contrast-enhancing, high-grade tumors. In nonenhancing, low-grade tumors, high-field systems surely provide an improved spatial resolution. Yet, the question of whether high- and low-field iMRI differs in terms of patient benefit or clinical outcome remains unanswered. This, however, is a crucial concern, especially when looking at the set-up and installation costs of the different available iMRI systems.

◆ Future Perspectives

Advances in technology have improved the precision of intracranial surgery, and iMRI is the latest development in this field. The potential impact on the management of patients with brain tumors is obvious. The use of low-field MRI scanners in glioma surgery is safe, reliable, and most useful in assessing the extent of resection of intrinsic, infiltrating brain tumors whose boundaries cannot be clearly distinguished by the surgeon. Although several retrospective analyses have documented the benefit of implementing iMRI into the neurosurgical routine in glioma surgery by means of increasing the extent of resection, prospective randomized studies are still lacking that might prove the benefit of iMRI compared with the standard microneurosurgical resection of brain tumors. Further, use of iMRI itself has not been proven to prolong survival in patients with glial tumors. Although beneficial effects are suggested by previous studies, there is no level I evidence to promote the use of iMRI today, and pursuant studies are needed.

One clear advantage over the administration of fluorescent porphyrins to visualize tumor tissue intraoperatively is the usability of iMRI in low-grade gliomas and its implementation of functional anatomic data. In the future, preoperative functional MRI datasets may be incorporated into neuronavigation, as well as intraoperative diffusion weighted imaging to depict white matter tracts. Both concepts are feasible in high-field and low-field iMRI systems.[48–50]

For obvious reasons, glioma patients will not be cured by neurosurgical intervention. Additional treatment modalities are and will remain mandatory to prolong survival and to maintain quality of life for these patients. However, maximum tumor resection without induction of disabling neurologic deficits appears to be one of the strongest predictive factors. Therefore, the neurosurgeon's abilities and the advances of modern aides such as iMRI will certainly translate into benefit for our patients.

References

1. Albert FK, Forsting M, Sartor K, Adams HP, Kunze S. Early postoperative magnetic resonance imaging after resection of malignant glioma: objective evaluation of residual tumor and its influence on regrowth and prognosis. Neurosurgery 1994;34(1):45–60, discussion 60–61

2. McGirt MJ, Chaichana KL, Gathinji M, et al. Independent association of extent of resection with survival in patients with malignant brain astrocytoma. J Neurosurg 2009;110(1):156–162

3. Stummer W, Pichlmeier U, Meinel T, Wiestler OD, Zanella F, Reulen HJ; ALA-Glioma Study Group. Fluorescence-guided surgery with 5-aminolevulinic acid for resection of malignant glioma: a randomised controlled multicentre phase III trial. Lancet Oncol 2006;7(5):392–401

4. Stummer W, Reulen HJ, Meinel T, et al; ALA-Glioma Study Group. Extent of resection and survival in glioblastoma multiforme: identification of and adjustment for bias. Neurosurgery 2008;62(3):564–576, discussion 564–576

5. Sanai N, Berger MS. Glioma extent of resection and its impact on patient outcome. Neurosurgery 2008;62(4):753–764, discussion 264–266

6. Claus EB, Horlacher A, Hsu L, et al. Survival rates in patients with low-grade glioma after intraoperative magnetic resonance image guidance. Cancer 2005;103(6):1227–1233

7. Hall WA, Liu H, Martin AJ, Truwit CL. Intraoperative magnetic resonance imaging. Top Magn Reson Imaging 2000;11(3):203–212

8. Black PM, Moriarty T, Alexander E III, et al. Development and implementation of intraoperative magnetic resonance imaging and its neurosurgical applications. Neurosurgery 1997;41(4):831–842, discussion 842–845

9. Seifert V, Zimmermann M, Trantakis C, et al. Open MRI-guided neurosurgery. Acta Neurochir (Wien) 1999;141(5):455–464

10. Tronnier VM, Wirtz CR, Knauth M, et al. Intraoperative diagnostic and interventional magnetic resonance imaging in neurosurgery. Neurosurgery 1997;40(5):891–900, discussion 900–902

11. Wirtz CR, Bonsanto MM, Knauth M, et al. Intraoperative magnetic resonance imaging to update interactive navigation in neurosurgery: method and preliminary experience. Comput Aided Surg 1997;2(3-4):172–179

12. Bohinski RJ, Kokkino AK, Warnick RE, et al. Glioma resection in a shared-resource magnetic resonance operating room after optimal image-guided frameless stereotactic resection. Neurosurgery 2001;48(4):731–742, discussion 742–744

13. Muragaki Y, Iseki H, Maruyama T, et al. Usefulness of intraoperative magnetic resonance imaging for glioma surgery. Acta Neurochir Suppl (Wien) 2006;98:67–75

14. Schulder M, Sernas TJ, Carmel PW. Cranial surgery and navigation with a compact intraoperative MRI system. Acta Neurochir Suppl (Wien) 2003;85:79–86

15. Schulder M, Salas S, Brimacombe M, et al. Cranial surgery with an expanded compact intraoperative magnetic resonance imager. Technical note. J Neurosurg 2006;104(4):611–617

16. Senft C, Seifert V, Hermann E, Franz K, Gasser T. Usefulness of intraoperative ultra low-field magnetic resonance imaging in glioma surgery. Neurosurgery 2008; 63(4, Suppl 2)257–266, discussion 266–267

17. Oh DS, Black PM. A low-field intraoperative MRI system for glioma surgery: is it worthwhile? Neurosurg Clin N Am 2005;16(1):135–141

18. Nimsky C, Ganslandt O, Tomandl B, Buchfelder M, Fahlbusch R. Low-field magnetic resonance imaging for intraoperative use in neurosurgery: a 5-year experience. Eur Radiol 2002;12(11):2690–2703

19. Wirtz CR, Knauth M, Staubert A, et al. Clinical evaluation and follow-up results for intraoperative magnetic resonance imaging in neurosurgery. Neurosurgery 2000;46(5):1112–1120, discussion 1120–1122

20. Nimsky C, Ganslandt O, Fahlbusch R. Comparing 0.2 tesla with 1.5 tesla intraoperative magnetic resonance imaging analysis of setup, workflow, and efficiency. Acad Radiol 2005;12(9):1065–1079

21. Zimmermann M, Seifert V, Trantakis C, et al. Open MRI-guided microsurgery of intracranial tumours. Preliminary experience using a vertical open MRI-scanner. Acta Neurochir (Wien) 2000;142(2):177–186

22. Rohde V, Rohde I, Thiex R, Küker W, Ince A, Gilsbach JM. The role of intraoperative magnetic resonance imaging for the detection of hemorrhagic complications during surgery for intracerebral lesions an experimental approach. Surg Neurol 2001;56(4):266–274, discussion 274–275

23. Samdani AF, Schulder M, Catrambone JE, Carmel PW. Use of a compact intraoperative low-field magnetic imager in pediatric neurosurgery. Childs Nerv Syst 2005;21(2):108–113, discussion 114

24. Kremer P, Tronnier V, Steiner HH, et al. Intraoperative MRI for interventional neurosurgical procedures and tumor resection control in children. Childs Nerv Syst 2006;22(7):674–678

25. Black PM, Alexander E III, Martin C, et al. Craniotomy for tumor treatment in an intraoperative magnetic resonance imaging unit. Neurosurgery 1999;45(3):423–431, discussion 431–433

26. Metzger AK, Lewin JS. Optimizing brain tumor resection. Low-field interventional MR imaging. Neuroimaging Clin N Am 2001;11(4):651–657, ix

27. Knauth M, Wirtz CR, Tronnier VM, Aras N, Kunze S, Sartor K. Intraoperative MR imaging increases the extent of tumor resection in patients with high-grade gliomas. AJNR Am J Neuroradiol 1999;20(9): 1642–1646

28. Hadani M, Spiegelman R, Feldman Z, Berkenstadt H, Ram Z. Novel, compact, intraoperative magnetic resonance imaging-guided system for conventional neurosurgical operating rooms. Neurosurgery 2001;48(4):799–807, discussion 807–809

29. Ram Z, Hadani M. Intraoperative imaging—MRI. Acta Neurochir Suppl (Wien) 2003;88:1–4

30. Ntoukas V, Krishnan R, Seifert V. The new generation PoleStar n20 for conventional neurosurgical operating rooms: a preliminary report. Neurosurgery 2008; 62(3, Suppl 1)82–89, discussion 89–90

31. Hinks RS, Bronskill MJ, Kucharczyk W, Bernstein M, Collick BD, Henkelman RM. MR systems for image-guided therapy. J Magn Reson Imaging 1998;8(1):19–25

32. Lewin JS. Interventional MR imaging: concepts, systems, and applications in neuroradiology. AJNR Am J Neuroradiol 1999;20(5):735–748

33. Schulder M, Carmel PW. Intraoperative magnetic resonance imaging: impact on brain tumor surgery. Cancer Control 2003;10(2):115–124

34. Knauth M, Wirtz CR, Aras N, Sartor K. Low-field interventional MRI in neurosurgery: finding the right dose of contrast medium. Neuroradiology 2001;43(3):254–258

35. Nimsky C, Ganslandt O, Buchfelder M, Fahlbusch R. Glioma surgery evaluated by intraoperative low-field magnetic resonance imaging. Acta Neurochir Suppl (Wien) 2003;85:55–63

36. Roberts DW, Hartov A, Kennedy FE, Miga MI, Paulsen KD. Intraoperative brain shift and deformation: a quantitative analysis of cortical displacement in 28 cases. Neurosurgery 1998;43(4):749–758, discussion 758–760

37. Bergsneider M, Sehati N, Villablanca P, McArthur DL, Becker DP, Liau LM. Mahaley Clinical Research Award: extent of glioma resection using low-field (0.2 T) versus high-field (1.5 T) intraoperative MRI and image-guided frameless neuronavigation. Clin Neurosurg 2005;52: 389–399

38. Tronnier VM, Bonsanto MM, Staubert A, Knauth M, Kunze S, Wirtz CR. Comparison of intraoperative MR imaging and 3D-navigated ultrasonography in the detection and resection control of lesions. Neurosurg Focus 2001;10(2):E3

39. Erdoğan N, Tucer B, Mavili E, Menkü A, Kurtsoy A. Ultrasound guidance in intracranial tumor resection: correlation with postoperative magnetic resonance findings. Acta Radiol 2005;46(7):743–749

40. Rygh OM, Selbekk T, Torp SH, Lydersen S, Hernes TA, Unsgaard G. Comparison of navigated 3D ultrasound findings with histopathology in subsequent phases of glioblastoma resection. Acta Neurochir (Wien) 2008;150(10):1033–1041, discussion 1042

41. Buchfelder M, Fahlbusch R, Ganslandt O, Stefan H, Nimsky C. Use of intraoperative magnetic resonance imaging in tailored temporal lobe surgeries for epilepsy. Epilepsia 2002;43(8):864–873

42. Hirschberg H, Samset E, Hol PK, Tillung T, Lote K. Impact of intraoperative MRI on the surgical results for high-grade gliomas. Minim Invasive Neurosurg 2005;48(2):77–84

43. Schneider JP, Trantakis C, Rubach M, et al. Intraoperative MRI to guide the resection of primary supratentorial glioblastoma multiforme—a quantitative radiological analysis. Neuroradiology 2005;47(7): 489–500

44. Bernstein M, Al-Anazi AR, Kucharczyk W, Manninen P, Bronskill M, Henkelman M. Brain tumor surgery with the Toronto open magnetic resonance imaging system: preliminary results for 36 patients and analysis of advantages, disadvantages, and future prospects. Neurosurgery 2000;46(4):900–907, discussion 907–909

45. Zimmermann M, Seifert V, Trantakis C, Raabe A. Open MRI-guided microsurgery of intracranial tumours in or near eloquent brain areas. Acta Neurochir (Wien) 2001;143(4):327–337

46. Szelényi A, Gasser T, Seifert V. Intraoperative neurophysiological monitoring in an open low-field magnetic resonance imaging system: clinical experience and technical considerations. Neurosurgery 2008; 63(4, Suppl 2)268–275, discussion 275–276

47. Trantakis C, Winkler D, Lindner D, et al. Clinical results in MR-guided therapy for malignant gliomas. Acta Neurochir Suppl (Wien) 2003; 85:65–71

48. Schulder M, Azmi H, Biswal B. Functional magnetic resonance imaging in a low-field intraoperative scanner. Stereotact Funct Neurosurg 2003;80(1-4):125–131

49. Nimsky C, Ganslandt O, Hastreiter P, et al. Preoperative and intraoperative diffusion tensor imaging-based fiber tracking in glioma surgery. Neurosurgery 2007; 61(1, Suppl)178–185, discussion 186

50. Ozawa N, Muragaki Y, Nakamura R, Lseki H. Intraoperative diffusion-weighted imaging for visualization of the pyramidal tracts. Part II: clinical study of usefulness and efficacy. Minim Invasive Neurosurg 2008;51(2):67–71

12

Intraoperative MRI Scanning in High-Grade Gliomas

Hubertus Maximillian Mehdorn, Arya Nabavi, Felix Schwartz, and Lutz Dörner

Neurosurgical resection of intracranial glioma is the first and most crucial step in treating patients with intrinsic brain tumors: it provides for a correct histologic diagnosis and by debulking the tumor, raised intracranial pressure can be reduced. In the presence of space-occupying low-grade gliomas usually the goal of surgery is to remove the tumor as radically as possible to prevent or to delay recurrence. Previously for high-grade glioma (HGG), both astrocytoma WHO grade III and glioblastoma multiforme (GBM) WHO grade IV, a wait-and-see attitude, biopsy, or removal of a minor part of the tumor have been suggested, followed by radiotherapy with or without chemotherapy. Recently,[1] however, it has been posited that surgery would only be useful in cases of massive space-occupying lesions. The surgery would not really affect patient survival because only a portion of the tumor cells would be removed, leaving the rest of the active tumor in the brain. There are times one has to advocate to perform only a brain biopsy to establish a correct diagnosis. Median survival rates for GBM range from 41 to 53 weeks.[2–4] Also, infiltration of functionally relevant structures both at the brain surface and in the white matter by the malignant tumor carries the risk of major permanent worsening of neurologic status and thereby quality of life—factors that have been closely related to overall survival following tumor diagnosis and surgery.[2,5] This was certainly true with diagnostic imaging based on computed tomography (CT) or even earlier angiography, scintigraphy, and other procedures. Now, with the use of preoperative magnetic resonance imaging (MRI), better delineation of tumor margins can be achieved, as well as the ("microscopic") extension of tumor beyond the contrast-enhancing tumor margins as seen on contrast-enhanced T1-weighted images (T1WIs).[6,7] Further refinement including MR spectroscopy (MRS) helps to better elucidate tumor biology. Also, the tumor can be correlated to functionally relevant brain areas both by the use of functional MRI (fMRI) and diffusion weighted imaging (DWI), allowing for delineation of the pyramidal tract or intercenter fiber tracts, a process called fiber-tracking.[8,9]

Over the years, more evidence has accumulated that the most complete tumor removal possible improves a patient's survival chances. By undergoing radical removal based on MRI criteria, the contrast-enhancing part of the tumor is completely removed as witnessed on an early (maximal 72 hours) postoperative MRI scan, with the understanding that this contrast-enhancing area comprises only part of the tumor and that further malignant tumor spread cannot be ruled out.

Jeremic et al[10] have shown in a group of 86 patients with GBM that patients treated with more radical surgery had a survival of 56 weeks versus 26 weeks for those who had undergone only biopsy. Also, progression-free survival at 1 year was higher in those radically resected (20% versus 0%). Similarly, Yoshida et al[11] showed that besides age, histology, and type of adjuvant therapy, radical resection had a high impact on survival rates. The group of patients who had undergone gross total tumor resection or had experienced a complete response to adjuvant therapy showed survival rates of 42% at 3 years and 24% at 5 years. In a phase II study of multimodal therapy of recurrent malignant gliomas, Rostomily et al[12] found in a multivariate analysis that greater surgical debulking and smaller postoperative tumor volumes were associated with prolonged median time to progression (MTP) but not median survival time (MST), which rather was related to a lobar versus deep tumor location. Obwegeser et al[13] performed a multivariate analysis in 157 patients with malignant tumors and showed a significant effect of survival after radical macroscopic surgery ($p = 0.005$), postoperative radiotherapy ($p < 0.001$), and chemotherapy ($p < 0.01$). More recently, in our institution a multivariate analysis confirmed these results in a larger cohort and particularly stressed the indication for surgery independent of the patient's chronologic age;[14] however, a Finnish group[15] did not show a surgical benefit in older patients. Other groups have demonstrated this beneficial effect of radical removal as well.[16,17] Also in a malignant gliomas in childhood study (Childrens Cancer Group Study CCG 945), radical surgical resection (defined as greater than 90% resection as seen on imaging studies – mostly MRI) was shown to be the most powerful predictor of outcome.[18] The authors also point to the importance of training of the neurosurgeon in either adult or pediatric neurosurgery.

To select GBM patients who might be suitable for radical surgical resection, Shinoda et al[19] suggested a topographical grading system based on tumor location, size, and eloquence of adjacent brain as seen on MRI. They found in a multivariate analysis that gross total resection in stage I patients was an independent good prognostic factor. Many techniques have been developed with the aim to support maximal tumor removal.

◆ Awake Craniotomy

Aggressive tumor removal is usually hindered by the neurosurgeon's fear of creating a major neurologic and permanent deficit when removing tissue from eloquent areas. Therefore, early in modern neurosurgery and with the refinement of anesthesia and local anaesthetics, awake craniotomy was undertaken with the patient's cooperation by talking to him or her and making him or her perform voluntary movements during surgery. Details of this technique have been described elsewhere.[20,21] Many groups now use this technique on a routine basis. The results reported show that a more radical tumor removal can be achieved using this technique for tumors in eloquent areas. Our group[21] recently has reported a 77% complete resection rate for tumor surgery in the motor areas using awake craniotomy compared with only 33% when the patient was operated under general anesthesia. This technique has also been implemented in the setting of high-field intraoperative MRI (iMRI) by our group since early 2006: this is reviewed in Chapter 17.

◆ Neuronavigation

Preoperative imaging provides a good picture of brain anatomy and the tumor; images both from CT and MRI (best in the format of magnetization-prepared rapid gradient echo [MP-RAGE]) can be used for neuronavigation and allow a more-targeted approach to the tumor. However, this method of targeting can be used safely only in skull base surgery and to a minor extent once the dura has been opened. Once the dura is opened, brain shift occurs initially due to release of cerebrospinal fluid (CSF) from the subarachnoid spaces, such as the sylvian fissure and the basal cisterns, and secondarily due to tumor removal.[22,23] Best surgical judgment needs to be implemented when proceeding with surgery of a tumor located in the white matter. The location of anatomic structures needs to be taken into consideration, especially the distance of the brain surface from the dura, which depends initially on the position of the patient's head and may vary

considerably from location to location due to inherent brain firmness – "elasticity"– altered by the tumor and the extent of tumor removal. In view of the brain shift it is understandable that only a few groups[24] have reported that neuronavigation per se did improve survival of GBM patients (13.4 months versus 10.3 months), whereas our group[25] as well as others[26] recently had not shown a benefit. However, Wirtz et al[24] stated that they had achieved radical resection as defined by postoperative MRI in 31% of all cases, an improvement when compared to 19% in conventional operations.

◆ Aminolevulinic Acid Fluorescence

Aminolevulinic acid (ALA) fluorescence has been studied extensively in many phase I to III studies and has been shown to effectively increase the percentage of radical resections in high-grade glioma (HGG) surgery as proven by postoperative MRI scans,[27–29] thus prolonging the recurrence-free survival interval. It is now commercially available in Europe as Gliolan (Medac, Wedel, Germany). This technique can safely be applied both in primary and recurrent HGGs. It requires oral application of Gliolan some 3 to 4 hours prior to initiating surgery, and a special microscope lamp producing filtered, violet–blue excitation light for visualizing fluorescence is required. The lamps are available on Zeiss (Carl Zeiss AG, Oberkochen, Germany), Möller-Wedel (Wedel, Germany), and Leica (Sols, Germany) microscopes. The ALA is absorbed by tumor cells and is converted into protoporphyrin IX, which can be detected by utilizing this special light. After regular tumor exposure using white light, the borders of the HGG are delineated by switching to fluorescence mode, and the tumor can be resected using an ultrasound aspirator, guided by the intense red light to depict the highly cell-dense tumor. Vessel damage can also be prevented because arteries and veins show up as pale blue-green structures. Fluorescence is only visible from tissue not immersed in fluids such as blood and CSF. Once the tumor has been removed up to its borders, fluorescence fades away and gives way to a light red (salmon-like) color.

The advantage of ALA fluorescence guidance is that it is relatively cheap and highly effective; it guides the surgeon in a rapidly repeatable manner during surgery, and can also be used in recurrent HGG surgery with good accuracy. The problem obviously is that it registers only surface fluorescence: it is impossible to look around corners or underneath the surface. This limitation — together with good surgical judgment not to touch/resect eloquent brain areas — would also explain why using ALA did not give nearly 100% radical resection in the major studies. On the other hand, this technique can also be used on recurrent HGG surgery.

◆ Intraoperative Ultrasound

Intraoperative ultrasound has been advocated and elaborated by some groups[30,31] to intraoperatively enhance surgeons' vision of tumor borders, and is regularly used in many centers, even coupled to navigation devices. Its advantage again is high flexibility, but its disadvantage is that it is, to a certain degree as all ultrasound devices, a highly subjective method requiring intensive training. With this in mind, it should carry the same radical resection rate as low-field iMRI scanning[32]

◆ Intraoperative Magnetic Resonance Imaging

The introduction of MRI into a surgical operating room was what seems today the logical extension of improving preoperative imaging and making it available for intraoperative control in glioma surgery. To be a valuable adjunct for HGG surgery, an iMRI machine needs to have the same scanning properties as commercially available MRI scanners used routinely pre- and postoperatively for all parts of the body.

Schwartz[33] in Boston, Hall[34,35] in Minneapolis, Knauth[36] in Heidelberg, and Fahlbusch[37] in Erlangen together with various MRI equipment manufacturers were the first to report the implications of iMRI around 1996. Low- and midfield machines were in many sites followed by high-field MRI equipment.[38] Many obstacles needed to be overcome such as geometric distortion,[39] and the values of various field strengths were repeatedly discussed.[40-42] Having overcome initial problems based on the hardware and the magnetic field that prevents the use of regular surgical instruments within it, all groups focused on what patients might benefit the most from iMRI. Those patients requiring radical tumor resection, namely patients with low-grade gliomas (LGG) and pituitary adenomas, were determined to benefit the most from this new applied procedure.

Knauth et al[36] reported that the extent of glioma resection was more radical ("complete" in 75.6%) using iMRI, in this case a 0.2 tesla (T) machine, as compared to 36.6% in matching patients operated without iMRI. Claus et al[43] have reported longer survival rates in a higher percentage of LGG patients operated under iMRI.

Only a few reports have been published by the groups mentioned to support the use of iMRI in HGG surgery. Martin et al[44] reported on the use of a 1.5 T machine during glioma surgery in 30 patients and found a low frequency of complications while achieving a radiologically complete tumor resection in 80% of the patients. They found it difficult to read the images of contrast-enhancing tumors intraoperatively. This lesson was different from the one learned when operating on LGG; Schneider et al[45] reported a good correlation (10 of 12 tumors, the remaining 2 being on the border zone of the LGG) of residual tumor suspected on iMRI using a 0.5 T machine and neuropathologic examination of this area. This group[46] also reported a higher resection rate in HGG: a decrease of residual tumor from 29% at first control to 10% at final imaging.

Knauth et al[47] addressed the problem of delineating a contrast-enhancing lesion (both metastasis and HGG) on the basis of their 0.2 T MRI scanner, comparing the results with those obtained using a standard 1.5 T MRI scanner preoperatively.

Based on a "normal" referral basis to a tertiary referral center in a university hospital, we have confirmed that patients harboring HGGs are more common than LGG patients. From September 2005 through May 2009, we operated on 24 astrocytomas WHO grade II, 60 astrocytomas WHO grade III, and on 140 glioblastomas WHO grade IV. In the remainder of this chapter, we will focus on the treatment of HGG patients using iMRI based on our experience over the last 4 years.

Technique

Operating Room Setting

Details of the operating room setup have been published in previous articles from our group[48,49] and are also presented in chapters of this book.

We have adapted the iMRI setting from the Minneapolis group,[34,35] using a short-bore Philips Intera 1.5 T MRI scanner (Philips Healthcare, Andover, MA), but in a dedicated MRI operating room (OR) that was designed specifically for this purpose when we constructed a new building with four ORs for our department. From September 2005 until May 2009, we have treated 426 patients in this MRI-OR. Patients presented with a variety of disease entities: mostly HGG (n = 200), followed by pituitary adenomas (n = 64) and LGG (n = 24). Meningiomas, metastases, and cavernomas were rarely seen, and spinal tumors were rarer still. This setting is also used for preoperative stereotactic imaging for deep brain stimulation (DBS).

Patient Positioning and Safety

Because iMRI surgery may last longer than regular surgery, special care should be given to patient comfort and safety. Positioning the head in a fixed optimal position is achieved using a Mayfield three-pin (amagnetic head pins; Integra Neurosciences, Plainsboro, NJ) head clamp made of carbon fiber material (Promedics GmbH, Düsseldorf, Germany), and the headholder is attached to the rails of the MRI table (modified Angio DIAGNOST 5 Syncra Tilt Patient Support; Philips Healthcare). The cranial end of the table may be raised or lowered, but it may not be tilted along its long axis. The head position is optimized to allow for the most vertical access to the lesion with special care to avoid the surrounding structures. Patient positioning takes some time because the head needs to be fixed in a position with the Mayfield clamp so that the surgical field is above the level of the heart valves and the head fits into the tunnel of the magnet. The flexible circular surface coils (Sense flex large, diameter 20 cm; Flexicoils, Philips Healthcare) are placed below and above the head accordingly allowing extended access to the surgical field. The patient is covered with a warmtouch mattress (Mallinckrodt WarmTouch Convective Air Warming System, Tyco Healthcare Group, Albertville, AL) to prevent the body from cooling down during the surgery. The warming tube connecting the heating apparatus to the mattress is disconnected while the patient is brought into the magnet for scanning. The mattress itself is compatible with the MRI environment. This setting also allows enough patient comfort to perform a glioma operation under local anesthesia (awake craniotomy), which is discussed in Chapter 17.

Scanning

The software we used was based on actual Philips software release versions up to 12.1. Flexicoils are used intraoperatively. Once this is achieved, the patient is positioned for MRI scanning in the tunnel, care being taken to accommodate the long tubing and lines for anesthesia. In this initial position, only a fast T2-weighted image (T2WI) is taken to see that everything is in order, and the patient is taken out of the scanner and brought into the operating position by turning the table approximately 30 degrees. Neuronavigation is registered in a standard fashion (BrainLab VectorVision, Heimstetten, Germany) based on preoperatively acquired MRI or CT scans, the later being fused to the standard MRI scans and using iPlan cranial software (BrainLab).

As opposed to the Siemens system (Siemens AG, Erlangen, Germany) incorporating automatic registration, our system requires an amagnetic reference tool (BrainLab iopStar), which is firmly attached to the Mayfield clamp, but can be removed during scanning. The head is referenced in the usual manner, allowing for targeting the tumor and optimizing access to the lesion while sparing eloquent structures. Once the tumor approach is delineated, sterile prepping is done and the complex procedure of draping is performed. To accommodate rescanning, the surgical draping should keep the surgical field and its surroundings sterile, but not hinder the ability to move the patient into the MRI tunnel.

Surgical Procedure

Surgery is performed outside the 5-gauss line; therefore, all the usual neurosurgical instruments including the surgical microscope may be used. Standard neuronavigation is used as required. When the tumor has been exposed, ALA-fluorescence (Gliolan) guidance is used to maximize surgical tumor resection. Once ALA fluorescence has suggested that the HGG has been removed completely or nearly completely, the surgical field is covered with a sterile drape and the patient is turned, on the operating table, into the gantry of the MRI scanner. Bringing the patient from the surgical to the scanning position usually takes no more than 4 minutes.

Scanning is started with T2 sequences usually in all three planes, and depending on the information required additional scans and sequences are performed. Once the morphologic configuration of the surgically created tumor cavity suggests that the tumor has been indeed nearly completely removed, T1WIs without and with contrast are performed. The complete intraoperative imaging protocol includes an axial T2W sequence (repetition time/echo-time [TR/TE] = 4840/110; slice thickness 5 mm), diffusion-weighted imaging (TR/TE = 3900/84; echo-planar imaging [EPI] factor 15;

high b value = 1000 mm^2/s; low b value = 0 mm^2/s; slice thickness 5 mm), and T1WIs (TR/TE = 400/15; slice thickness 3.5–5 mm) in three planes before administering the contrast agent (20 mL gadolinium-DTPA; Schering, Berlin, Germany).

Subtraction images derived from this sequence allow for delineation of enhancing tumor remnants. These datasets can be transferred into the neuronavigation computer and used for rereferencing the surgical site and compensate for the brain-shift. In a further refinement, perfusion studies are also performed, which may show additional evidence of tumor remnants in repeat intraoperative studies.[50] This information may be used to better target tumor remnants. It depends on the software used whether the perfusion studies can be used immediately during continued surgery or afterward.

Once the patient is turned again into the operating position, another layer of sterile drapes is placed carefully, and surgery is continued. In most patients using combined ALA-fluorescence and iMRI, it is sufficient to perform one additional MRI study to see that the tumor has been completely removed. An additional series is needed only in cases involving a difficult tumor location and/or extension.

Because the entire surgery from induction of anesthesia until the end usually takes approximately 4 to 5 hours, secondary repeat scanning can be hindered by working hours; therefore, in about half of the patients the "very last" scan confirming radical removal of any contrast-enhancing lesion cannot be performed, so a control postoperative MRI scan is performed the next day.

If a complete scan is performed with wound closed and Mayfield clamp removed, the patient is scanned in the SENSE head coils (Philips Healthcare). This may be particularly helpful in patients operated on before a weekend or holidays.

Figure 12.1 demonstrates a right-handed patient with a left temporomesial GBM undergoing iMRI-guided resection to show the benefits and pitfalls of iMRI. Surgery was performed under general anesthesia as speech areas and fiber tracts demonstrated that no eloquent structures would be touched.

Results

The benefit of iMRI scanning in HGG patients is prolonged overall tumor-free survival with a high quality of life. However, this still needs to be proven by a randomized controlled possibly multicenter prospective trial. When we started using iMRI in our department, we used it in the initial phase preferentially in patients presenting with "difficult tumors" – mostly tumors located in the dominant hemisphere, close to eloquent areas, both in primary HGG and recurrent tumors – in addition to regular microsurgical techniques and neuronavigation. We continued to use regular microsurgical procedures and neuronavigation in the rest of our patients, when no surgical team familiar with the iMRI setting was available or in cases of emergency craniotomies.

In total, in the first period between September 2005 and October 2007, we performed 193 operations for gliomas. The patient population with the first surgery included 75 WHO grade IV gliomas and 28 WHO grade III gliomas. Among these 103 primary operations, 60 operations were performed using iMRI and 43 operations were performed using regular microsurgical techniques. The patients were analyzed retrospectively with regard to radicality of resection, and were followed prospectively in a regular fashion as outpatients, some of whom underwent second surgery as well.[51]

The degree of radical resection was higher using iMRI than not using it. Among 40 patients in whom iMRI surgery

was performed with the intention to radically remove the HGG, this was achieved in 37 cases (92.5%). This compared favorably to the 22 out of 27 (81, 4%) patients in whom radical resection was intended but not achieved, using regular microsurgical techniques.

All patients with HGG underwent conventional radiotherapy and additional chemotherapy with temozolomide (TMZ). No differences were discovered with regard to dosing TMZ. Kaplan-Meier survival curves were calculated for HGG (WHO grades III and IV) and for GBM patients WHO grade IV.

From **Fig. 12.2A** it is obvious that iMRI brings a significant benefit of a higher total survival time when HGG III and IV

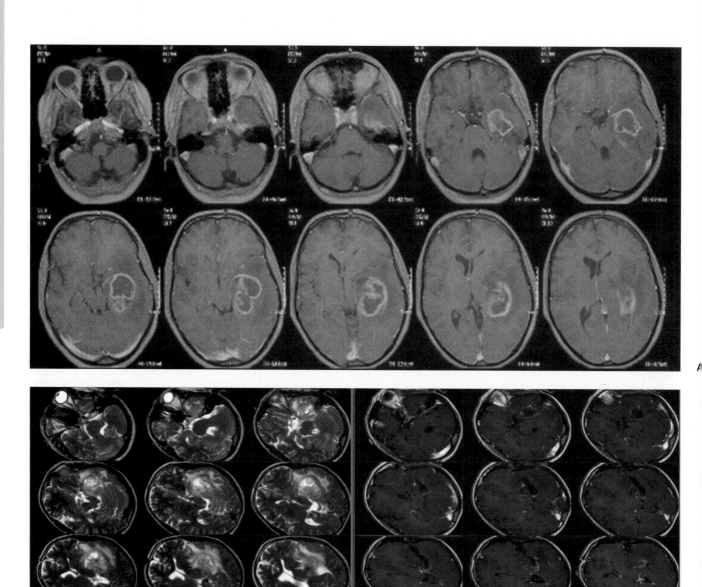

Fig. 12.1 Course of a patient with left temporal glioblastoma. Initially, she presented with headaches and speech disturbances. **(A)** Preoperative contrast-enhanced T1-weighted magnetic resonance imaging (T1W MRI) **(B)** iMRI: T2W MRI before opening the dura and contrast-enhanced T1W MRI after nearly complete tumor removal through transsylvian

approach. Some enhancing tumor remnants were removed until on aminolevulinic acid (ALA) fluorescence, no further tumor was seen. Histology confirmed glioblastoma multiforme (GBM); MGMT status negative, treatment with radiotherapy and temozolomide according to Stupp schema.

are pooled together. The median survival time increases from 10 to 37 months to 20 to 37 months. Nearly twice as many survivors at 36-month follow-up are noted in the iMRI group when compared with the non-iMRI patients.

However, this benefit is less clear, but still obvious when comparing only GBM patients (**Fig. 12.2B**). Nearly 17 (16 to 53) months of median survival in the iMRI group compare favorably to the 9 to 43 months of median survival in the non-iMRI group, but at 2-year follow-up both curves cross at 20% survival.

This, in our opinion, indicates that iMRI is definitely helpful in the initial phase when radical resection is of primary importance to obtain an early and intermediate good survival, but long-term treatment options need to be optimized to provide for long-term survival rates, and further therapies are required in this regard.

The radicality of surgical resection has always been linked to more neurologic impairment. Therefore, we also looked at the Karnofsky performance score (KPS) for our patients. Although KPS preop was slightly higher in the iMRI group than in the non-iMRI patients (83.02 ± 13.64 versus $75.56 \pm$), it fell to 74.44 ± 15.22 in the iMRI group as compared with 72.44 ± 20.02 in the non-iMRI patients. This means that KPS is not significantly different for either group.

The benefit of iMRI in the setting of recurrent HGG surgery is less clear. A reason may be – besides a smaller number leading to less statistically relevant conclusion— that radical tumor removal in recurrent HGG would result

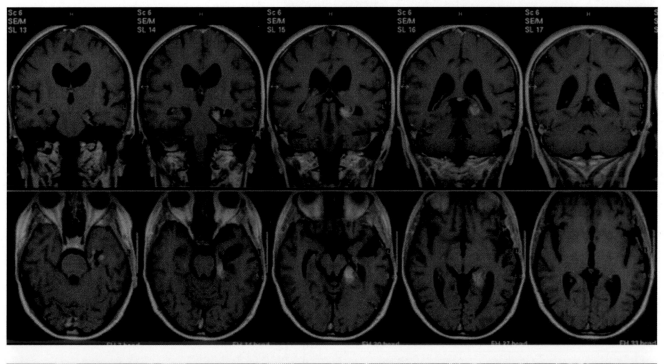

C

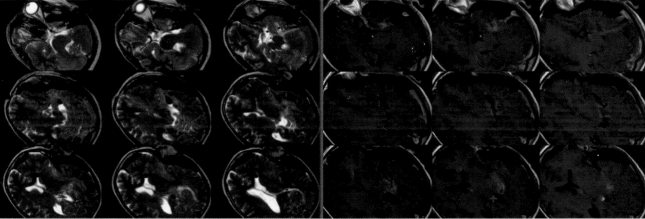

D

Fig. 12.1 (*Continued*) Course of a patient with left temporal glioblastoma. **(C)** Six months later on routine control, tumor enhancement was seen posterior to the initial tumor; neurologically normal. **(D)** Second surgery was suggested to the patient, again with iMRI and ALA fluorescence; and was performed using the same approach as previously: intermediate iMRI with T2W and T1W images, the later showing diffuse contrast enhancement making it difficult to distinguish tumor remnants, so tumor remnants were carefully removed until no further ALA fluorescence was seen.   (*Continued on page 114*)

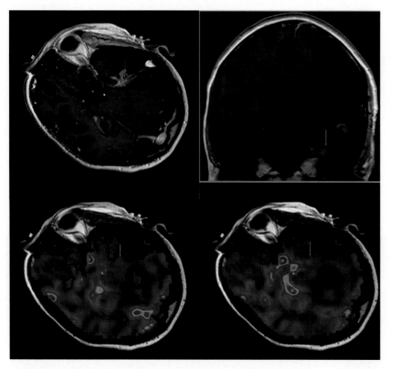

Fig. 12.1 (*Continued*) Course of a patient with left temporal glioblastoma. **(E)** Susceptibility contrast-weighted (iDSC-) MRI based on the final perfusion images shows tumor remnants better than regular contrast-enhanced T1W images both on cerebral blood volume (CBV) and cerebral blood flow (CBF). This correlates well with small contrast enhancing lesion on MRI 24 hours postoperatively: upper left iMRI, upper right post coronal section; below iCBV and CBF calculations of tumor remnant (thanks to Dr. Ulmer, Dept. of Neuroradiology, University Hosp Kiel.)

E

in a high number of patients with increased neurologic impairment.

Pitfalls and Questions

Repeat Scanning

The main question is how often an iMRI scan and what sequences should be performed. Using the Boston version of the low-field system ("double donut") where the surgeons stand in the scanner, or the Odin (now PoleStar, Medtronic Navigation, Inc., Louisville, CO) system, which can easily be brought up to the surgical field, frequent use during surgery is feasible, showing phenomena such as brain-shift and step-wise tumor removal. Using high-field systems this may be more cumbersome, and therefore one tries to limit the number of intraoperative scans to minimize surgical time while not limiting the benefit. Also the sequences used need to be defined. Obviously, it would be ideal to perform a standard set of sequences once the surgeon has felt that he has removed the glioma as radically as possible. If there are still some unexpected tumor remnants, after having removed

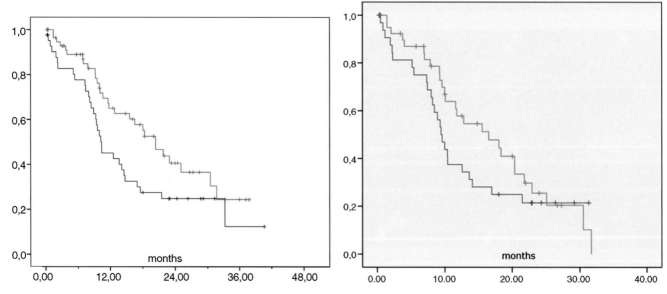

Fig. 12.2 Kaplan-Meier survival curves calculated based 103 primary HGG patients. *Green line* indicates use of intraoperative MRI (iMRI), *blue line* indicates no iMRI used; time line in months. **(A)** Grade III and IV patients pooled together. **(B)** Grade IV patients.

them as well, another set of sequences should be performed to prove the progress with repetition until "complete removal" has been achieved. However, besides the extension of precious surgical time and a certain risk of infection due to changing/adding drapes another problem might arise.

Repeat Contrast Application

Standard MRI scans with T1WI and T2WI, as well as DWI and PWI can be performed depending on the length of time that is deemed necessary to obtain adequate imaging. In patients with pituitary adenoma, the first intermediate scans can safely be obtained using only T2WIs because the diaphragma–chiasm relation can well be demonstrated in this modality. In HGG, contrast enhancement in T1WIs correlates well with active tumor and also with strong fluorescence under ALA; hence its disappearance is used to define radical tumor resection. As has been previously described by the Heidelberg group,[36] repeat contrast injection may hinder evaluation of contrast enhancement because contrast may diffuse into surrounding tissue over time, mainly due to surgical manipulations and an open blood–brain barrier. This time dependent phenomenon is shown in **Fig. 12.1D**. A technique with the potential to overcome this problem is dynamic susceptibility contrast weighted (iDSC-) MRI, based on a dynamic perfusion study (**Fig. 12.1E**).We

have used this protocol in a series of patients and were able to demonstrate even small tumor remnants.[50] When a bolus injection is given to the patient and a perfusion study is performed, tumor remnants can be well seen even in a second intraoperative imaging at a time distance of 1 hour or so. Special software (nordicICE; NordicNeuroLab, Bergen, Norway) on a dedicated computer is required, which then needs to be transferred back into the neuronavigation computer because the standard software on the Philips MRI scanner console is not sufficient to provide these calculations. Repeat performance should be possible, but has not yet been necessary in our limited series of patients.

Rereferencing

To overcome the problem of brain-shift (**Fig. 12.3**), iMRI is helpful; the data from repeat scanning need to be imported into the neuronavigation device. This sometimes cumbersome step entails image-fusion of the old and the new scans, which needs to be performed manually, for example, in turning the head in the first step before allowing automated rereferencing. This may be difficult for the computer software of the neuronavigation device; therefore, close attention must be given to this process before using the rereferenced data set for further surgery. Otherwise, the orientation of the fused scans may be useless.

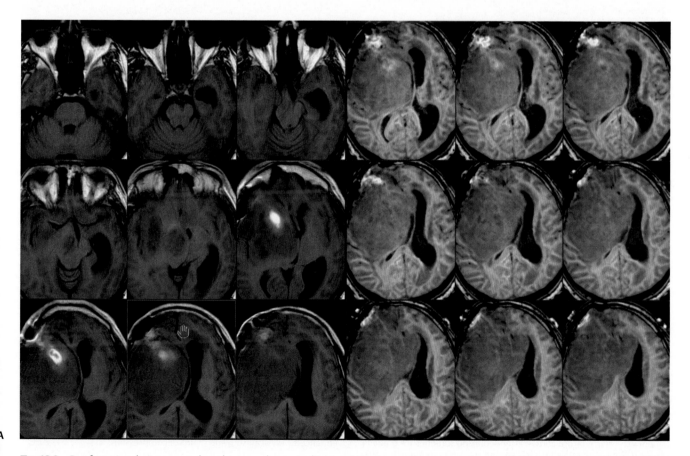

Fig. 12.3 Rereferencing during surgery based on a newly acquired intraoperative magnetic resonance imaging (iMRI) scan. Patient was referred from abroad after debulking surgeries for grade III glioma. **(A)** Preoperative T1-weighted (T1W) MRI and fiber tracking of pyramidal tract. *(Continued on page 116)*

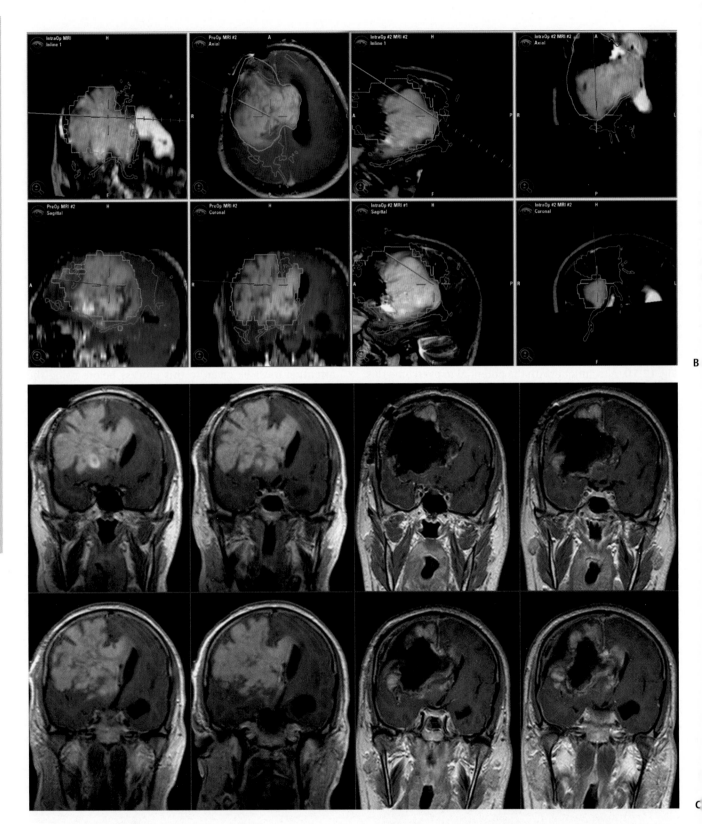

B

C

Fig. 12.3 (*Continued*) Rereferencing during surgery based on a newly acquired intraoperative magnetic resonance imaging (iMRI) scan. Patient was referred from abroad after debulking surgeries for grade III glioma. **(B)** Intraoperative first and second scans for rereferencing after initial debulking; pointer on the right side close to the pyramidal tract. **(C)** Preoperative and postoperative coronal sections on contrast-enhanced T1W scan showing major decompression.

Repeat Application of Diffusion Tensor Imaging

Although we routinely use the preoperatively acquired DTI datasets to define and integrate fiber tracts into surgical approach planning (**Fig. 12.3**), we have so far not applied repeat DTI[52–54] acquisition due to software deficits on our machine, which will be overcome shortly. It will be interesting to see what impact this technology may have upon surgery and its results on HGG. Hopefully, it will further the extent of radical resection while preserving the functions.

Safety and Comfort Issues

Although surgery may last a bit longer than usual, in our experience repeat MRI scanning is feasible with no additional harm to the patient with respect to infections due to turning the patient and bringing him or her into a basically unsterile MRI tunnel environment. The obstacle is overcome by a dedicated surgical team applying careful repeat draping. This can even be performed in patients undergoing awake craniotomy, although the warming effect of several layers of sterile drapes may be very unpleasant to the awake patient lying in the tunnel of the MRI scanner. This issue of patient safety and comfort has been addressed in a careful neuropsychological study from our group by Göbel et al[55] showing that attention to the patients' needs and caring for them before, during, and after surgery is of utmost importance. Our youngest patient who underwent awake craniotomy and iMRI was 15 years old and tolerated the procedure quite well. We even had patients undergoing repeat awake craniotomy with iMRI for tumor recurrence, but such a seemingly heroic approach is only suggested to a well-informed and cooperative patient and depends clearly on an excellent patient–surgeon relationship.

◆ Discussion

The experience gained by our group and our data as well as that of others clearly show that iMRI scanning is easily integrated into the setting of surgery for high-grade glioma. We have also shown the benefit of this additional technical adjunct even in high-grade glioma patients, improving short-term survival for those patients while preserving function and quality of life. Of course, the question arises whether the investment both in machine hardware and additional surgical time is worth it and to what extent it can be justified. We feel that this important question must be answered by each single institution and country depending on the economic situation. Also, low-field systems may find their place in HGG surgery, although high-field systems certainly offer better imaging qualities and additional options as outlined. More intelligent solutions may be found in the future such as multiuser MRI-rooms, more rapid surgical standard preparations, better dedicated software easing image fusions, perfusion studies, DTI integration into navigation,[52–54] modifications of surgically applicable contrast media – all finally leading to an economically optimized multifaceted surgicomedical approach to HGG. However, it is anticipated that the benefit of iMRI will become standard in a few years in specialized centers as has the use of the surgical microscope in the 20 years after its introduction into neurosurgery,[56] and more recently with neuronavigation, further improving the short-term survival for patients with high-grade gliomas and the long-term survival for low-grade glioma patients. Additional research is needed to better define indications for the use of iMRI in the setting of various gliomas and other surgical entities and to expand it into spine surgery. High-field MRI will become, on the other hand, a very useful tool to explore further surgical options such as guidance for catheter placement in the setting of convection-enhanced delivery of interstitially applicable drugs, to name only one promising example. More controlled multicenter studies might be helpful to get more precise information concerning the benefit of these advanced techniques using iMRI. The final fate of patients with intrinsic brain tumors, however, may depend on the progress of understanding tumor biology and the role of molecular markers such as p53, MGMT receptors, and others to develop adequate local therapy[57] without the side effects inherent in present day chemotherapies.

References

1. Mitchell P, Ellison DW, Mendelow AD. Surgery for malignant gliomas: mechanistic reasoning and slippery statistics. Lancet Neurol 2005;4(7):413–422
2. Kowalczuk A, Macdonald RL, Amidei C, et al. Quantitative imaging study of extent of surgical resection and prognosis of malignant astrocytomas. Neurosurgery 1997;41(5):1028–1036, discussion 1036–1038
3. Laws ER, Parney IF, Huang W, et al; Glioma Outcomes Investigators. Survival following surgery and prognostic factors for recently diagnosed malignant glioma: data from the Glioma Outcomes Project. J Neurosurg 2003;99(3):467–473
4. Durmaz R, Erken S, Arslanta_ A, Atasoy MA, Bal C, Tel E. Management of glioblastoma multiforme: with special reference to recurrence. Clin Neurol Neurosurg 1997;99(2):117–123
5. Stark AM, Nabavi A, Mehdorn HM, Blömer U. Glioblastoma multiforme-report of 267 cases treated at a single institution. Surg Neurol 2005;63(2):162–169, discussion 169
6. Pauleit D, Langen KJ, Floeth F, et al. Can the apparent diffusion coefficient be used as a noninvasive parameter to distinguish tumor tissue from peritumoral tissue in cerebral gliomas? J Magn Reson Imaging 2004;20(5):758–764
7. Jenkinson MD, Du Plessis DG, Walker C, Smith TS. Advanced MRI in the management of adult gliomas. Br J Neurosurg 2007;21(6): 550–561 Review
8. Gössl C, Fahrmeir L, Pütz B, Auer LM, Auer DP. Fiber tracking from DTI using linear state space models: detectability of the pyramidal tract. Neuroimage 2002;16(2):378–388
9. Le Bihan D, Mangin JF, Poupon C, et al. Diffusion tensor imaging: concepts and applications. J Magn Reson Imaging 2001;13(4):534–546 Review
10. Jeremic B, Grujicic D, Antunovic V, Djuric L, Stojanovic M, Shibamoto Y. Influence of extent of surgery and tumor location on treatment outcome of patients with glioblastoma multiforme treated with combined modality approach. J Neurooncol 1994;21(2):177–185
11. Yoshida J, Kajita Y, Wakabayashi T, Sugita K. Long-term follow-up results of 175 patients with malignant glioma: importance of radical tumour resection and postoperative adjuvant therapy with interferon, ACNU and radiation. Acta Neurochir (Wien) 1994;127(1-2): 55–59
12. Rostomily RC, Spence AM, Duong D, McCormick K, Bland M, Berger MS. Multimodality management of recurrent adult malignant gliomas: results of a phase II multiagent chemotherapy study and analysis of cytoreductive surgery. Neurosurgery 1994;35(3):378–388, discussion 388

13. Obwegeser A, Ortler M, Seiwald M, Ulmer H, Kostron H. Therapy of glioblastoma multiforme: a cumulative experience of 10 years. Acta Neurochir (Wien) 1995;137(1-2):29–33

14. Stark AM, Hedderich J, Held-Feindt J, Mehdorn HM. Glioblastoma—the consequences of advanced patient age on treatment and survival. Neurosurg Rev 2007;30(1):56–61, discussion 61–62

15. Vuorinen V, Hinkka S, Färkkilä M, Jääskeläinen J. Debulking or biopsy of malignant glioma in elderly people - a randomised study. Acta Neurochir (Wien) 2003;145(1):5–10

16. Salcman M. Surgical resection of malignant brain tumors: who benefits? Oncology (Williston Park) 1988;2(8):47–56, 59–60, 63 (Williston Park)

17. Pang BC, Wan WH, Lee CK, Khu KJ, Ng WH. The role of surgery in high-grade glioma—is surgical resection justified? A review of the current knowledge. Ann Acad Med Singapore 2007;36(5):358–363 Review

18. Finlay JL, Wisoff JH. The impact of extent of resection in the management of malignant gliomas of childhood. Childs Nerv Syst 1999;15(11-12):786–788

19. Shinoda J, Sakai N, Murase S, Yano H, Matsuhisa T, Funakoshi T. Selection of eligible patients with supratentorial glioblastoma multiforme for gross total resection. J Neurooncol 2001;52(2):161–171

20. Tonn JC. Awake craniotomy for monitoring of language function: benefits and limits. Acta Neurochir (Wien) 2007;149(12):1197–1198

21. Pinsker MO, Nabavi A, Mehdorn HM. Neuronavigation and resection of lesions located in eloquent brain areas under local anesthesia and neuropsychological-neurophysiological monitoring. Minim Invasive Neurosurg 2007;50(5):281–284

22. Nimsky C, Ganslandt O, Cerny S, Hastreiter P, Greiner G, Fahlbusch R. Quantification of, visualization of, and compensation for brain shift using intraoperative magnetic resonance imaging. Neurosurgery 2000;47(5):1070–1079, discussion 1079–1080

23. Nabavi A, Black PM, Gering DT, et al. Serial intraoperative magnetic resonance imaging of brain shift. Neurosurgery 2001;48(4):787–797, discussion 797–798

24. Wirtz CR, Albert FK, Schwaderer M, et al. The benefit of neuronavigation for neurosurgery analyzed by its impact on glioblastoma surgery. Neurol Res 2000;22(4):354–360

25. Engelland K. Influence of the use of neuronavigation upon the clinical course and quality of life in patients with intrinsic brain tumors. Diss., Medical Fac Kiel: 2001

26. Litofsky NS, Bauer AM, Kasper RS, Sullivan CM, Dabbous OH; Glioma Outcomes Project Investigators. Image-guided resection of high-grade glioma: patient selection factors and outcome. Neurosurg Focus 2006;20(4):E16

27. Stummer W, Novotny A, Stepp H, Goetz C, Bise K, Reulen HJ. Fluorescence-guided resection of glioblastoma multiforme by using 5-aminolevulinic acid-induced porphyrins: a prospective study in 52 consecutive patients. J Neurosurg 2000;93(6):1003–1013

28. Stummer W, Pichlmeier U, Meinel T, Wiestler OD, Zanella F, Reulen HJ; ALA-Glioma Study Group. Fluorescence-guided surgery with 5-aminolevulinic acid for resection of malignant glioma: a randomised controlled multicentre phase III trial. Lancet Oncol 2006;7(5):392–401

29. Stummer W, Reulen HJ, Meinel T, et al; ALA-Glioma Study Group. Extent of resection and survival in glioblastoma multiforme: identification of and adjustment for bias. Neurosurgery 2008;62(3):564–576, discussion 564–576

30. Lindner D, Trantakis C, Renner C, et al. Application of intraoperative 3D ultrasound during navigated tumor resection. Minim Invasive Neurosurg 2006;49(4):197–202

31. Rasmussen IA Jr, Lindseth F, Rygh OM, et al. Functional neuronavigation combined with intra-operative 3D ultrasound: initial experiences during surgical resections close to eloquent brain areas and future directions in automatic brain shift compensation of preoperative data. Acta Neurochir (Wien) 2007;149(4):365–378

32. Tronnier VM, Bonsanto MM, Staubert A, Knauth M, Kunze S, Wirtz CR. Comparison of intraoperative MR imaging and 3D-navigated ultrasonography in the detection and resection control of lesions. Neurosurg Focus 2001;10(2):E3

33. Schwartz RB, Hsu L, Kacher DF, et al. Intraoperative dynamic MRI: localization of sites of brain tumor recurrence after high-dose radiotherapy. J Magn Reson Imaging 1998;8(5):1085–1089

34. Hall WA, Martin AJ, Liu H, et al. High-field strength interventional magnetic resonance imaging for pediatric neurosurgery. Pediatr Neurosurg 1998;29(5):253–259

35. Hall WA, Martin AJ, Liu H, Nussbaum ES, Maxwell RE, Truwit CL. Brain biopsy using high-field strength interventional magnetic resonance imaging. Neurosurgery 1999;44(4):807–813, discussion 813–814 Review

36. Knauth M, Wirtz CR, Tronnier VM, Aras N, Kunze S, Sartor K. Intraoperative MR imaging increases the extent of tumor resection in patients with high-grade gliomas. AJNR Am J Neuroradiol 1999;20(9):1642–1646

37. Fahlbusch R, Ganslandt O, Nimsky C. Intraoperative imaging with open magnetic resonance imaging and neuronavigation. Childs Nerv Syst 2000;16(10-11):829–831

38. Nimsky C, Ganslandt O, Von Keller B, Romstöck J, Fahlbusch R. Intraoperative high-field-strength MR imaging: implementation and experience in 200 patients. Radiology 2004;233(1):67–78

39. Archip N, Clatz O, Whalen S, et al. Compensation of geometric distortion effects on intraoperative magnetic resonance imaging for enhanced visualization in image-guided neurosurgery. Neurosurgery 2008;62(3, Suppl 1)209–215, discussion 215–216

40. Oh DS, Black PM. A low-field intraoperative MRI system for glioma surgery: is it worthwhile? Neurosurg Clin N Am 2005;16(1):135–141 Review

41. Schulder M, Carmel PW. Intraoperative magnetic resonance imaging: impact on brain tumor surgery. Cancer Control 2003;10(2):115–124

42. Schulder M, Salas S, Brimacombe M, et al. Cranial surgery with an expanded compact intraoperative magnetic resonance imager. Technical note. J Neurosurg 2006;104(4):611–617

43. Claus EB, Horlacher A, Hsu L, et al. Survival rates in patients with low-grade glioma after intraoperative magnetic resonance image guidance. Cancer 2005;103(6):1227–1233

44. Martin AJ, Hall WA, Liu H, et al. Brain tumor resection: intraoperative monitoring with high-field-strength MR imaging-initial results. Radiology 2000;215(1):221–228

45. Schneider JP, Schulz T, Schmidt F, et al. Gross-total surgery of supratentorial low-grade gliomas under intraoperative MR guidance. AJNR Am J Neuroradiol 2001;22(1):89–98

46. Schneider JP, Trantakis C, Schulz T, Dietrich J, Kahn T. [Intraoperative use of an open mid-field MR scanner in the surgical treatment of cerebral gliomas]. Z Med Phys 2003;13(3):214–218

47. Knauth M, Wirtz CR, Aras N, Sartor K. Low-field interventional MRI in neurosurgery: finding the right dose of contrast medium. Neuroradiology 2001;43(3):254–258

48. Nabavi A, Dörner L, Stark AM, Mehdorn HM. Intraoperative MRI with 1.5 Tesla in neurosurgery. Neurosurg Clin N Am 2009;20(2):163–171

49. Nabavi A, Goebel S, Doerner L, Warneke N, Ulmer S, Mehdorn M. Awake craniotomy and intraoperative magnetic resonance imaging: patient selection, preparation, and technique. Top Magn Reson Imaging 2009;19(4):191–196

50. Ulmer S, Helle M, Jansen O, Mehdorn HM, Nabavi A. Intraoperative dynamic susceptibility contrast weighted magnetic resonance imaging (iDSC-MRI) - Technical considerations and feasibility. Neuroimage 2009;45(1):38–43

51. Schwartz F, Dawirs N, Hedderich D, Nabavi A, Mehdorn HM. The effect of ioMRI on survival of high grade glioma patients. In preparation (2009)

52. Nimsky C, Ganslandt O, Fahlbusch R. Implementation of fiber tract navigation. Neurosurgery 2006; 58(4 Suppl 2)ONS-292–ONS-303

53. Nimsky C, Ganslandt O, Hastreiter P, et al. Preoperative and intraoperative diffusion tensor imaging-based fiber tracking in glioma surgery. Neurosurgery 2007; 61(1, Suppl)178–185, discussion 186

54. Ozawa N, Muragaki Y, Nakamura R, Lseki H. Intraoperative diffusion-weighted imaging for visualization of the pyramidal tracts. Part II: clinical study of usefulness and efficacy. Minim Invasive Neurosurg 2008;51(2):67–71

55. Goebel S, Nabavi A, Schubert S, Mehdorn HM: Patient perception of combined awake brain tumour surgery and intraoperative 1.5-T-MRI: The Kiel experience. Submitted to Neurosurgery; 2009)

56. Yasargil MG. Microsurgery Applied to Neurosurgery. New York: Thieme Medical Publishers; 1967

57. Hall WA. Extending survival in gliomas: surgical resection or immunotherapy? Surg Neurol 2004;61(2):145–148

13

Pituitary Tumor Resection–iMRI in Transsphenoidal Surgery

Rudolf Fahlbusch and Vincenzo Paternó

Despite ongoing advances in pharmacologic treatment and radiotherapeutic management, especially of hormonally active pituitary adenomas, surgery remains the therapy of choice for the large majority of these tumors and it is the first treatment of choice in hormonally inactive tumors. Among the advanced technologies in transsphenoidal surgery, neuronavigation,[1–6] endoscopy,[7,8] and especially intraoperative magnetic resonance imaging (iMRI)[1,9–16] are remarkable adjuvant techniques that have been introduced into the operating room (OR) in recent years. Intraoperative imaging is used as an immediate intraoperative quality control, evaluating the extent of tumor removal during the surgical procedure and allowing us to extend resections in those cases where tumor remnants are documented.[9–12,14–16] Using low-field and especially high-field 1.5 tesla (T) iMRI scanners during the surgical treatment, it's possible to find that up to one-third of pituitary macroadenomas, suprasellar tumor remnants as small as 3 to 4 mm, as well as larger adenoma remnants were hidden to the surgeon's eye in folds of the descending sellar diaphragm.

The first intraoperative imaging modality used during transsphenoidal surgery was x-ray fluoroscopy,[17] limited by the fact that only bony structures of the cranium were visible. In an early attempt to estimate indirectly the extent of tumor removal, intraoperative gas cisternography was used. First attempts for a direct evaluation of the effects of transsphenoidal surgery started in the 1980s with the application of ultrasound[18,19] and computed tomography (CT).[20] Unfortunately, these early attempts were not encouraging because of the restricted quality of the intraoperative images. In the mid-1990s, the development of an open MRI system made iMRI possible for the first time. This application was pioneered by Black et al,[21] who operated in a continuously running magnetic field using the so-called double doughnut system. In the 0.2 tesla open-MRI installations in Erlangen and Heidelberg, the patient was transported into the magnet, while surgery was performed outside the strong magnetic field. The evolution from low-field MRI scanners to high-field MRI scanners definitely revolutionized intraoperative imaging in transsphenoidal surgery with regard to resection control and high-quality intraoperative images. High-field MRI has a clear advantage in image quality compared with the intraoperative low- and midfield MRI systems (0.12–0.5 T).[22]

Not only patients with large tumors but also smaller adenomas, especially developing against and into the cavernous sinus can profit from iMRI control.

Morphologically radical tumor resection is a prerequisite for endocrine remission in normally smaller hormonally active tumors, in acromegaly, and Cushing disease.

iMRI increases the rate of complete tumor removal and endocrine normalization and improves endocrine outcome to "nearly normalization."[23] In the case of a biochemical cure of growth hormone secreting tumors in acromegaly, follow-up MRI scans may not even be required if endocrine parameters are controlled because no tumor remnant will be visible.[24] In nonfunctioning tumors, there are no hormonal markers available that would allow an early prognosis of outcome. A morphologic assessment of the radicality of the tumor resection is still required as the most sensitive diagnostic tool. Because of immediate postoperative artifacts, this information can only be gained some 2 to 3 months after the operation.[25]

◆ Operating Room Set-up

Today different industry companies offer low-field (0.15 T – Medtronic Navigation, Inc., Louisville, CO; 0.2 T – Siemens AG, Erlangen, Germany), mid-field (0.3 T – Hitachi Medical Corp., Tokyo, Japan; 0.5 T – General Electric Medical Systems, Waukesha, WI), high-field (1.5 T – General Electric,

Philips Healthcare, Andover, MA], Siemens), and ultra-high-field (3.0 T – General Electric, Philips, Siemens).

The senior author (RF) started with 0.2 T system (Magnetom Open, Siemens) in 1996, followed by 1.5 T system (Sonata, Siemens) in 2002 in Erlangen.

We now present our actual system, the INI Brain Suite, an operating theater with a 1.5 T Magnetom Espree scanner (Siemens), which was installed in 2006/2007 at the International Neuroscience Institute INI (Hannover, Germany).

This is a high-field MRI scanner with a superconductive 1.5 T magnet with a length of 160 cm and an inner bore diameter of 70 cm equipped with a gradient system with a field strength of up to 40 millitesla per meter (mT/m; effective 69 mT/m) and a slew rate of up to 200 T/m/s effective. This was the first "open" 1.5 T MRI, used for therapeutic purposes.

A rotatable surgical table (Trumpf, Saalfeld, Germany) is adapted to the scanner to allow for a special surgical MRI tabletop. This surgical table can be locked into various positions. The principal surgical position is at 160 degrees with the patient's head at the 5 gauss (G) line (distance of 4 meters to the center of the scanner). As soon as the rotating mechanism has been locked, the height of the table, the angle of tilt, and the lateral tilt can be modified. The table movements are controlled remotely. Only the rotation about the table axis to turn the table into the axis of the scanner is performed manually, for safety reasons.

MRI-compatible ventilation (Aestiva 5/MRI, General Electric, Hannover, Germany) and MRI-compatible monitoring are available for control of anesthesia and for wireless 2.4 GHz data transfer from the radiofrequency- (RF-) shielded cabin. The perfusion and infusion pumps are shielded for MRI compatibility.

After starting with the NC4 Zeiss Multivision microscope, which was installed at the left side of the head, outside of the 5 G line, we are working now with the ceiling mounted Pentero C Multivision microscope (Zeiss, Oberkochen, Germany). The holding device is placed in the middle line within the 5 G line, the microscope itself can have a flexible position in connection with the preferred position of the operating field (to the best of our knowledge, we tested this MRI-compatible ceiling-mounted Zeiss Pentero system for the first time).

If navigation is indicated in transsphenoidal surgery (encased arteries, loss of anatomic landmarks in second operation), we use the BrainLab integrated VectorVision Sky Navigation System (BrianLab, Heimstetten, Germany) with roof-fixed infrared camera and touch screen display. The patient is fixed in a special ceramic head holding system (**Fig. 13.1A**) and the registration is done automatically through an integrated special coils system. A fiberoptic connection ensures MRI-compatible integration into the RF room. The camera used to monitor the positions of the microscope and other instruments is ceiling-mounted, as is the touch screen, which is used to operate the navigation system. Two 50-inch flat-screen monitors (Braco) mounted on the left wall of the Brain Suite are available for viewing the images from the microscope and the MRI console, as well as various software applications. The microscope videos are documented using Medimage software (Vepro, Pfungstadt, Germany) and in parallel in the MRI control room. The electric current to the microscope and to other devices that may interfere with the MRI signal is automatically switched off during MR imaging. The 0.5 mT and 20 mT lines are marked on the floor. The 20 mT line also is marked with a raised stainless steel strip as a physical threshold. The instruments table and the various rotating stools (Trumpf) are fully MRI compatible. The procedures for emergency magnet quenching and for monitoring of oxygen levels in the operating room are the same as those in standard clinical MRI installations.

◆ Transsphenoidal Surgery and iMRI

In general, the great majority of tumors operated via transsphenoidal approach do not require head fixation. Imaging is performed using a standard U-shaped large flexible coil that is adapted and draped to the head (**Fig. 13.1B**). The surgeon, who prefers Cushing's positioning for transsphenoidal surgery, is standing behind the patient's head in **Fig. 13.1C**. A schematic outline of the operating room was published previously.[11,26]

The whole transsphenoidal procedure is identical to that performed in regular operating rooms. Besides the sublabial and unilateral paraseptal approach to the sphenoidal sinus, we prefer in general the direct pernasal transsphenoidal approach with endoscope assistance. Porcelain-coated drills are used—especially to avoid metal artifacts during imaging—to open the sphenoidal sinus and to remove the sellar floor. Transsphenoidal surgery is routinely accompanied by endonasal endoscope using 0 degree and 30 degree, 4-mm rigid endoscopes by visualizing the surgical site on a ceiling-mounted monitor or in the eyepiece of the microscope. Selective adenomectomy was performed in all patients. In general, regular operating micro instruments are used during the transsphenoidal surgery at the 5 G line. In contrast to earlier years when we used MRI-compatible nasal speculum for intraoperative imaging, the direct endoscopic-assisted endonasal approach allows us examinations without the speculum, just installing simple cotton as a place holder in the nasal cavity. If necessary, especially in cases with defects of diaphragm sellar and cerebrospinal fluid (CFS) leaks, the sellar floor was covered at the end of surgery with muscle fascia and/or subcutaneous fat tissue, which was obtained during the same surgical session from the right thigh positioned at the border of the 5 G perimeter. Therefore, in the case of intraoperative CSF leakage, a transitory lumbar drainage was administered. In direct pernasal surgery, no nasal packing is necessary.

The timing of intraoperative imaging is decided by the neurosurgeon; intraoperative imaging is performed either when he has the impression of complete tumor removal or, in the case of incomplete tumor removal, when he thinks no further removal at this stage of surgery is possible using the transsphenoidal approach. Just before intraoperative imaging, the opened sellar floor is covered with a flat piece of bone

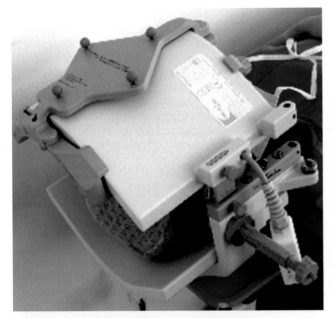

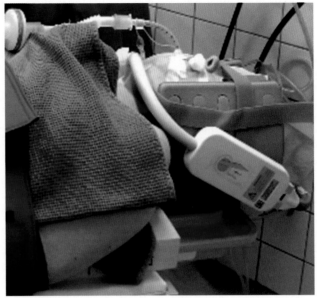

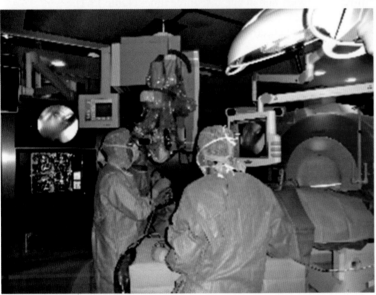

Fig. 13.1 **(A)** Rigid navigated magnetic resonance (MR) coil is used to fix the head during all surgical procedures. **(B)** Flexible MR coil is placed around the head, so the head can be moved during surgery without restrictions; a coil-preamplifier is attached to the flexible coil with tape. **(C)** Intraoperative scenario of our MR imaging (MRI-) operating room for microneurosurgical procedures. The head is placed at the 5 gauss red line; the surgeon is standing behind the head (Cushing's position). The microscope and its associated monitor are fixed on the roof of the operating theater, on the left side of the surgeon; the instrument tables with endoscope and as well the nurses are stationed on the right side of the surgeon. The anesthesiologist's workstation is located in the right corner of the operating theater, opposite the MRI table end. The circuit for the endotracheal tube is connected to an MRI-compatible anesthesia machine. Many standard surgical instruments can be used between the 5- and 20-gauss magnetic field lines. Two 50´ plasma monitors are collocated on the left wall of the operating theater. A movable MRI-compatible navigation monitor and infrared navigation arm is located close to the left middle part of right wall of the operating theater. An extra 21´ liquid crystal display (LCD) monitor is fixed on the roof on the left side of the operating theater.

wax for better delineation of the sellar outlines in the intraoperative images, minimizing artifacts caused by blood from the sphenoid sinus or the nasal cavity. Then, the surgical site is covered with a sterile drape, and the MRI table is rotated 160 degrees into the scanner. The time between the decision for iMRI and the actual start of imaging is ~2 minutes.

After the patient is moved into the center of the scanner, certain circuits are switched off, including the fluorescent lamps and the operating microscope. The imaging starts with a localizer sequence (field of view [FOV]: 280 mm; repetition time [TR]: 20 milliseconds; time [TE]: 50 milliseconds; scan time: 9 seconds). T2-weighted (T2W) half Fourier single-shot turbo spin echo sequences (slice thickness: 5 mm; FOV: 230 mm; TR: 1000 milliseconds; TE: 89 milliseconds; scan time: 25 seconds at five acquisitions) in coronal and sagittal orientation are measured next to

give a quick overview. Afterward, T1-weighted (T1W) coronal and sagittal spin echo sequences are applied (slice thickness: 3 mm; FOV: 270 mm; TR: 450 milliseconds; TE: 12 milliseconds; scan time: 4 minutes 57 seconds at four acquisitions). In addition, high-resolution T2W turbo-spin echo sequence with an in-plane resolution of 0.6 × 0.4 mm are measured (slice thickness: 3 mm; FOV: 230 mm; TR: 4000 milliseconds; TE: 97 milliseconds; scan time: 6 minutes 6 seconds at 3 acquisitions).

If the intraoperative imaging depicts some remaining tumor (which was not detected by endoscopic inspection before) that appears to be accessible for further resection, surgery is continued. After further resection, a repeated iMRI scan is performed before closure. The identical imaging protocol is applied for preoperative, as well as postoperative imaging in the first week after surgery and after 3 months.

Scanning at the identical pre- and intraoperative image slice position allowed a good comparison of pre- and intraoperative images in a side-by-side display. So fibrin glue, applied for hemostasis, could be identified and differentiated from tumor remnants. Furthermore, the use of porcelain-coated drills prevented extensive drilling artifacts, which would otherwise obscure image interpretation. Because T2W imaging proved to be superior in the identification of tumor remnants and additional T1W imaging did not provide any further information, T1W imaging was omitted from the intraoperative imaging protocol in most of the patients.

The criteria for selecting these patients were pituitary macroadenoma with or without suprasellar extension. All patients had preoperative high-field MRI, contrast-enhanced scans focused on the sellar region to diagnose the extent of tumor growth and invasion of adjacent structures.

In tumors with parasellar extension, we differentiated between (a) displacement of the cavernous sinus, (b) focal invasiveness with focal protrusion through the middle wall of the cavernous sinus, and (c) general invasiveness. Tumor parts located in the lateral part of the cavernous sinus, lateral from the carotid artery were regarded as not total resectable (NTR).

Patients with nonsecreting residual tumor remnants were followed closely with postoperative MRI; if tumor growth was detected, patients were scheduled for stereotactic radiosurgery. In patients with secreting tumors, further medical and/or stereotactic radiosurgery was recommended.

Although various pathologic process in the parasellar region, for example craniopharyngioma, are profiting from iMRI control during and after resection, be it via a frontolateral craniotomy or a transsphenoidal approach.

Here we will mainly focus on transsphenoidal resection of pituitary adenomas.

◆ Current Results

Between February 2007 and March 2009, a consecutive series of 38 patients (12 female and 26 male; 10 to 84 years of age) with pituitary macroadenomas underwent transsphenoidal surgery at the International Neuroscience Institute. To evaluate the extent of tumor removal, high-field MRI was performed during sella exploration once in 25 cases, in 10 cases twice, and in one case three times (**Table 13.1**).

All patients underwent a sophisticated preoperative and postoperative endocrinologic and ophthalmologic evaluation.

Table 13.1 Preoperative and Postoperative Endocrinologic and Ophthalmologic Evaluation of Patients with Pituitary Macroadenomas

P	Age/ sex	Tumor size	Tumor type	CSI	Pr.op/rec.	Goal	iop1 MRI	iop2 MRI	TR	Post PF	PG
1	34/M	40 mm	Atyp GH-PRL	R	/	NTR	r-CS	NTR	NTR	N	L
2	30/W	25 mm	PRL	N	/	TR	l-SS	TR	TR	PI	N
3	84/W	21 mm	Apo-NS	B	/	NTR	SS/CS	/	NTR	N	L
4	65/M	23 mm	Apo-NS	N	/	TR	aS/bD	TR	TR	PI	L
5	60/M	25 mm	NS	N	/	TR	rL/mCS	/	TR	PI	N
6	56/M	18 mm	NS	R	+	NTR	NTR	NTR	NTR	PI	L
7	34/M	21 mm	NS	N	/	TR	NTR	TR	TR	N	L
8	20/M	62 mm	PRL	L	+	NTR	NTR	/	NTR	PI	R
9	36/W	12 mm	GH-NS	R	+	NTR	NTR	/	NTR	PI	L
10	57/W	18 mm	NS	N	/	TR	TR	/	TR	PI	LP
11	23/M	15 mm	GH	R	+	NTR	NTR	NTR	NTR	PI	L
12	16/W	16 mm	NS	N	+	NTR	NTR	/	NTR	PI	/
13	52/M	83 mm	PRL	L	/	NTR	TR	/	TR	PI	R
14	60/M	27 mm	NS	L	+	NTR	TR	/	TR	PI	R
15	59/W	29 mm	NS	R	+	NTR	NTR	/	NTR	PI	L
16	10/M	10 mm	GH-PRL	B	/	NTR	NTR	/	NTR	PI	R
17	36/M	18 mm	PRL	L	/	NTR	NTR	/	NTR	PI	R
18	59/M	40 mm	NS	R	/	NTR	NTR	/	NTR	N	L
19	59/M	25 mm	NS	R	/	NTR	NTR	/	NTR	PI	L
20	51/M	15 mm	GH-PRL	B	/	TR	TR	/	TR	PI	MF
21	44/M	15 mm	GH-PRL	R	/	TR	TR	/	TR	PI	L
22	48/M	14 mm	GH	N	/	TR	TR	/	TR	PI	L

P	Age/ sex	Tumor size	Tumor type	CSI	Pr.op/rec.	Goal	iop1 MRI	iop2 MRI	TR	Post PF	PG
23	37/W	15 mm	GH	N	+	TR	NTR	TR	TR	PI	L
24	44/M	38 mm	NS	N	/	TR	NTR	TR	TR	PI	L
25	68/M	62 mm	NS	N	/	TR	TR	/	TR	PI	N
26	62/W	30 mm	NS	R	/	TR	NTR	TR	TR	PI	ML
27	60/M	80 mm	Atyp-NS	B	/	TR	NTR	NTR/TR	TR	PI	ML
28	48/M	30 mm	NS	R	+	TR	NTR	TR	TR	PI	ML
29	60/W	17 mm	NS	N	/	TR	TR	/	TR	PI	M
30	60/M	17 mm	ACTH	R	/	TR	TR	/	TR	PI	L
31	51/M	30 mm	NS	R	/	TR	TR	/	TR	PI	M
32	59/M	37 mm	NS	N	/	TR	TR	/	TR	PI	N
33	55/M	10 mm	GH	R	/	TR	TR	/	TR	PI	ssL
34	60/W	42 mm	NS	N	/	TR	TR	/	TR	ND	L
35	37/W	10 mm	PRL	N	/	TR	TR	/	TR	PI	L
36	66/M	20 mm	NS	N	+	TR	TR	/	TR	PI	ssR

Abbreviations: P, patient; Tumor size, the largest adenoma extension in one direction; Tumor type, the clinical function status of the adenoma; NS, no secreting, LH–FSH subtype included; GH, growth hormone secreting adenoma; PR, prolactin secreting adenoma; Apo, apoplexy; Atyp, atypical; CSI, cavernous sinus invasion; N, no invasion; R, right invasion; L, left invasion; B, bilateral invasion; Pre.op/rec, previous operation/ recurrence): / (no previous operation) and + (previously operated / recurrence); Goal, preoperative surgical goals; TR, total tumor removal; NTR, no total tumor removal; iop1 MRI, first intraoperative magnetic resonance imaging control; r/l CS, right/left cavernous sinus remnant tumor; – r/l SS, right/left suprasellar remnant tumor; SS/CS, suprasellar-lateral cavernous sinus remnant tumor; rL/mCS, lateral right remnant tumor in a dissenting fold of the diaphragm sellar and in the upper middle wall of the cavernous sinus; aS/bD, anterior to the sellar and below the diaphragm); iop2 MRI, second intraoperative magnetic resonance imaging control; TR, total tumor removal; NTR, no total tumor removal; TR, tumor resection; TR, total tumor removal; NTR, no total tumor removal; Post-PF, postoperative pituitary function; N, normal; PI, partial insufficiency; TI, total insufficiency; DI, diabetes insipidus; PG, pituitary gland collocation in the sella region; N, normal collocated; L, shift of the pituitary to the left; R, shift of the pituitary to the right; ML, mediolateral; SS-R, (suprasellar on the right) – / (not defined).

Endocrinologic findings were documented as partial pituitary functions (hypogonadism, hypothyroidism, hypocortisolism, and diabetes insipidus).

Before surgery, all patients gave their informed consent for iMRI.

Tumor visualization with the high-field 1.5 tesla iMRI Espree scanner under anesthesia showed a very good, even better congruency with the preoperative high-field MRI (1.5 tesla) and ultra high-filed MRI (3.0 tesla) scans.

Preoperatively we distinguished between totally and nontotally resectable tumors. Nontotal resection was defined in tumors, invading the lateral wall of the cavernous sinus, in asymmetrical and suprasellar tumors, as well as generally invasive pituitary adenomas. In eight patients (21%), in which tumors had encased carotid arteries and/or the sphenoid sinus was only poorly pneumatized, we used the integrated navigation system for the surgical approach and tumor removal intraoperative guidance.

Figure 13.2 gives an overview of the results and consequences of intraoperative MRI in all 36 patients. In this series, 20 of 38 patients (53%) had uni- or bilateral cavernous sinus invasion on preoperative MRI. Therefore, intended complete resection was considered to be possible only in 26 of 38 patients (68%). According to tumor residuals, detected by iMRI, surgery was continued in 11 of these 38 patients (29%). An additional tumor resection

was possible in 8 of 24 patients (33.3%) with intended complete tumor resection. In 2 of 13 patients (15.4%), in whom incomplete tumor resection was initially planned, total resectability was achieved; depending on the intraoperative finding, no extensive invasion but displacement of the cavernous sinus was found.

In 11 patients (29%), iMRI control showed accessible residual tumors leading to further resection, 8 of them achieved a complete resection. After tumor resection, the final iMRI scan documented adequate decompression of the optic pathway in all the patients (100%).

Implementation of iMRI led to an increased operation time of 20 or 40 minutes, depending on one or two MRI control procedures, respectively.

Sensitivity of the iMRI was 100% for suprasellar, intrasellar, right and left parasellar regions.

In five patients (13%), the intraoperative interpretation of iMRI was equivocal; thus it was difficult to distinguish between very small tumor remnants and perioperative changes such as artifacts (blood, fibrin glue).

Comparison of high-field MRI performed intraoperatively and 3 months later demonstrated very high predictive value that was already on intraoperative examination (preoperative = intraoperative = 3-months postoperative MRI). This includes our current experience that postoperative MRI scans, performed 3 months after the operation, are for the

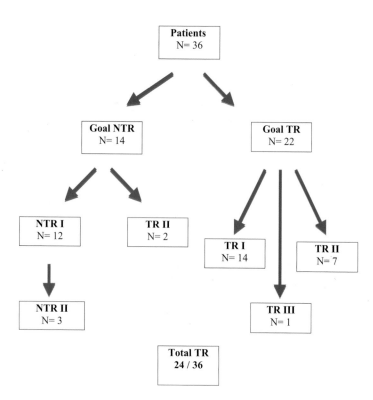

Fig. 13.2 Overview of the result of the 36 patients undergoing high-field intraoperative magnetic resonance imaging (iMRI). In a group of 36 patients, we planned preoperatively to achieve total tumor resection (TR) in 22 cases. After the first iMRI control, we achieved our goal in 14 and 12 cases, respectively; we were also able to improve our goal, obtaining total tumor removal in two patients, who were preoperatively scheduled in the nontotal tumor resectable (NTR) group. After the second iMRI control, we achieved our goal in 7 and 2 cases, respectively; and we needed a third iMRI control to achieve the last total tumor resection. In our series, we achieved total tumor resection in two-thirds of patients.

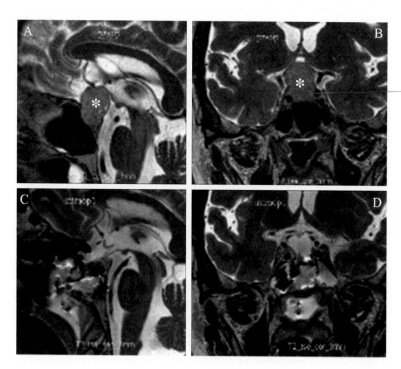

Fig. 13.3 (A,B) Preoperative: Intra- and suprasellar hormone inactive pituitary adenoma (*). (C,D) Intraoperative: Complete tumor removal.

majority of patients with complete resected pituitary adenomas no longer necessary.

Illustrative examples for primary totally and nontotally tumor resection are depicted in **Figs. 13.3, 13.4, 13.5, 13.6, 13.7, 13.8, 13.9**.

In our experience intraoperative high-field MRI in transsphenoidal surgery is a safe and reliable technique. We did not observe any infection in this series and no adverse events related to intraoperative high-field MRI such as accidents caused by the ferromagnetic instruments.

◆ Discussion

Brain MRI is considered to be the standard diagnostic tool for intra- and parasellar structures. There is no doubt that preoperative high-resolution MRI of the sellar and

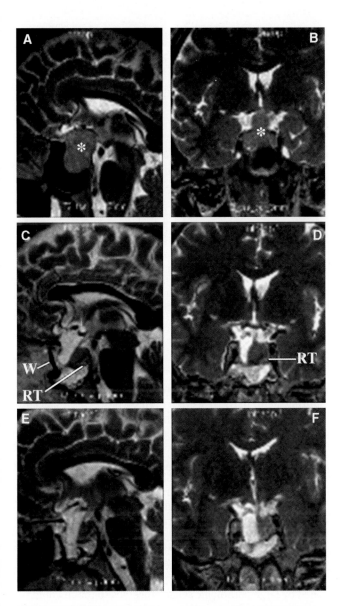

Fig. 13.4 **(A,B)** Preoperative: Intra- and suprasellar hormone inactive pituitary adenoma (*). Chiasm syndrome and secondary hypogonadism. It is difficult in obtain complete surgical tumor removal in the narrow neck to the suprasellar space. **(C,D)** Intraoperative 1: Small remnant tumor (RT) left dorsolateral. W, wax. **(E,F)** Intraoperative 2: Complete selective adenomectomy different signal (Special case: pituitary gland in the midline position).

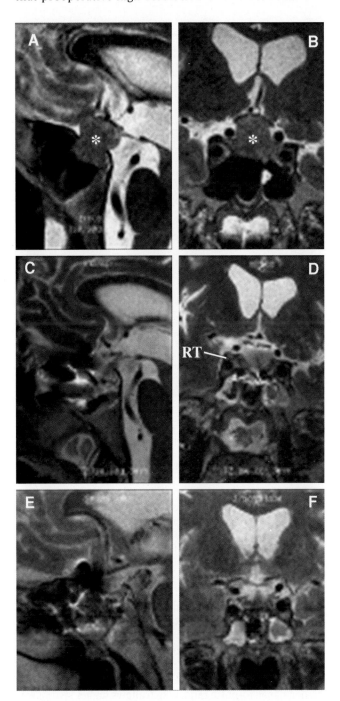

Fig. 13.5 **(A,B)** Preoperative: Intrasellar and irregular suprasellar hormonally inactive pituitary adenoma (*). It is difficult to obtain complete surgical tumor removal in the irregular suprasellar part of the tumor. **(C,D)** Intraoperative: Lateral right small remnant tumor (RT) in a dissenting fold of the diaphragm sellar and in the upper middle wall of the cavernous sinus. **(E,F)** Postoperative: Complete tumor removal successfully documented 3 months after surgery.

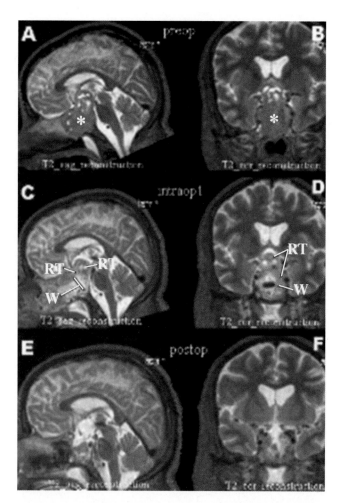

Fig. 13.6 **(A,B)** Preoperative: Intra-, para-, suprasellar, and sphenoidal sinus invasive macroadenoma (*). Direct transnasal transsphenoidal microscopic-, endoscopic-, and neuronavigation-assisted approach. **(C,D)** Intraoperative: Remnant tumor (RT) intra- and suprasellar involving the left cavernous sinus wall. **(E,F)** Postoperative: After complete tumor removal.

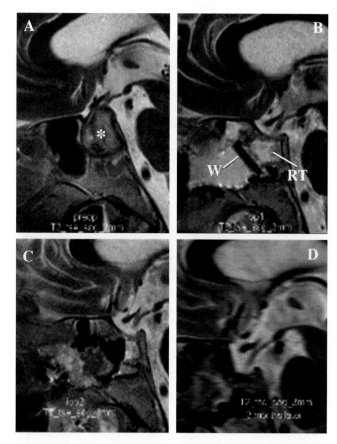

Fig. 13.7 **(A)** Preoperative: Pituitary apoplexy in necrotic hormonally inactive pituitary adenoma (*). Immunohistochemically focal luteinizing hormone and follicle-stimulating hormone expression. **(B)** Intraoperative 1: Small tumor remnant (RT) anteriorly to the sellar and below the diaphragm. W, wax. **(C)** Intraoperative 2: After complete tumor removal. **(D)** 3 Months later: Descent of the diaphragm with the residual pituitary gland, no tumor remnant.

parasellar structures may improve intraoperative neuronavigational guidance for microsurgical and/or endoscopic tumor resection.

For more than 10 years, several neurosurgical departments in Europe and the United States have been acquiring experience in an intraoperative MRI theater starting with low-field MRI. High-field MR (1.5 tesla) and ultra high-field MR (3.0 tesla) iMRI scanners are already becoming available from most manufacturers for clinical applications. Compared with low-field (0.15 and 0.2 tesla) and midfield (0.5 tesla),[22] conventional high-field MRI units offer the advantage of a higher signal-to-noise ratio, which allows higher spatial resolution providing images with details approaching those of a histologic specimen.[27]

The currently established low-field to high-field MR images have certain drawbacks in the visualization of sellar lesions for diagnosis and surgery. These drawbacks include lateral extension into the parasellar spaces, which occurs in

30 to 45% of pituitary adenomas and is the most common limiting factor in the resection of these processes, especially in the case of invasion. The invasive parasellar growth of sellar lesions, through the medial border of the cavernous sinus must be taken into account for surgical planning, but visualization of the fine structure of the medial cavernous sinus border is often unsatisfactory with standard MRI. Therefore, prediction of cavernous sinus invasion based on MR images may rely on indirect signs such as encasement of the intracavernous internal carotid artery (ICA), replacement of the medial cavernous sinus compartment by tumor tissue or tumor growth beyond tangents joining the intracavernous and supraclinoid segments of the ICA. Another drawback is that the normal pituitary gland may be flattened by large pathologic sellar processes so that it could be difficult to recognize it on preoperative conventional MR images. The preoperative knowledge of its position in relation to the lesion may be crucial for preserving its integrity and function.

Due to its higher resolution, 3.0 tesla MRI may allow the delineation of parasellar anatomy in such detail that a medial

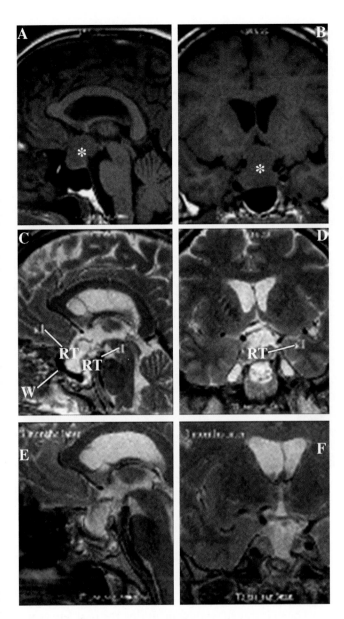

Fig. 13.8 **(A,B)** Preoperative: Intra-, para-, and irregular suprasellar invasive hormonal inactive pituitary macroadenoma (*). Chiasm syndrome and secondary hypogonadism. **(C,D)** Intraoperative: Small remnant tumor (RT) anteriorly and posteriorly between bone and descending capsule. W, wax. **(E,F)** 3 Months later: Complete selective adenomectomy.

cavernous sinus border may be visible, which is particularly important for surgery of laterally invasive sellar lesions. It also provides optimal imaging during intraoperative navigation.[27]

However, there are no convincing data available that intraoperatively, the 3.0 tesla MRI is superior to 1.5 tesla iMRI in the imaging of pituitary lesions. This could be solved by the introduction of useful head coils and solving the current problem of geometric distortion as a routine procedure.

The intraoperative assessment of the completeness of tumor resection is often very difficult. It is based on routine visualization as well as on the surgeon and his or her experience. The relative smallness of the operative field, the extensive recesses of the sella that are beyond the visibility of expert neurosurgeons applying modern endoscopic techniques are reasons for incomplete tumor resection.

The application of all this technology minimally increases the operation time, a small trade-off considering that a short interruption of surgery for scanning offers the chance for improved cure rates. The learning curve of the operating team is such that more frequent use of iMRI clearly improves scanning time and reduces unnecessary delays. Techniques in positioning and optimizing image quality are similarly gained with experience.

The ability of iMRI to assess the extent of resection of pituitary macroadenomas depends also on the ability to obtain technically adequate images for interpretation during an operation; so that it can be more or less possible to differentiate residual tumor from adjacent anatomic structures (e.g., optic chiasm, infundibulum, and normal gland) and from hyperacute changes during open surgery. We prefer initially T2WIs for quick information on a large remnant and to continue with surgery without having the whole battery of information received with a T1 sequence.

The application of a piece of bone wax at the position of the removed sellar floor and irrigation with saline, which remained in the intrasellar cavity during imaging, prevented problems with image interpretation like blood mimicking tumor remnants. Other practices to define the tumor cavity by implantation of Gelfoam (Pfizer Pharmaceuticals, New York, NY) are in discussion.[24,28]

The knowledge of the exact localization of the remaining tumor, originally overlooked, hidden in a fold of the descending diaphragm sellae, allows the surgeon to remove the remaining tumor tissue by a well-directed approach.

High-field iMRI scanning increased the rate of complete tumor removal, so that we jumped from 50 to 80% in the resectable tumors in whom complete tumor removal seemed to be possible via the transsphenoidal approach. In our actual series of 22 total resectable and 14 nontotal resectable pituitary adenomas, we could improve the rate of total resections in the first series from 63 to 100% (from 14 to 22 cases), in both groups together from 44 to 66% (from 16 to 24 cases).

In the literature improvement rates for total resections are described in up to 30 to 40% of the cases.[20,22,26] Higher resection rates are reported in series using high-field MRI in contrast to lower resection rates in series, performing low-field iMRI.[9,22]

From our point of view and personal experience, early postoperative MRI can be helpful in selected cases, when fortunately – and in general surprisingly – no early artifacts are visible; however, it is no alternative to intraoperative imaging. Normally, too many artifacts (blood, plastic material, etc.) interfere with image interpretation. Only images performed 2 to 3 months after surgery provide reliable information about the extent of resection. The main disadvantage is the missed chance of continuing tumor resection immediately. Comparing the result of intraoperative imaging and scanning after 3 months, the rate of false-positives was very low at 6%; there were no false-negative intraoperative findings.

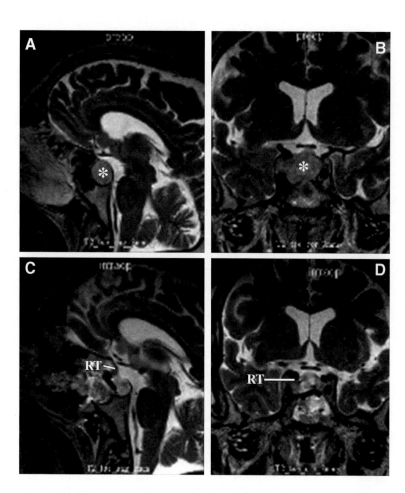

Fig. 13.9 **(A,B)** Preoperative: Intra-, irregular supra-, and parasellar hormonally inactive pituitary adenoma (*).
(C,D) Intraoperative: Small remnant tumor (RT) in the right dorsolateral sinus cavernosus. No complete tumor removal.

The importance of iMRI in pituitary surgery, reflected by experienced neurosurgeons in the literature, will have even more importance for neurosurgeons with less experience in this field.

The implementation of iMRI calls for many ergonomic and financial considerations. The question (i.e., which iMRI system has the optimal cost/benefit ratio for a given hospital) has to be answered with regard to the capability of reconstruction measures and shielding of the operating room, the available investment budget to purchase the iMRI system, and the requirements to use the scanner either strictly for intraoperative scans or for diagnostic purposes as well. A shared-resource MRI operating suite that facilitates performance of both neurosurgical and diagnostic procedures in a single unit, greatly improves the cost-benefit ratio.[29] Only a few 1.5 T and even fewer 3.0 T MRI (Instabul, Prague, etc.) systems are currently used in patients with pituitary tumors and of course, such a huge investment is only reasonable if such an installation is used intensively. After installation of such a system, the additional costs for a single surgical procedure are low.

Arguments for iMRI scanning are as follows. Intraoperative imaging results in immediate intraoperative quality control; immediately after surgery, the surgical result is obvious. During the postoperative phase, there is no psychological stress for the patient and no waiting time, which is normally 3 months, to obtain an artifact-free MRI scan. In case of persistent tumor, immediate planning for further management is possible so that the surgical procedure can be continued or planned for surveillance, transcranial resection, treatment with maintenance drugs, or radiotherapy.

However, an increasing number of low-field scanners have been installed worldwide during the past few years; this has proved to the useful.[30] The visualization of the suprasellar space is to some extent comparable in low- and high-field MRI; nevertheless, high-field imaging is clearly superior in the evaluation of the cavernous sinus area due to its limited field of view and the imaging resolution characteristic of low-field strength.[31]

Whatever the future development of intraoperative imaging of pituitary surgery offers, even today there are efficient tools available to improve traditional surgical results significantly.

References

1. Anand VK, Schwartz TH, Hiltzik DH, Kacker A. Endoscopic transsphenoidal pituitary surgery with real-time intraoperative magnetic resonance imaging. Am J Rhinol 2006;20(4):401–405
2. Elias WJ, Chadduck JB, Alden TD, Laws ER Jr. Frameless stereotaxy for transsphenoidal surgery. Neurosurgery 1999;45(2):271–275, discussion 275–277

3. Jane JA Jr, Thapar K, Alden TD, Laws ER Jr. Fluoroscopic frameless stereotaxy for transsphenoidal surgery. Neurosurgery 2001;48(6):1302–1307, discussion 1307–1308

4. Knosp E, Steiner E, Kitz K, Matula C. Pituitary adenomas with invasion of the cavernous sinus space: a magnetic resonance imaging classification compared with surgical findings. Neurosurgery 1993;33(4):610–617, discussion 617–618

5. Lasio G, Ferroli P, Felisati G, Broggi G. Image-guided endoscopic transnasal removal of recurrent pituitary adenomas. Neurosurgery 2002;51(1):132–136, discussion 136–137

6. Walker DG, Ohaegbulam C, Black PM. Frameless stereotaxy as an alternative to fluoroscopy for transsphenoidal surgery: use of the InstaTrak-3000 and a novel headset. J Clin Neurosci 2002;9(3):294–297

7. Cappabianca P, Cavallo LM, Colao A, de Divitiis E. Surgical complications associated with the endoscopic endonasal transsphenoidal approach for pituitary adenomas. J Neurosurg 2002;97(2):293–298

8. Jho HD, Alfieri A. Endoscopic endonasal pituitary surgery: evolution of surgical technique and equipment in 150 operations. Minim Invasive Neurosurg 2001;44(1):1–12

9. Bohinski RJ, Warnick RE, Gaskill-Shipley MF, et al. Intraoperative magnetic resonance imaging to determine the extent of resection of pituitary macroadenomas during transsphenoidal microsurgery. Neurosurgery 2001;49(5):1133–1143, discussion 1143–1144

10. Dort JC, Sutherland GR. Intraoperative magnetic resonance imaging for skull base surgery. Laryngoscope 2001;111(9):1570–1575

11. Fahlbusch R, Ganslandt O, Buchfelder M, Schott W, Nimsky C. Intraoperative magnetic resonance imaging during transsphenoidal surgery. J Neurosurg 2001;95(3):381–390

12. Martin CH, Schwartz R, Jolesz F, Black PM. Transsphenoidal resection of pituitary adenomas in an intraoperative MRI unit. Pituitary 1999;2(2):155–162

13. Nimsky C, Ganslandt O, Hofmann B, Fahlbusch R. Limited benefit of intraoperative low-field magnetic resonance imaging in craniopharyngioma surgery. Neurosurgery 2003;53(1):72–80, discussion 80–81

14. Okudera H, Takemae T, Kobayashi S. Intraoperative computed tomographic scanning during transsphenoidal surgery: technical note. Neurosurgery 1993;32(6):1041–1043

15. Pergolizzi RS Jr, Nabavi A, Schwartz RB, et al. Intra-operative MR guidance during trans-sphenoidal pituitary resection: preliminary results. J Magn Reson Imaging 2001;13(1):136–141

16. Schulder M, Sernas TJ, Carmel PW. Cranial surgery and navigation with a compact intraoperative MRI system. Acta Neurochir Suppl (Wien) 2003;85:79–86

17. Hardy J, Wigser SM. Trans-sphenoidal surgery of pituitary fossa tumors with televised radiofluoroscopic control. J Neurosurg 1965;23(6):612–619

18. Arita K, Kurisu K, Tominaga A, et al. Trans-sellar color Doppler ultrasonography during transsphenoidal surgery. Neurosurgery 1998;42(1):81–85, discussion 86

19. Doppman JL, Ram Z, Shawker TH, Oldfield EH. Intraoperative US of the pituitary gland. Work in progress. Radiology 1994;192(1):111–115

20. Nimsky C, von Keller B, Ganslandt O, Fahlbusch R. Intraoperative high-field magnetic resonance imaging in transsphenoidal surgery of hormonally inactive pituitary macroadenomas. Neurosurgery 2006;59(1):105–114, discussion 105–114

21. Black PM, Moriarty T, Alexander E III, et al. Development and implementation of intraoperative magnetic resonance imaging and its neurosurgical applications. Neurosurgery 1997;41(4):831–842, discussion 842–845

22. Nimsky C, Ganslandt O, Fahlbusch R. Comparing 0.2 tesla with 1.5 tesla intraoperative magnetic resonance imaging analysis of setup, workflow, and efficiency. Acad Radiol 2005;12(9):1065–1079

23. Fahlbusch R, Keller B, Ganslandt O, Kreutzer J, Nimsky C. Transsphenoidal surgery in acromegaly investigated by intraoperative high-field magnetic resonance imaging. Eur J Endocrinol 2005;153(2):239–248

24. Zirkzee EJ, Corssmit EP, Biermasz NR, et al. Pituitary magnetic resonance imaging is not required in the postoperative follow-up of acromegalic patients with long-term biochemical cure after transsphenoidal surgery. J Clin Endocrinol Metab 2004;89(9):4320–4324

25. Dina TS, Feaster SH, Laws ER Jr, Davis DO. MR of the pituitary gland postsurgery: serial MR studies following transsphenoidal resection. AJNR Am J Neuroradiol 1993;14(3):763–769

26. Nimsky C, Ganslandt O, Von Keller B, Romstöck J, Fahlbusch R. Intraoperative high-field-strength MR imaging: implementation and experience in 200 patients. Radiology 2004;233(1):67–78

27. Wolfsberger S, Ba-Ssalamah A, Pinker K, et al. Application of three-tesla magnetic resonance imaging for diagnosis and surgery of sellar lesions. J Neurosurg 2004;100(2):278–286

28. Kiliç T, Ekinci G, Seker A, Elmaci I, Erzen C, Pamir MN. Determining optimal MRI follow-up after transsphenoidal surgery for pituitary adenoma: scan at 24 hours postsurgery provides reliable information. Acta Neurochir (Wien) 2001;143(11):1103–1126

29. McPherson CM, Bohinski RJ, Dagnew E, Warnick RE, Tew JM. Tumor resection in a shared-resource magnetic resonance operating room: experience at the University of Cincinnati. Acta Neurochir Suppl (Wien) 2003;85:39–44

30. Schwartz TH, Stieg PE, Anand VK. Endoscopic transsphenoidal pituitary surgery with intraoperative magnetic resonance imaging. Neurosurgery 2006;58(1, Suppl)ONS44–ONS51, discussion ONS44–ONS51

31. Gerlach R, du Mesnil de Rochemont R, Gasser T, et al. Feasibility of Polestar N20, an ultra-low-field intraoperative magnetic resonance imaging system in resection control of pituitary macroadenomas: lessons learned from the first 40 cases. Neurosurgery 2008;63(2):272–284, discussion 284–285

14

Functional Magnetic Resonance Imaging-Guided Brain Tumor Resections

Peter D. Kim, Charles L. Truwit, and Walter A. Hall

Intraoperative magnetic resonance imaging (iMRI) was developed to allow neurosurgeons near-real time visual feedback during surgery. Applications of this technology have included image-guided biopsy, drainage of cysts, instillation of therapeutic agents, thermal ablations, laminectomies,[1,2] and the most obvious application, the resection of brain tumors. Prognosis after the resection of high grade glial tumors is in part dependent upon the extent of resection;[3,4] therefore maximal resection is likely worth the extra time and cost of intraoperative imaging.[5,6] The relationship between prognosis and the extent of resection is somewhat more controversial in low grade glial tumors[7,8] but is still likely to be directly related. Furthermore, the control of seizures, which are often present with low-grade tumors, can be related to extent of resection.[9] The margins of low-grade tumors are often less distinct than those of high grade tumors, and adjacent structures may therefore be at greater risk for injury if resection is performed without some form of image guidance. iMRI can provide the surgeon with direct evidence of whether or not there is a radiographically complete resection prior to leaving the operating room (**Figs. 14.1** and **14.2**). Radiographic evidence that a gross total resection has been accomplished not only provides assurance of maximal resection, but also allows the surgeon to avoid unnecessary further resection of normal cortex adjacent to a tumor. In many cases, the limiting factor in an aggressive surgical resection of tumors is the presence of nearby functional cortex. For obvious reasons, accomplishing a maximal resection with minimal disruption of normal brain parenchyma is particularly relevant to the surgical treatment (biopsy or resection) of these tumors located near eloquent parts of the brain.

Multiple strategies have been employed to assist the surgeon in the resection of tumors near eloquent cortex. Traditional neuronavigation techniques have allowed surgeons to operate with smaller, more accurate surgical corridors, whereas techniques such as direct cortical stimulation, other forms of neuromonitoring and performance of tumor resection while the patient is awake allow for some degree of real

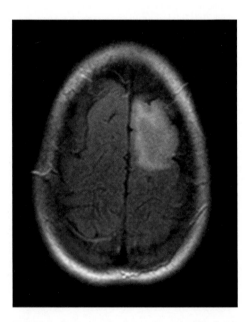

Fig. 14.1 Preoperative 1.5 tesla axial turbo fluid-attenuation inversion recovery magnetic resonance imaging (FLAIR MRI) scan of a left frontal low-grade glioma before surgical manipulation of the brain or the occurrence of brain-shift. The brain activation scan for this patient is shown in **Fig. 14.4** and demonstrates that the cortical location of finger tapping function was posterior to the tumor. (From Hall W, Kim P, Truwit C, Functional Magnetic Resonance Imaging-Guided Brain Tumor Resection. Philadelphia: Lippincott Williams and Wilkins; 2008. Reprinted with permission.)

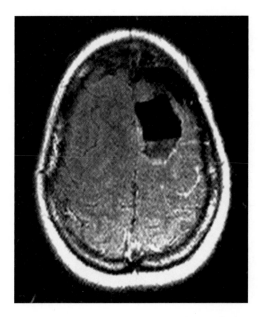

Fig. 14.2 Intraoperative 1.5 tesla axial turbo fluid-attenuation inversion recovery magnetic resonance imaging (FLAIR MRI) scan of the patient displayed in **Fig. 14.1** that demonstrates that the entire preoperative tumor imprint has been resected and the goal of surgery has been achieved. (From Hall W, Kim P, Truwit C, Functional Magnetic Resonance Imaging-Guided Brain Tumor Resection. Philadelphia: Lippincott Williams and Wilkins; 2008. Reprinted with permission.)

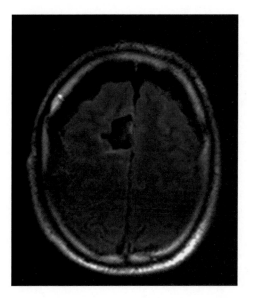

Fig. 14.3 Intraoperative turbo fluid-attenuation inversion recovery magnetic resonance imaging (FLAIR MRI) scan that was obtained at 1.5 tesla showing a complete radiographic resection of a right frontal low-grade glioma. The surgical cavity is filled with air and pneumocephalus is present over both frontal lobes. Brain-shift has resulted from the egress of cerebrospinal fluid during the surgical procedure. (From Ulmer S, Jansen O. FMRI – Basics and Clinical Applications. New York: Springer Science + Business Media; 2009. Reprinted with permission.)

time or near-real time feedback regarding the integrity of surrounding eloquent areas. Frameless neuronavigation provides the neurosurgeon with precise data at the beginning of a procedure and thus is an excellent tool for planning a surgical corridor; however, as the surgery progresses, there may be a shift of normal brain tissue into the surgical bed as tumor is resected, or away from the surgical site if there is significant egress of cerebrospinal fluid (CSF) out of the cranium.[10,11] Removal of the calvarium at the time of craniotomy combined with the loss of CSF when the dura mater is opened can result in significant amounts of brain shift within the cranium (**Fig. 14.3**). The result of this shifting of the brain is that the images that are used in determining completeness of resection (and the safety of further resection) may be inaccurate leading either to unexpected residual tumor or surgical incursion into functional areas of normal brain, depending upon the direction of the shift. Attempts that have been described to quantify and compensate for brain shift have utilized ultrasound or vascular markers.[12] Cortical stimulation and other neuromonitoring techniques and awake neurosurgery allow for some degree of near-real time feedback regarding the integrity of functional areas during surgery. These techniques, however, require limitations to anesthesia, do not provide the neurosurgeon with image guidance, and often do not provide meaningful feedback until eloquent cortex has been breached. Furthermore, these techniques, while useful in preserving eloquent areas of brain, offer no information concerning the completeness of resection.

◆ Functional MRI

Functional magnetic resonance imaging (fMRI) is a technique in which patients undergo MRI while performing particular tasks to map precisely those areas of the brain that are being activated. Functional MRI is a noninvasive but also indirect method of mapping eloquent cortex. The mechanism that allows for the generation of fMRI is complex and depends upon the delivery, volume, and fractional oxygenation of blood.[13] As discrete cortical areas are activated during each specific task, metabolic activity increases and oxygen is therefore extracted from hemoglobin molecules to an extent that is increased over baseline. The loss of the oxygen results in a focal increase in intracellular deoxyhemoglobin, with its unpaired iron electrons within the hemoglobin molecule, thus altering the local magnetic field, and a signal change relative to adjacent tissues on suitably tailored MR images. Cortical activation also results in an increase in local blood flow which compensates for this effect. Because of this combination of antagonistic effects, the degree of activation is not measured in fMRI. Unlike data from neurophysiologic techniques, fMRI data can be directly applied to preoperative imaging studies, allowing for determination of the surgical goals prior to taking the patient to the operating suite. The surgeon is additionally provided with a visual representation of the position eloquent cortex and its relationship to the tumor, which aids in both the preoperative and intraoperative surgical decision making (**Fig. 14.4**).

fMRI has previously been used in conjunction with neuronavigation, and functional images can be coregistered

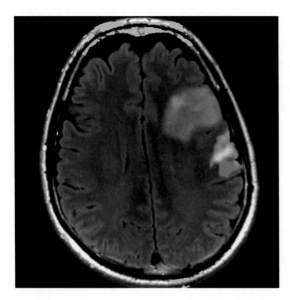

Fig. 14.4 Axial turbo fluid-attenuation inversion recovery magnetic resonance imaging (FLAIR MRI) scan demonstrating a left frontal low-grade glioma. This brain activation study was performed at 3.0 tesla and the task being performed was finger tapping of the right hand. (From Ulmer S, Jansen O. FMRI – Basics and Clinical Applications. New York: Springer Science + Business Media; 2009. Reprinted with permission.)

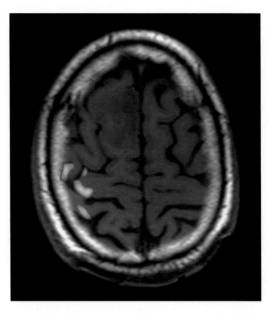

Fig. 14.5 Axial T1-weighted brain activation study performed at 3.0 tesla showing the area for finger tapping of the left hand. The tumor that is planned to be resected surgically is just anterior and medial to the cortical area for brain activation. The posterior aspect of the tumor is nicely delineated by a medial and lateral sulcus. (From Ulmer S, Jansen O. FMRI – Basics and Clinical Applications. Philadelphia: Lippincott Williams and Wilkins; 2008. Reprinted with permission.)

with those that are used for neuronavigation. Because of the limitations caused by brain shift, as described above, fMRI used in this way was not fully protective against iatrogenic neurologic deficit. To provide more accurate delineation of functional areas during surgery, functional MRI has been combined with intraoperative scanning. In this chapter, the technique of intraoperative MRI (iMRI) with fMRI is described.

Functional imaging as a surgical modality allows for the delineation of eloquent brain areas prior to surgery (**Fig. 14.5**). The identification of the location of brain function in turn allows surgery to be performed without particular consideration to the type of anesthesia used and without the need to spend additional time defining functional areas during surgery. Furthermore, the tasks performed during fMRI acquisition may be more complex than those tasks performed during awake craniotomy. Our paradigm for combining functional imaging with iMRI has been the preoperative acquisition of fMRI combined with surgical resection or biopsy using iMRI at high field strength (1.5 tesla).

As with all imaging modalities, functional MRI and iMRI do not replace meticulous surgical planning and execution. The surgeon utilizing the algorithm described above must mentally extrapolate the relevant blood oxygen level-dependent (BOLD) fMRI to iMRI scans. Critical to the success of iMRI is the neurosurgeon's ability to determine when intraoperative scanning should take place, based upon his or her recognition that a critical juncture in the procedure has been reached. Furthermore, he or she must be cognizant of underlying white matter tracts, which may be encroached upon while a surgeon is operating far from areas of brain activation. Diffusion tensor imaging (DTI) is a relatively new MRI modality

that allows for the mapping of the location of white matter tracts and may be useful in combination with fMRI when it is felt that there is a high risk of undermining white matter tracts during the removal of a particular tumor.

◆ Patient Selection

Ideal candidates for fMRI-guided brain tumor resection are those patients who harbor tumors that are located adjacent to eloquent cortex, who are able to cooperate with the tasks associated with brain activation, and who have minimal or no neurologic deficits caused by the tumor. Patients with significant preoperative neurologic deficits due to infiltration of tumor tissue into functional brain areas are not optimal candidates for fMRI-guided resection. Similarly, patients who are severely claustrophobic and thus require strong sedation for MRI are not candidates for fMRI-guided neurosurgery. Although seizure activity affects BOLD imaging, a history of seizures is not a contraindication to fMRI.

Low-grade and high-grade glial tumors, as well as metastatic lesions, have all been resected using our paradigm of iMRI with fMRI. Of the original 346 procedures performed at the University of Minnesota using iMRI, 103 were craniotomies with resection of brain tumors. Of these cases, 14 (14%) were deemed to be close enough to eloquent cortex to necessitate preoperative fMRI. Additionally, we have used fMRI preoperatively to determine whether a patient is not a candidate for image-guided resection, choosing iMRI-guided brain biopsy instead (**Fig. 14.6**).

◆ Technical Aspects

The ideal magnetic field strength for iMRI-guided surgery has been debated. The first iMRI-guided surgical system used a 0.5 tesla (T) scanner. The generation of T1- and T2-weighted images (T1WIs, T2WIs) is necessary for any iMRI scanner, however advanced applications such as magnetic resonance angiography (MRA), diffusion weighted images (DWI), magnetic resonance spectroscopy (MRS) and MR perfusion studies require high field strength (1.5T). Increasing the field strength requires greater caution with regard to ferromagnetic compatibility. Low-field (< 0.5 T) scanners have been utilized with success and we have described extensive experience with high-field scanning at 1.5 T and 3.0 T.[1,14] fMRI requires a field strength of at least 1.5 T and we have published results using both 1.5 T and 3.0 T fMRI. The initial experience with fMRI utilized the same 1.5 T scanner that was used intraoperatively for preoperative BOLD fMRI studies. Subsequently, we have used a 3.0 T scanner that is separate from the iMRI suite to perform fMRI. The 3.0 T MRI allows for higher resolution fMRI on multiple slices, which in turn provides the neurosurgeon with a greater three-dimensional (3D) characterization of brain activation areas (**Fig. 14.7**). Because the fMRI studies are acquired prior to surgery, ferromagnetic compatibility concerns are no more of an issue than they are with routine diagnostic imaging.

For iMRI, the choice between having a dedicated iMRI scanner or a conventional diagnostic MRI scanner placed in

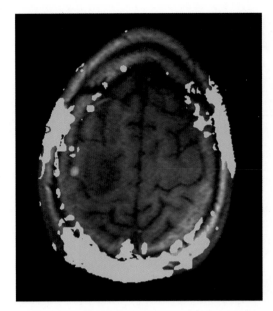

Fig. 14.6 Axial fluid-attenuation inversion recovery magnetic resonance imaging (FLAIR MRI) brain activation scan for left finger tapping at 3.0 tesla demonstrating the activation is immediately lateral to a presumed low-grade glioma. Based on the results of the brain activation study, the patient underwent an MRI-guided brain biopsy, which disclosed an astrocytoma. Because of the infiltrative nature of this tumor type, the patient was subsequently treated with adjuvant radiation therapy. (From Hall W, Kim P, Truwit C, Functional Magnetic Resonance Imaging-Guided Brain Tumor Resection. Philadelphia: Lippincott Williams and Wilkins; 2008. Reprinted with permission.)

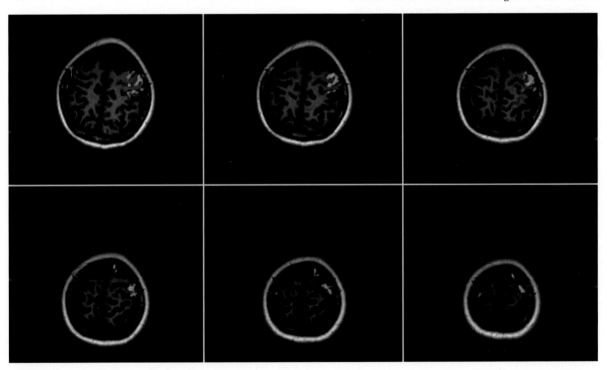

Fig. 14.7 A 3.0 tesla brain activation scan showing the location of the motor cortex after right finger tapping was performed. Axial T1-weighted magnetic resonance image showing multiple sequential brain slices displayed from an inferior to a superior direction, each demonstrating brain activation. The brain tumor is clearly anterior to the area of brain activation and was found to be an oligodendroglioma at surgery. (From Hall W, Kim P, Truwit C, Functional Magnetic Resonance Imaging-Guided Brain Tumor Resection. Philadelphia: Lippincott Williams and Wilkins; 2008. Reprinted with permission.)

a modified operating room is also a subject of debate. Dedicated scanners offer a more seamless transition between surgery and image acquisition. The original 0.5 T scanner described for iMRI use was a double-donut design in which the neurosurgeon operated between two magnetic coils, allowing for continuous scanning during the entire surgical procedure.[15] Other dedicated low-field iMRI systems allow for the rapid conversion from surgery to imaging.

We have previously argued that a high-field diagnostic scanner located within a modified operating suite is relatively affordable, simple to develop, and efficacious. In our experience, the time and effort required to shift from surgery to intraoperative imaging is short, with no more than 10 to 15 minutes of additional anesthesia time resulting from each intraoperative scan obtained. Furthermore, if the surgical procedure can be performed entirely within the MRI environment with MRI-compatible instruments, as is necessary when operating using the 3.0 T magnet, then patient transport into the bore of the magnet for scanning is possible within minutes. Intraoperative MRI using fMRI-guidance may be performed with either strength scanner, and our experience with the 1.5 T diagnostic scanner is described here.

◆ Preoperative fMRI Acquisition

Patients are usually brought to the scanner before the day of surgery where preoperative fMRI is performed. On a rare occasion a patient will have their fMRI performed immediately before the induction of general anesthesia. Areas that are activated during the task and therefore functionally relevant are determined using BOLD MRI. Patients perform specific tasks at a self-paced rate with intervening periods of rest. We have used fMRI to map speech, motor function, and short-term memory. To map language function, patients perform silent speech since actual verbalization results in movement of the head which will result in the misrepresentation of the area of brain activation for language (**Fig. 14.8**). Patients are instructed to think of the names of animals beginning at the start of the alphabet. List retention is used to map short term memory and finger and toe tapping are used for motor function brain activation. These images are reviewed by the neurosurgeon prior to planning of the surgery.

The original 1.5 T MRI system we have used for brain activation studies was a short bore scanner (Gyroscan ACS-NT; Philips Healthcare, Andover, MA) with strong imaging gradients (23 millitesla per meter [mT/m], 105 mT/m per millisecond) necessary to permit echo planar imaging (EPI) used for brain activation studies. For the fMRI protocol at 1.5 T we use is a single-shot EPI scan (repetition time/ echo-time [TR/TE]: 3000/40 ms; field of view [FOV]: 210 mm) with a 64 × 64 image matrix and 7 mm thick slices with 1 mm intersection gap. Acquisition is repeated 72 times over 4 minutes in sequential fashion. A wave pattern is overlaid upon a linear graph that indicates when the activity is and is not being performed, thus providing a measure of test accuracy (**Fig. 14.9**). High-quality fMR images are made available

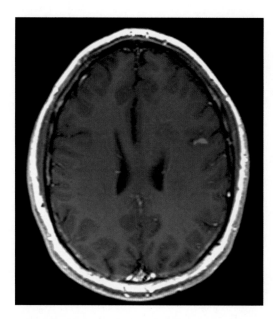

Fig. 14.8 Axial T1-weighted contrast-enhanced brain activation scan performed at 3.0 tesla demonstrating the area for cortical localization of silent speech. The tumor is not visible on this scan slice because it is anterior and superior to the area of brain activation (From Hall W, Kim P, Truwit C, Functional Magnetic Resonance Imaging-Guided Brain Tumor Resection. Philadelphia: Lippincott Williams and Wilkins; 2008. Reprinted with permission.)

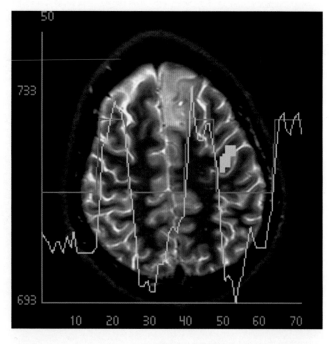

Fig. 14.9 For the functional magnetic resonance imaging (fMRI) protocol at 1.5 T we use is a single-shot echo-planar image (EPI) scan. A wave pattern is overlaid upon a linear graph that indicates when the activity is and is not being performed, thus providing a measure of test accuracy. This axial T2-weighted MR image shows that the left frontal tumor is just anterior to the area of brain activation. The task being performed by the patient is finger tapping of the right hand.

on liquid crystal display (LCD) monitors in the iMRI suite adjacent to the scanner. These can be viewed at any time during the operative procedure. Rigid cranial fixation allows for sequential scanning at an identical plane thus allowing the surgeon to interpret whether residual tumor is present and if there is integrity of the functional cortex between pre- and intraoperative scans.

Two different 3.0 T scanners have been used. The first 3.0 T scanner was another short bore scanner (Intera; Philips Healthcare, Andover, MA) with strong imaging gradients (33 mT/m, 180 mT/m per millisecond) allowing for generation of EPI sequences. The length of this system is 157 cm and the inner bore diameter measures 60 cm. The 5 gauss footprint measures 5.8 × 7.0 m. Software for BOLD imaging was provided by Philips Healthcare. The protocol for acquisition of fMRI is a single shot EPI scan (TR/TE: 3000 ms/35 ms; FOV: 230 mm) with 4-mm-thick slices, a 1-mm intersection gap, and an 80 × 128 image matrix. A 7-minute imaging interval is used with acquisition repeated sequentially 100 times. The second 3.0 T scanner (Siemens AG, Erlangen, Germany) uses a single-shot EPI sequence (TR/TE, 2660 ms/30 ms; FOV, 192 mm) for fMRI. There was a 64 × 64 image matrix with 3-mm-thick scan slices and a 0.8-mm intersection gap. For this scanner, a 3-minute imaging interval with acquisition repeated 60 times was used.

The iMRI suite consists of a scanner that may be used for conventional diagnostic studies between surgeries, contained within a fully operational surgical suite. The scanner is a 1.5 T short bore scanner (Gyroscan ACS-NT; Philips Healthcare, Andover, MA) with 100 cm flared openings that facilitate transport into the magnet. The inner bore of the scanner measures 60 cm and the total length is 180 cm. The main field magnet is actively shielded and the resulting 5 gauss (G) line covers a "peanut-shaped" area of ∼7.8 × 5.0 meters. The 5 G line must be well demarcated to avoid mishaps related to the inadvertent entry of ferromagnetic objects into the iMRI suite. Not only is the floor marked by brightly colored tape, but we also have a mechanical screen that can be lowered to the floor from the ceiling. A rotating pedestal table that serves as the operating table is positioned in line with the scanner and can be docked to the scanner table when intraoperative images are desired. The scanner table will also extend up to 40 cm beyond the far opening of the magnet allowing for surgery to be performed within the 5 G line, at the opposite end of the magnet. The operating microscope, as well as all anesthesia equipment and monitors, craniotome, and fiberoptic headlight are all MRI-compatible. The evening before the suite is to be used for surgery it is meticulously cleaned and subsequently treated as a sterile operative environment. Pocketless color-coded scrubs are required for all personnel within the iMRI suite to prevent members of the team from inadvertently entering with ferromagnetic objects. Our experience and that of others has suggested that high-field MRI may be safely integrated within an operating suite. At the University of Minnesota, the iMRI suite has been used for over 1000 procedures without a significant magnet-related mishap.

◆ Operative Procedure

Prior to their arrival in the iMRI operating suite, patients are placed under general anesthesia, and appropriate monitoring lines are placed including an arterial line. MRI visible markers are placed on the head to localize the lesion with respect to the cranial opening to minimize the length of the planned incision as well as the size of the hair shave. The patient's head is then fixed in a Malcolm-Rand carbon fiber head frame (Elekta, Decatur, GA), which allows for the repetition of scans at exactly reproduced scan planes. A head coil that consists of two circular loops arranged as a phased array is also placed in a manner that will not interfere with the surgical access. This array provides imaging of high-quality similar to that obtained with conventional diagnostic head coils. A neuroradiologist is present for each case to optimize the imaging strategy.

MRI is performed prior to the onset of the procedure. This provides a preoperative image of the tumor in the same orientation and scan projections that will be obtained with iMRI during the procedure. The tumor is localized using the previously placed markers, and the surgical trajectory is planned. After the initial imaging, patients are removed from the magnet still in cranial fixation with the head coil in place over the operative site. They are then transferred to the operating table and prepped and draped for surgery. Surgery is generally performed at the near end of the room outside the 5 G line, but may alternately be performed on the opposite side of the magnet within the magnetic field using all MRI-compatible materials.

Craniotomy is performed in the standard fashion up until the time that the surgeon desires iMRI. Tumor margins that are located away from functional brain tissue are identified using direct visualization and surgical judgment. Specifically, tissue that appears to be grossly abnormal is removed by simple suction or using an ultrasonic aspirator until normal appearing brain tissue is identified. The consistency of normal brain tissue compared with residual brain tumor must be well known to the neurosurgeon and a decrease in the degree of hemorrhage and the vascularity of the tissue being resected will often indicate that the tumor margin has been reached. In the direction toward functional brain tissue a more conservative approach is taken with the neurosurgeon relying on the iMRI to demonstrate that the tumor margin has been exposed. For low-grade gliomas the distinction between normal and abnormal tissue may be very subtle in which case the surgeon is guided by anatomic landmarks and the preoperative MRI.

Intraoperative scans are performed to assess the presence of residual disease as well as the proximity to eloquent areas as defined by fMRI, at the discretion of the surgeon. Generally, a scan is obtained when based on operative findings the surgeon feels that the resection is complete or that a maximal safe resection has been accomplished (**Fig. 14.10**). The number of intraoperative scans varies depending on the complexity of the surgery and the histologic composition of the tumor. In our experience, scans are generally not performed within an hour of one another, and the time of scanning is usually not more than 10 minutes to obtain the necessary images for

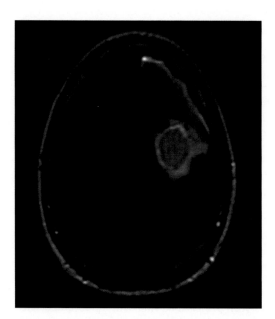

Fig. 14.10 Intraoperative 1.5 tesla axial turbo fluid attenuation inversion recovery magnetic resonance imaging (FLAIR MRI) scan of a patient with a left frontal astrocytoma that is adjacent to the cortical area for right-hand motor activation. An area of increased signal around the resection cavity is suggestive of the presence of residual tumor. The central sulcus is seen posterior to the resection cavity, and the area of increased signal was felt by the surgeon to possibly be infiltrating into the motor cortex, which resulted in the discontinuation of the tumor resection. (From Hall W, Kim P, Truwit C, Functional Magnetic Resonance Imaging-Guided Brain Tumor Resection. Philadelphia: Lippincott Williams and Wilkins; 2008. Reprinted with permission.)

review. In cases where the tumor is particularly close to eloquent cortex, one or more intermediate scans are usually obtained. The choice of imaging sequence is determined by the neuroradiologist in conjunction with the neurosurgeon. For low-grade gliomas, T2 FLAIR (fluid-attenuated inversion recovery) or HASTE (half-Fourier-acquisition single-shot turbo-spin echo) images are most often used. When surgery

is performed on enhancing lesions, contrast is reserved until there is either a great degree of certainty as to the completeness of the resection or a complex point of the surgery mandates administration of contrast before continuing. Contrast is withheld as long as possible largely because the premature administration of contrast will result in diffusion or imbibition of contrast into the surgically violated, peritumoral brain around the resection cavity making it difficult to interpret subsequent contrast scans.

Prior to scanning, all surgical instruments that are not MRI-compatible are removed from the operative field. These instruments include scalpel blades, suture needles, retraction devices, and any wires that could lead to a thermal injury. Once MRI is completed, the scans are reviewed by both the neurosurgical team and the neuroradiologist to confirm the completeness of the tumor resection. Once the decision is made that the tumor resection is complete, the scalp is closed. The cranial bone flap is secured to the skull with an MRI-compatible titanium plating system and the incision is closed using interrupted absorbable sutures. A running nonabsorbable suture is used to close the skin. ChloraPrep (CareFusion, San Diego, CA) is placed over the surgical incision and a sterile dressing is left in place for 48 hours. The wound is kept dry for 3 days, after which it can become wet and come in contact with soap or shampoo.

Prior to leaving the iMRI suite, one final sequence of MRI scans is obtained to exclude the presence of hemorrhage that could have occurred during the closure. Hyperacute blood can be difficult to detect because oxyhemoglobin has not yet converted to deoxyhemoglobin; therefore, it is necessary to combine HASTE, gradient echo (GE)-T2*, and turbo FLAIR scan sequences to accurately identify intraoperative hemorrhage (**Fig. 14.11**). If there is any concern that there may be blood at the surgical site, the set of three scans is repeated 15 to 20 minutes after the first postresection scans.

Postoperatively patients are monitored initially in an intensive care unit setting. Blood pressure is monitored using an arterial line and is titrated using an antihypertensive agent such as nicardipine. Subsequently, patients are advanced in

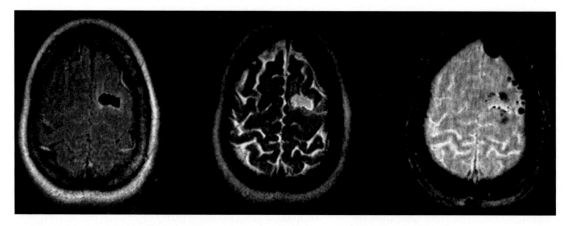

Fig. 14.11 Postresection turbo-FLAIR (fluid-attenuation inversion recovery) (left), T2-weighted HASTE (half-Fourier single-shot turbo spin echo) (middle), and T2*-weighted fast low-angle shot gradient-echo (right) imaging demonstrates an absence of an intraoperative hemorrhage in the tumor resection cavity. (From Hall W, Liu H, Truwit C. Functional magnetic resonance imaging–guided resection of low-grade gliomas. Surg Neurol 64:20–27; 2005. Reprinted with permission.)

their activity level and discharged home once they are ambulating independently, tolerating a regular diet, and their incisional pain is well controlled. There is no need for postoperative scanning because of the quality of the intraoperative imaging that demonstrates the completeness of the surgical resection prior to leaving the iMRI suite. A shortened hospital stay and the lack of a need for postoperative imaging both contribute to a reduction in medical costs, which justifies this cost-effective approach to brain tumor surgery.

◆ Previous Results of fMRI-Guided Tumor Surgery

The results obtained with fMRI-guided brain tumor resection using the previously described brain activation paradigms have been encouraging. In one surgical series, 16 patients with low-grade glial tumors near eloquent cortex were planned for resection using preoperative fMRI and iMRI at 1.5 T.[16] In one patient, surgical resection was not attempted after it was determined that the tumor was located within the motor cortex responsible for tongue function (**Fig. 14.12**). Of those 15 patients undergoing resection, gross total resection was achieved in 10, whereas residual tumor was intentionally left in the other five cases. Residual tumor was not removed because of extension into motor cortex in four patients and areas for speech activation in the other patient. Of the 10 patients with a gross total resection followed for a mean duration of 27 months, there was no recurrence in this series (range of follow up, 14 to 87 months). A series of patients undergoing ioMRI tumor resection at 1.5 T after fMRI at 3.0 T has also been reported.[17] Both low-grade and high-grade glial tumors were included in this series, as well as three patients with meningiomas. In this series of 13 patients, 12 underwent resection and one had a biopsy after it was determined that the tumor was surrounded by areas of brain activation for motor movement of the hand. Gross total resection was accomplished in 10 of these patients, whereas the other two patients had aggressive subtotal resections performed where the residual tumor was intentionally left behind because of infiltration into functional areas. In these two series of

patients, there were no lasting postoperative neurologic deficits. In those patients experiencing transient neurologic deficits, most were felt to be due to postoperative edema adjacent to the resection cavity extending into functional areas of the brain. Two of the 15 patients in the first series had transient deficits, which consisted of hemiparesis in one patient and a motor apraxia in the second patient. Five of 12 patients had postoperative transient neurologic deficits in the second series, which consisted of speech apraxia in two patients, motor apraxia in two patients, and both speech and motor apraxia in one patient. As we have reported with other patients having iMRI-guided surgery, there have been no adverse events related to ferromagnetic instrumentation. iMRI-guidance resulted in the subsequent further resection of tumor tissue in several cases and also led to the decision to discontinue further tumor resection.

The relatively high incidence of transient postoperative deficits may be upon first examination somewhat alarming; however, we believe that this is evidence of the need for fMRI in these patients. The ability to monitor simultaneously, the extent of the tumor resection and the preservation of functional areas adjacent to the surgical site allowed for maximally aggressive resections that would not have been attempted in other circumstances. Therefore, the presence of transient neurologic deficits represents, in our view, validation of this approach. Furthermore, it is our belief that neuronavigation would be subject to the effects of brain shift after a significant amount of tumor has been resected and would therefore not permit safe but aggressive tumor resections in this setting. Cortical stimulation and awake craniotomy have also been used to preserve eloquent cortex during maximally aggressive tumor resections; however, both of these techniques can be subject to postoperative swelling leading to new neurologic deficits. Finally, although direct cortical stimulation can only provide surface mapping of eloquent areas of brain, our paradigm of fMRI with iMRI could easily be combined with diffusion tensor imaging for the delineation and subsequent preservation of white matter tracts.

A 3.0 T iMRI scanner has been installed and early surgical results have been reported.[17] Although scanning at this field strength does pose new challenges, it also offers superior

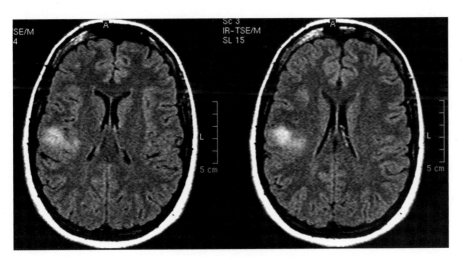

Fig. 14.12 In this patient with a biopsy-proven astrocytoma, surgical resection was not attempted after it was determined that the tumor was located within the motor cortex responsible for tongue function based on brain activation studies performed in three different scan planes.

imaging to that of the 1.5 T MRI scanner. In addition to the enhanced detail that may make possible applications such as placement of deep brain stimulator electrodes, the 3.0 T iMRI scanner would also allow the neurosurgeon to obtain multiple slice fMRI immediately prior to the induction of general anesthesia in the operative suite, thus saving the patient time and transportation costs.

◆ Conclusions

Although generally not acquired intraoperatively, fMRI can play an important role in iMRI-guided neurosurgery. In addition to the coregistration of fMRI images for use with traditional neuronavigation techniques, a relatively simple paradigm for the preoperative acquisition of fMRI combined with iMRI to determine the extent of resection and the preservation of eloquent areas has been demonstrated to provide an effective means of maximizing safe removal of tumor. Increasing magnet field strength combined with other MRI pulse sequences such as diffusion tensor imaging and when appropriate, frameless neuronavigation, likely represents the future evolution of this technique. Careful preoperative planning, astute surgical judgment, an awareness of the surgical findings and meticulous neurosurgical technique will always be mainstays of safe and successful tumor surgery.

References

1. Hall WA, Liu H, Martin AJ, Truwit CL. Intraoperative magnetic resonance imaging. Top Magn Reson Imaging 2000;11(3):203–212 Review
2. Chu RM, Tummala RP, Hall WA. Intraoperative magnetic resonance-guided neurosurgery. Neurosurg Q 2003;13(4):234–250
3. Buckner JC. Factors influencing survival in high-grade gliomas. Semin Oncol 2003; 30(6, Suppl 19)10–14 Review
4. Lacroix M, Abi-Said D, Fourney DR, et al. A multivariate analysis of 416 patients with glioblastoma multiforme: prognosis, extent of resection, and survival. J Neurosurg 2001;95(2):190–198
5. Hall WA, Kowalik K, Liu H, Truwit CL, Kucharezyk J. Costs and benefits of intraoperative MR-guided brain tumor resection. Acta Neurochir Suppl (Wien) 2003;85:137–142
6. Kucharczyk J, Hall WA, Broaddus WC, Gillies GT, Truwit CL. Cost-efficacy of MR-guided neurointerventions. Neuroimaging Clin N Am 2001; 11(4):767–772, xii
7. Berger MS, Deliganis AV, Dobbins J, Keles GE. The effect of extent of resection on recurrence in patients with low grade cerebral hemisphere gliomas. Cancer 1994;74(6):1784–1791
8. Claus EB, Horlacher A, Hsu L, et al. Survival rates in patients with low-grade glioma after intraoperative magnetic resonance image guidance. Cancer 2005;103(6):1227–1233
9. Chang EF, Potts MB, Keles GE, et al. Seizure characteristics and control following resection in 332 patients with low-grade gliomas. J Neurosurg 2008;108(2):227–235
10. Nimsky C, Ganslandt O, Hastreiter P, Fahlbusch R. Intraoperative compensation for brain shift. Surg Neurol 2001;56(6):357–364, discussion 364–365
11. Reinges MH, Nguyen HH, Krings T, Hütter BO, Rohde V, Gilsbach JM. Course of brain shift during microsurgical resection of supratentorial cerebral lesions: limits of conventional neuronavigation. Acta Neurochir (Wien) 2004;146(4):369–377, discussion 377
12. Rasmussen IA Jr, Lindseth F, Rygh OM, et al. Functional neuronavigation combined with intra-operative 3D ultrasound: initial experiences during surgical resections close to eloquent brain areas and future directions in automatic brain shift compensation of preoperative data. Acta Neurochir (Wien) 2007;149(4):365–378
13. Brown GG, Perthen JE, Liu TT, Buxton RB. A primer on functional magnetic resonance imaging. Neuropsychol Rev 2007;17(2):107–125
14. Truwit CL, Hall WA. Intraoperative magnetic resonance imaging-guided neurosurgery at 3-T. Neurosurgery 2006; 58(4, Suppl 2)ONS338–ONS345
15. Black PM, Moriarty T, Alexander E III, et al. Development and implementation of intraoperative magnetic resonance imaging and its neurosurgical applications. Neurosurgery 1997;41(4):831–842, discussion 842–845
16. Hall WA, Liu H, Truwit CL. Functional magnetic resonance imaging-guided resection of low-grade gliomas. Surg Neurol 2005;64(1):20–27, discussion 27
17. Hall WA, Truwit CL. 3-Tesla functional magnetic resonance imaging-guided tumor resection. Int J CARS 2006;1(4):223–230

15

Diffusion Tensor Imaging-Guided Resection

Christopher Nimsky

An important add-on to intraoperative imaging is the use of navigation, allowing preserving neurologic function despite increased resections. The integration of functional data from functional magnetic resonance imaging (fMRI) and magnetoencephalography (MEG) identifying cortical eloquent brain areas into standard three-dimensional (3D) anatomic datasets is known as functional navigation.[1–3] Functional eloquent structures, such as the motor strip- or language-related areas can be identified during surgery by visualizing their position using the microscope heads-up display technology. Functional navigation allows resection of tumors close to eloquent brain areas with low postoperative deficits; intraoperative imaging ensures that the maximum extent of a resection can be achieved. The concept of functional navigation was expanded by the integration of further data leading to so-called multimodal navigation. fMRI and MEG only identify cortical eloquent brain areas. To prevent postoperative neurologic deficits it is also mandatory to preserve the major white matter tracts that are connected to these eloquent brain areas, such as the pyramidal tract for the motor system.

Major white matter tracts can be reconstructed and visualized applying techniques based on diffusion weighted imaging (DWI). DWI depicts differences in tissue anisotropy by measuring the self-diffusion properties, i.e., the Brownian motion of water molecules. Diffusion is anisotropic – orientation-dependent – in areas with a strong aligned microstructure, including cell membranes and the myelin sheath surrounding myelinated white matter, causing impediment of the water motion, so that a differentiation between white and gray matter becomes possible.[4]

DWI gives only a rough estimation of the localization of major white matter tracts by depicting the differences in anisotropy.[5,6] Because only areas of an aligned microstructure are identified, no directional information, which would facilitate the identification of clinically relevant white matter bundles, is available. That is why the definition of major white matter tracts based on DWI relies to a great extent on individual anatomic knowledge and therefore is much user dependent. In case of large space-occupying lesions a reliable identification of these structures may not be possible at all.

Diffusion tensor imaging (DTI) is based on measuring multiple diffusion weighted images in different gradient directions to resolve the orientation of the white matter tracts. Isotropic diffusion can be graphically represented as a sphere, whereas anisotropic diffusion can be graphically expressed as an ellipsoid, with the water molecules moving along the long axis of a fiber bundle and less movement perpendicularly. To estimate the nine tensor matrix elements required for a gaussian description of water mobility, the diffusion gradient must be applied to at least six non-collinear directions. The eigenvalues represent the three principal diffusion coefficients measured along the three coordinate directions of the ellipsoid. The eigenvectors represent the directions of the tensor.

Thus DTI can resolve the dominant fiber orientation in each voxel element. The direction of greatest diffusion measured by DTI parallels the dominant orientation of the tissue structure in each voxel, representing the mean longitudinal direction of axons in major white matter tracts. DTI provides information about the normal course, the displacement, or interruption of white matter tracts around a tumor, as well as a widening of fiber bundles due to edema or tumor infiltration can be detected.[7–15]

◆ DTI Visualization Strategies

Fractional Anisotropy Maps

The diffusion tensor information can be represented as color-encoded fractional anisotropy (FA) maps, which are generated by mapping the principal eigenvector components into red, green, and blue color channels, weighted by fractional anisotropy. Assuming the patient is lying in a supine position and the head is not tilted, then the color mapping defines white matter tracts oriented in an anterior/posterior direction in green, a left/right direction in red, and a superior/inferior direction in blue.[16]

Glyph Representations

The simplification of a tensor to a scalar metric reduces the amount of information contained in the tensor. A possibility to show the entire information of the second-order tensors is to use glyphs.[17] Several shapes have been proposed for representing tensors using glyphs. A popular approach is to use ellipsoids: the axes of the ellipsoid correlate with the directions of the eigenvectors and are scaled according to the corresponding eigenvalues (**Fig. 15.1A**). An advantage of tensor ellipsoids is that they can be rendered in real-time using graphics hardware. An even more satisfying shape for tensors are superquadric tensor glyphs, which provide a better and less-ambiguous spatial impression.[18] However, superquadrics are computationally much more expensive and are hard to achieve in real-time.

The advantage of glyph-based techniques is that the entire tensor information is visualized. Therefore, this visualization is especially appropriate for a detailed examination of the data. However, the results of this visualization approach are difficult to interpret in terms of underlying major white matter structures because no global connectivity information is provided. Consequently, a combination with other visualization techniques such as fiber tracking is recommended to obtain a meaningful representation. In addition, clipping or slice views of glyphs are necessary to avoid an overloading and cluttering of information in 3D.

Fiber Tracking

Fiber tracking is probably the most appealing and understandable technique for representing major white matter tracts and has been investigated by several groups. Various fiber tracking algorithms that compare local tensor field orientations measured by DTI from voxel to voxel have been implemented, allowing a noninvasive tracing of large fiber tract bundles in the human brain.[19–22] Fiber tracking has been used for preoperative visualization of major white matter tracts in patients with space-occupying lesions.[8,9,23] Commonly, the approaches are based on streamline techniques known from flow visualization (**Fig. 15.1B**). Thereby, the respective vector field is derived by taking the major eigenvector of each tensor. Fiber tracking algorithms often utilize thresholds, angle criterions, regularization techniques, and local filters to improve tracking results. In standard fiber tracking approaches the streamlines reconstructed by tracking algorithms are assumed to represent the most likely pathways through the tensor field. It is important to bear in mind that the term "fibers" is used for streamlines that actually do not represent the real anatomic fibers, but provide an abstract model of neural structures. Starting from seed voxels, the tracking is performed in a forward and backward

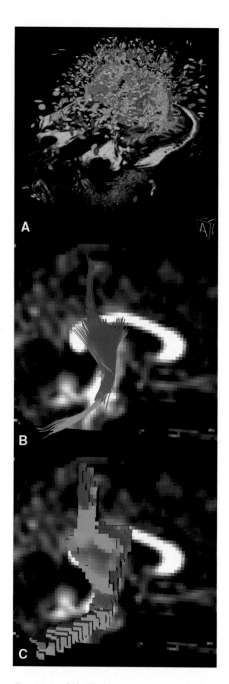

Fig. 15.1 **(A)** Glyph representation of the diffusion tensor imaging (DTI) data of the whole brain with coregistered three-dimensional T1-weighted magnetic resonance images; **(B)** streamline visualization of tracking result of the right pyramidal tract displayed along the B_0 diffusion data in sagittal view; **(C)** volume growing for visualizing the right pyramidal tract

direction with subvoxel precision. For the selection of seed voxels and for aborting the streamline propagation, FA is used as a threshold (**Fig. 15.2**). FA represents the degree of anisotropic diffusion and therefore is a proper measure for the probability of white matter. Following this assumption, voxels with high FA are used as seed voxels. If FA falls below a certain threshold, the tracking stops. Apart from the FA

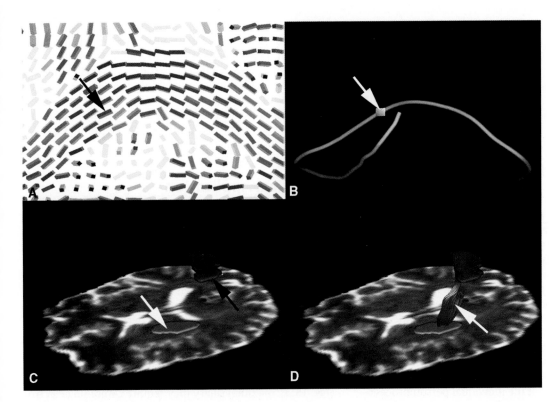

Fig. 15.2 Basic principle of fiber tracking. **(A)** Glyph-based fractional anisotropy map visualization; the black arrow depicts the seeding voxel for the tracking algorithm. **(B)** Single-fiber tracking starting from a single seeding voxel (*white arrow*); the reconstructed fiber tract is visualized as a streamtube. **(C)** Two regions of interest (ROI) approach for reconstruction of the left pyramidal tract; one ROI is placed in the internal capsule (*white arrow*), the other one in the motor cortex (*black arrow*). **(D)** Fibers passing through both ROIs are visualized (*white arrow*) representing the left pyramidal tract.

threshold for aborting fiber tracking, streamline propagation is aborted if it has reached a maximum length or if the angle between the last two steps is above a certain threshold. A further criterion for accepting a fiber is its length. Streamlines are rejected if they are below a minimum length. Besides these thresholds, the user may choose between a tracking encompassing the whole brain and tracking extracting fibers that run through user-defined regions of interest. The latter approach enables the reconstruction of separate tract systems, which is of special interest to actually delineate clinical relevant major white matter tracts. Meanwhile, standard fiber-tracking techniques provide a straightforward possibility to visualize major white matter tracts and their spatial relation to intracerebral lesions.[24–27] However, a lot of software tools allow only tracking combined with the display of the diffusion data; coregistration with standard anatomic data are a must for an intuitive analysis in space-occupying lesions.

Hulls

Unfortunately, most approaches do not satisfy the needs of neurosurgical planning. For clinical intraoperative use the actual border of a major white matter tract is of interest. A line representation like the visualization in standard fiber tracking lacks the ability to provide a border, so the user has to interpret the visualization as a model for the tract. The generation of hulls may overcome this drawback.[28] A surface is generated that wraps a particular subset of previously computed streamlines, representing a certain fiber tract bundle. The wrapping itself might be based on the determination of a centerline of the bundle and the subsequent construction of bounding curves around the set of corresponding lines. Finally, a mesh can be generated by connecting the curves, representing the surface of the fiber tract bundle model. The major advantage of this method is the intuitive visualization. The results may look like flexible tubes, which are closely related to the expected appearance of a major white matter bundle, or a complete 3D object is generated, which represents the major white matter tract of interest. The borders are depicted directly and the combination with volume rendering of anatomic magnetic resonance (MR) data provides a good spatial orientation. It must be noted that the surface is entirely dependent on the previously performed fiber tracking. Errors in the streamline calculation have an immediate influence on the resulting hull.

Alternatively, volume growing techniques are also possible to generate 3D objects representing major white tracts (**Fig. 15.1C**). In general, volume growing algorithms start from a predefined seed region and spread out within the volume until some terminating criterion is reached. Similar to region of interest-based fiber tracking, volume growing needs an initial region or volume of interest for starting the growing procedure. The algorithm then starts from each voxel within that region or volume and proceeds to neighboring voxels. In the same way as for fiber tracking, the growing process stops, as soon as a FA value below a specified threshold is reached. In addition, directional volume growing takes the shape of the local tensor, which controls the direction in which the process expands, and is taken into account.[29]

◆ Integration of DTI into Navigation

A major prerequisite of DTI-based navigation is the registration of the DTI data with standard 3D image data to define a common coordinate system.

As a first attempt to integrate information about major white matter tracts into a functional neuronavigation setup, diffusion data with limited directional information were used for a rough estimation of the course of the pyramidal tract and applied for intraoperative guidance during brain tumor resection.[5,6] These methods often required time-consuming preoperative manual data processing, such as the segmentation of the assumed major white matter tract in each single slice and subsequent image registration. The reliability of the reconstructed white matter tract depended mainly on the experience of the individual person processing the data.

The next step to actually integrate DTI data into navigational datasets was the registration of FA maps with the standard anatomic 3D images.[24,25,30] In contrast to the use of diffusion weighted images for the delineation of major white matter tracts, the manual segmentation in color-coded FA maps was more reliable and less user-dependent. However, still it was a time-consuming process that allowed only a rough estimation on the course of the pyramidal tract. Segmentation close to a lesion or a resection cavity was often not reliably possible.

Integration of tractography data into a stereotactic coordinate system was the next major step. Most of these applications and approaches however, were standalone applications developed for individual clinical sites.[24–27] A broad application for routine clinical use was not possible with the various prototype applications, and the missing standardization did not allow comparing the different approaches.

The implementation of a fiber-tracking algorithm into a standard navigation system, allowing routine usage and broad availability solved these restrictions.[31] Registration with standard anatomic image data greatly facilitated the generation and selection of the fibers of interest, and eased the delineation of the relationship of the tracked fibers to certain anatomic structures because the seed regions for the tracking algorithms could be defined in high-resolution 3D anatomic images. The implemented approach allows a straightforward definition of volumes of interest for selection of the fiber tracts of interest. Only two parameters, the FA threshold and the minimum length of the fibers that will be computed have to be selected by the user. The total generation of the fiber tracts, including image transfer, registration

of the diffusion data with the standard anatomic image data, tensor calculation, fiber tracking, and the final generation of a 3D object needs less than 10 minutes, depending to some extent on the individual strategy how the different seed volumes of interest during initiation of the tracking algorithm are selected.

Figure 15.3 depicts several screenshots of the planning software demonstrating how the right pyramidal tract is reconstructed and visualized.

◆ Clinical Application

Clinical results of using pyramidal tract navigation in a routine setting for glioma resection showed that the occurrence of unwanted neurologic sequelae could be reduced.

In a series of 70 patients where the pyramidal tract was visualized in the surgical field, in eight patients (11%) a new or aggravated postoperative paresis could be observed, which was transient in five of them. Thus, only in three patients (4.2%) there was a new permanent neurologic deficit.[32] These data clearly support the concept of functional neuronavigation (i.e., adding functional information to 3D anatomic datasets to reduce postoperative morbidity when operating on lesions close to eloquent brain areas) (**Fig. 15.3**). Maximal safety may require combining electrophysiologic brain mapping with functional navigation that integrates fMRI/MEG-data and DTI-based fiber tracking acquired before or during surgery. Like cortical eloquent brain areas can be identified by intraoperative electrophysiologic mapping; subcortical electrical stimulation helps to identify major white matter tracts intraoperatively.[33,34] Recent studies emphasize that functional neuronavigation and subcortical stimulation are complementary methods that may facilitate the preservation of pyramidal tracts.

Wu et al showed that DTI-based functional neuronavigation resulted in a significant decrease in postoperative neurological deficits, as well as in an improved 6-month Karnofsky Performance Scale score, when comparing a group of 118 glioma patients that were operated with DTI-based functional neuronavigation with a control group that was operated without DTI data.[35] Of course, the intraoperative knowledge of the exact position of the pyramidal tract does not prevent neurologic deficits per se; intraoperative events such as coagulation of small vessels close to the pyramidal tract may result in an injury of the pyramidal tract leading to neurologic deficits. The distance of how close a reconstructed major white matter tract can be approached is not yet clearly defined. Analyzing the DTI-based navigation data in regard to the distance between tumor and pyramidal tract revealed that a distance of 5 mm seems to be a critical distance, which should be taken into account as a safety margin. This corresponds well to an identical critical distance of ~5 millimeters when approaching functionally eloquent cortical brain areas delineated by fMRI or MEG data.[36,37]

Additional hulls around the reconstructed 3D objects representing major white matter tracts are a possibility to visualize these safety margins (**Fig. 15.4**). These encompassing

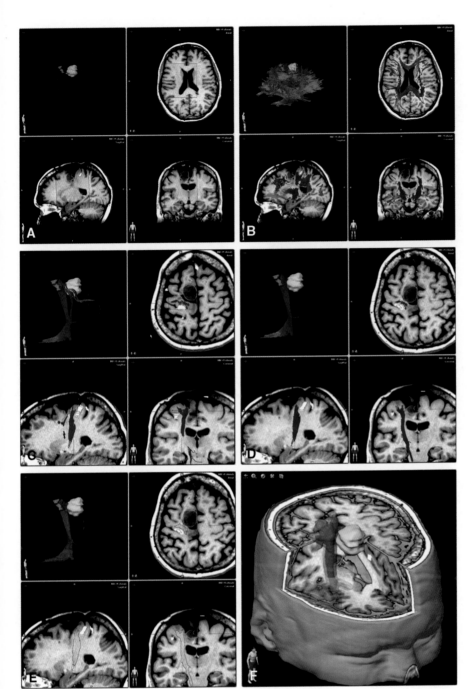

Fig. 15.3 Fiber-tracking software module integrated into navigation planning software. **(A)** Initially, a large volume of interest (VOI) is selected to start a whole head tracking; only fractional anisotropy and fiber length have to be adjusted by the user. Functional magnetic resonance imaging (fMRI) data are segmented in pink, the tumor in yellow. **(B)** Resulting whole head tracking. **(C)** As the next step, only fibers reaching the motor cortex, which is identified by fMRI, are selected. **(D)** Then some errant fibers are excluded, so that a fiber bundle representing the course of the right pyramidal tract results. **(E)** A three-dimensional (3D) hull wrapping the fibers of interest is generated automatically. **(F)** A safety margin of 5 mm is added as a transparent additional hull and can be visualized along the other 3D objects.

hulls ideally would vary in thickness respective to the quality and reliability of the reconstructed fiber bundle. In case of noisy unreliable data, a thick hull would be added, whereas in highly reliable data the hull would be thinner. The technical, as well as clinical definition of the extent of these safety margins has still to be established.

The integration of DTI data into a navigation environment offers the possibility to correlate DTI findings in a multimodal set-up; for example, correlations with MR spectroscopy and positron emission tomography (PET) become possible. Besides preservation of neurologic deficits, DTI navigation also allows for the correlation of histologic findings with DTI results. Thus tumor invasion of major white matter tracts can be detected and quantified.[38–42]

In glioma surgery DTI might also be used to predict a pattern of glioma recurrence, so that a better individualization of tumor management and stratification for randomized controlled trails might be possible.[43]

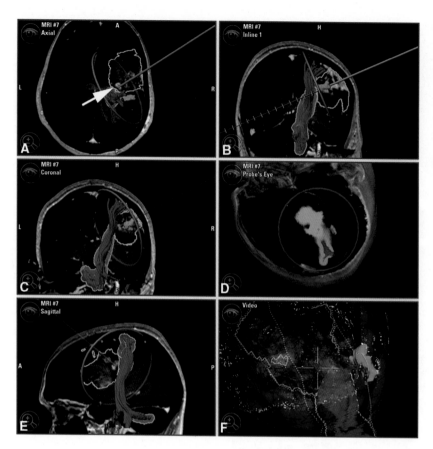

Fig. 15.4 Navigation screen in a patient with a right precentral anaplastic oligoastrocytoma. The microscope is focusing on the depth of the resection cavity at the end of tumor removal (*white arrow* in [A]) (the tumor is outlined in *yellow*, functional magnetic resonance imaging (fMRI) delineating the motor cortex in green, and the pyramidal tract in *blue*, the fiber tract bundle is visualized as three-dimensional object in *dark blue*, while the surrounding safety hull is visualized as two-dimensional contour in *light blue*). Views are (A) axial, (B) inline, (C) coronal, (D) probe's eye, (E) sagittal, and (F) microscope video with heads-up display visualizing the four objects.

Besides the pyramidal tract, the optic radiation as well as fibers connecting language-related areas are of special clinical interest.[44–48] Furthermore, it is possible to visualize structures like the fornix, which might be interesting in transventricular surgery and in attempts to correlate memory deficits when resecting large craniopharyngiomas to changes between pre- and postoperative reconstructions of the fornix.

The major question remains whether the tracking results actually reflect reality. A possible approach to decide this clinically is to correlate clinical findings with the effect on the results of DTI fiber tracking. Integration of the course of the pyramidal tract in the resection of supratentorial gliomas has resulted in reduced neurologic deficits, which can serve as a proof of concept. This is also supported by the results comparing pre- and postoperative reconstructions of major white matter structures in the brainstem which well correlated to clinical deficits (**Fig. 15.5**).[49] Visual field deficits in temporal lobe surgery for pharmaco-resistant epilepsy provide an ideal model to analyze the clinical validity of changes in fiber tracking by correlating the extent of visual field defects with the changes in pre- and intraoperative DTI-based reconstruction of the optic radiation. The significant correlation between postoperative visual field deficits and the extent of alterations of the optic radiation proved that reconstruction of major white matter tracts can be reliably used in a clinical setting.

◆ Intraoperative Fiber Tracking

Pre- and intraoperative DTI for tractography of major white matter tracts in glioma surgery was performed using a 1.5 tesla (T) MR scanner, which is placed in an operating theater.[50–53] Intraoperative fiber tract visualization using a software solution that was running on the MR scanner platform needed less than one minute, so that the whole evaluation could be performed during surgery (**Fig. 15.6**). The interactive 3D display with coregistered diffusion (B_0) images gave a quick and intuitive overview of the position of major white matter tracts. Thus fiber tracking is not only a method for preoperative neurosurgical visualization, but also for further intraoperative planning. Only in one patient was neurologic aggravation (2.7%) observed; it was probably not related to a misinterpretation of fiber tracking. The measured extent of shifting of the major white matter tracts in glioma surgery (+2.7 ± 6.0 mm) corresponded well to previous data on brain-shift of the so-called deep tumor margin, which was reported to be in a range of +4.4 ± 6.8 mm or +5.1 mm.[54,55] Furthermore, the individually unpredictable direction and great interindividual variability of white matter tract shifting confirmed these previous data.[54,56,57] The absolute amount of shifting correlated with the tumor volume: in larger tumors greater deformations were likely to occur. However, the direction of white matter tract shifting, whether in the outward or inward direction in respect to the craniotomy opening, seemed to

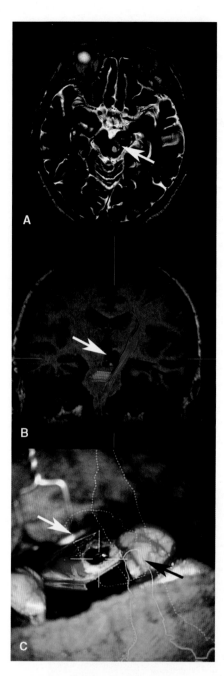

Fig. 15.5 Left-sided mesencephalic cavernoma (*white arrow* in **[A–C]**). **(A)** T2-weighted axial magnetic resonance (MR) image; **(B)** coronal T1-weighted MR image with three-dimensional visualization of the pyramidal tract (*black arrow*); **(C)** intraoperative view of the subtemporal approach, with the outlined cavernoma and course of the pyramidal tract (*white arrow*: cavernoma, *black arrow*: pyramidal tract).

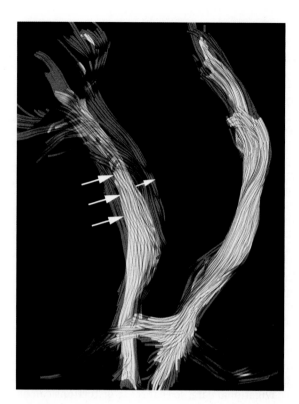

Fig. 15.6 Intraoperative imaging depicts a major shifting of the pyramidal tract during resection of a right temporal lobe tumor; pre- and intraoperative fiber tracking are overlaid. There is no shifting on the left side; however, a significant shifting on the right side (*small arrow* depicts the shifting of the mesial border of the pyramidal tract; the three *larger white arrows* depict the shifting of the outer border of the pyramidal tract at the depth of the resection cavity).

be unpredictable. Even the opening of the ventricular system was no reliable parameter to predict inward shifting due to the loss of cerebrospinal fluid (CSF).

The knowledge of the actual position of major white matter tracts during glioma resection helps to prevent too extensive resections, which could potentially damage major

white matter tracts and subsequently result in postoperative neurologic deficits. When data from fiber tracking are integrated into a navigational set-up, preferably with the simultaneous application of functional magnetic resonance imaging (fMRI) serving as seed regions for DTI fiber-tracking algorithms, it is essential that the effects of brain-shift, which clearly effect the spatial position of major white matter tracts, are compensated for. In contrast to mathematical models, which still have great restrictions simulating the brain-shift behavior for deep brain structures, intraoperative DTI is a reliable procedure used to obtain actual data for fiber tracking, representing the intraoperative situation after substantial parts of a glioma are removed and further guidance is needed.

The implementation of a DTI tracking algorithm in the navigation software allows for an intraoperative update of the navigation system with the intraoperative DTI data in less than 5 to 10 minutes, thus compensating for the effects of brain-shift not only for standard 3D anatomic data, but also for the position of major white matter tracts. This update possibility delineating the course of major white matter tracts based on intraoperative data, is a prerequisite for a real electrophysiologic validation of the white matter tract data. Reports on comparisons between subcortical electrical stimulations and preoperative DTI data showed some inconsistencies, which were probably due to the effects of brain-shift.[27,58]

◆ Challenges and Future Work

Due to the low resolution of DTI, anatomic structures are not available in great detail. In addition, DTI measurements based on echo planar imaging (EPI) suffer from imaging distortions, which can be attributed to the inhomogeneity of the magnetic field due to varying susceptibility within the measured tissue and to the small bandwidth of the EPI sequence in the phase-encoding direction. Susceptibility artifacts appear at the proximity of the skull base and near other air-filled spaces such as the brainstem and the frontal lobe and may cause severe distortions implying a displacement of anatomic structures, leading to a misregistration of anatomic and DTI data. Integrating tractography data into navigation actually is not trivial due to these image distortions inherent in EPI-based DTI data. There are several strategies to solve this problem: by measuring field maps describing image distortions, applying other MR sequence techniques that are less sensitive to distortions, or by performing a nonlinear registration of DTI and 3D navigational data, so that these distortions can be compensated for.[59]

A field map or distortion map provides additional experimental data obtained from a phantom and is used for scanner calibration. This information is used to partly compensate for the distortions of real image data. A major disadvantage of this approach is that distortion correction is limited only to field distortions independent of the subject's head geometry. For this reason, field maps are primarily restricted to eddy-current correction. Susceptibility artifacts cannot be compensated with field maps because it is impractical to build a phantom exactly duplicating the subject's anatomy. Presently, in modern functional scanning tools representing functional data in 3D anatomic datasets these field maps are implemented to identify and mark areas where the image information can no longer be trusted due to image distortions.

Alternative DTI sequences, such as stimulated acquisition mode (STEAM) sequences, are much less susceptible to imaging distortions.[31] Essentially, STEAM is insensitive to eddy currents, motion, and susceptibility gradients. However, it suffers from several drawbacks such as a coarser resolution and an increased measurement time, which still render its clinical use problematic. The STEAM approach is characterized by a lower signal-to-noise ratio than that of EPI. For this reason, EPI remains essential for clinical DTI on 1.5 T MR scanners, especially considering the intraoperative application due to the measurement time restrictions during a surgical procedure. Thus alternative strategies for distortion correction of DTI EPI data are still required.

Nonlinear registration schemes can be implemented to account for the spatial distortion of EPI when registering EPI to anatomic image data. A multiresolution approach using a high-order spline model for warping and a similarity measure

based on squared differences was proposed by Kybic et al.[60] Another approach estimated a deformation field with a hierarchical multigrid algorithm by minimizing a cost function based on mutual information.[61] Free-form deformation using 3D Bézier functions making extensive use of graphics hardware to accelerate the registration procedure is an alternative possibility.[62] In this approach that applies nonlinear registration using Bézier functions, the distortion of the pyramidal tract in the phase-encoding direction was most prominent at the cortex and the brainstem with a maximum of 15 and 11.5 mm, respectively (mean of 4.0 ± 2.8 mm and 3.2 ± 3.5 mm, respectively). However, in the area of interest—around the zone undergoing resection—the mean distortion was 2.4 ± 1.7 mm with a maximum of 9 mm.[59]

Distortion of echo planar images used for DTI-based fiber tracking can be evaluated by nonlinear registration. However, the implemented technique is still too time-consuming, so that it cannot be applied in a routine clinical setting. Rigid registration of EPI and standard anatomic images is still the clinical routine and it is important that the potential errors of image distortions are also known to the routine clinical user. Ideally, 3D hulls additionally encompassing the reconstructed fiber tracts would visualize the extent of these image distortions such as the degree of reliability and quality of the data (**Fig. 15.7**).

Besides progress in sequence development with reduced image distortion, de-noising, increased number of diffusion directions, and higher resolution of the raw data, further

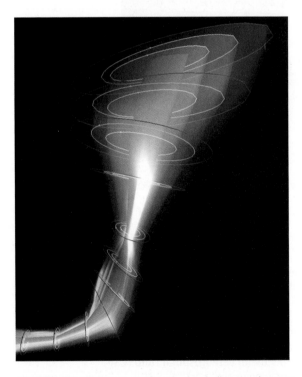

Fig. 15.7 Visualization concept of safety hulls around a reconstructed fiber tract system that vary in diameter, ideally reflecting the quality and reliability of the tracking result.

progress will also relate to a more accurate reconstruction of neural connectivity patterns. Correct identification of areas of fiber crossings is not possible by DTI because of its inability to resolve more than a single axon direction within each imaging voxel. Techniques that can resolve multiple axon directions within a single voxel may solve the problem of white matter fiber crossings, as well as white matter insertions into the cortex.[63]

Further challenges relate to the effects of edema surrounding a tumor where fiber tracking is attempted. Effects of edema and the tumor directly may impede the correct tracking so that either existing fibers are not visualized at all or even erroneous tracking may result. Multiregion of interest tracking approaches, as well as alternative tracking algorithms might help in this respect.

Alternative tracking strategies play a crucial role if more complex white matter tracts are to be reconstructed. Standard tracking algorithms might fail when white matter tracts connecting speech relevant areas are reconstructed. Tracking initialized from one speech area is not guaranteed to reach the second speech area at all. The reason is that fiber tracking is not goal oriented because regions of interest used in fiber tracking just serve as seed regions or to select fibers running through the region of interest. Additionally, imaging noise, integration errors, and partial volume effects may cause the fibers to miss the goal. A further aspect is that fiber-tracking algorithms are only able to progress as far as the certainty of the fiber direction represented by a strong anisotropy is sufficiently high. Near subcortical or cortical regions this effect forces the fiber propagation to terminate, so that it is a challenge to reconstruct a fiber bundle that connects Broca and Wernicke areas that are delineated by fMRI (**Fig. 15.8**). Pathfinding is a potential method to overcome these problems because it establishes a connection between two predefined areas and allows the calculation of the related probability. In artificial intelligence, pathfinding algorithms are commonly used for solving problems associated with such a state space search. These highly efficient algorithms are applied to derive a solution or path that connects an initial and final state corresponding to functional brain regions. The approach is thereby locally guided by cost functions based on the probability distribution function of each tensor. In this way, the uncertainty in path direction is modeled controlling the pathfinding procedure. Relative probabilities of different directions are taken into account, which guarantees the propagation of the path even if a voxel with low probability is encountered. The approach thus naturally handles imaging noise as well as branching, crossing, or kissing fibers. The probabilistic nature of the cost functions prevents the algorithm from drifting to errant routes. Additionally, the probabilities of each step can be recorded and visualized providing a connectivity estimate for the whole path.[64,65]

◆ Conclusion

DTI fiber-tracking data can be reliably integrated into navigational systems providing an intraoperative visualization of the major white matter tracts, allowing resection of

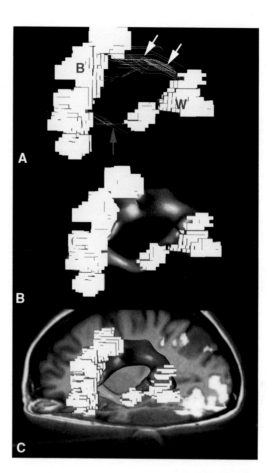

Fig. 15.8 Visualization of language-related fiber tracts by pathfinding connecting Broca (B) and Wernicke (W) areas, which are delineated by functional magnetic resonance imaging (fMRI). **(A)** Arcuate fasciculus (superior longitudinal fasciculus; *white arrows*) and inferior occipitofrontal fasciculus (*gray arrow*) are visualized as streamlines. **(B)** The reconstructed fibers are wrapped by a three-dimensional (3D) hull. **(C)** Both tract systems are visualized along a 3D T1-weighted MR image applying a side-cut view.

lesions adjacent to subcortical eloquent brain areas, that is the major white matter tracts, with low morbidity. Hulls wrapping the reconstructed fiber tract bundles can be used to visualize safety margins. Intraoperative imaging allows identifying the shifting of the major white matter tracts during surgery; the intraoperative image data can be used to update the navigation system, thus compensating for the effects of brain-shift. DTI is becoming increasingly important and has clinical implications in a variety of neurologic diseases, also in respect to a quantitative assessment of therapeutic regimens in time-course measurements. DTI data can also be applied to evaluate a neurologic deficit preoperatively, as well as to investigate changes in the peritumoral area, for example, that may have been caused by the invasion of gliomas.

Future advancements will be in the field of quantification and reduction of spatial inaccuracies of the raw DTI data, as well as in improvements in sequence design, tracking parameters, and algorithms.

References

1. Nimsky C, Ganslandt O, Kober H, et al. Integration of functional magnetic resonance imaging supported by magnetoencephalography in functional neuronavigation. Neurosurgery 1999;44(6):1249–1255, discussion 1255–1256

2. Ganslandt O, Fahlbusch R, Nimsky C, et al. Functional neuronavigation with magnetoencephalography: outcome in 50 patients with lesions around the motor cortex. J Neurosurg 1999;91(1):73–79

3. Kober H, Nimsky C, Möller M, Hastreiter P, Fahlbusch R, Ganslandt O. Correlation of sensorimotor activation with functional magnetic resonance imaging and magnetoencephalography in presurgical functional imaging: a spatial analysis. Neuroimage 2001;14(5):1214–1228

4. Basser PJ, Mattiello J, LeBihan D. MR diffusion tensor spectroscopy and imaging. Biophys J 1994;66(1):259–267

5. Coenen VA, Krings T, Mayfrank L, et al. Three-dimensional visualization of the pyramidal tract in a neuronavigation system during brain tumor surgery: first experiences and technical note. Neurosurgery 2001;49(1):86–92, discussion 92–93

6. Kamada K, Houkin K, Takeuchi F, et al. Visualization of the eloquent motor system by integration of MEG, functional, and anisotropic diffusion-weighted MRI in functional neuronavigation. Surg Neurol 2003;59(5):352–361, discussion 361–362

7. Beppu T, Inoue T, Shibata Y, et al. Measurement of fractional anisotropy using diffusion tensor MRI in supratentorial astrocytic tumors. J Neurooncol 2003;63(2):109–116

8. Clark CA, Barrick TR, Murphy MM, Bell BA. White matter fiber tracking in patients with space-occupying lesions of the brain: a new technique for neurosurgical planning? Neuroimage 2003;20(3):1601–1608

9. Hendler T, Pianka P, Sigal M, et al. Delineating gray and white matter involvement in brain lesions: three-dimensional alignment of functional magnetic resonance and diffusion-tensor imaging. J Neurosurg 2003;99(6):1018–1027

10. Lu S, Ahn D, Johnson G, Cha S. Peritumoral diffusion tensor imaging of high-grade gliomas and metastatic brain tumors. AJNR Am J Neuroradiol 2003;24(5):937–941

11. Price SJ, Burnet NG, Donovan T, et al. Diffusion tensor imaging of brain tumours at 3T: a potential tool for assessing white matter tract invasion? Clin Radiol 2003;58(6):455–462

12. Tummala RP, Chu RM, Liu H, Truwit CL, Hall WA. Application of diffusion tensor imaging to magnetic-resonance-guided brain tumor resection. Pediatr Neurosurg 2003;39(1):39–43

13. Wieshmann UC, Clark CA, Symms MR, Franconi F, Barker GJ, Shorvon SD. Reduced anisotropy of water diffusion in structural cerebral abnormalities demonstrated with diffusion tensor imaging. Magn Reson Imaging 1999;17(9):1269–1274

14. Witwer BP, Moftakhar R, Hasan KM, et al. Diffusion-tensor imaging of white matter tracts in patients with cerebral neoplasm. J Neurosurg 2002;97(3):568–575

15. Yamada K, Kizu O, Mori S, et al. Brain fiber tracking with clinically feasible diffusion-tensor MR imaging: initial experience. Radiology 2003;227(1):295–301

16. Pajevic S, Pierpaoli C. Color schemes to represent the orientation of anisotropic tissues from diffusion tensor data: application to white matter fiber tract mapping in the human brain. Magn Reson Med 1999;42(3):526–540

17. Pierpaoli C, Jezzard P, Basser PJ, Barnett A, Di Chiro G. Diffusion tensor MR imaging of the human brain. Radiology 1996;201(3):637–648

18. Kindlmann G. Superquadric tensor glyphs. In Proceedings of Eurographics – IEEE TCVG Symposium on Visualization. Piscataway, NJ: IEEE; 2004: 147–154

19. Basser PJ, Pajevic S, Pierpaoli C, Duda J, Aldroubi A. In vivo fiber tractography using DT-MRI data. Magn Reson Med 2000;44(4):625–632

20. Mori S, Crain BJ, Chacko VP, van Zijl PC. Three-dimensional tracking of axonal projections in the brain by magnetic resonance imaging. Ann Neurol 1999;45(2):265–269

21. Mori S, van Zijl PC. Fiber tracking: principles and strategies - a technical review. NMR Biomed 2002;15(7-8):468–480

22. Stieltjes B, Kaufmann WE, van Zijl PC, et al. Diffusion tensor imaging and axonal tracking in the human brainstem. Neuroimage 2001;14(3):723–735

23. Holodny AI, Schwartz TH, Ollenschleger M, Liu WC, Schulder M. Tumor involvement of the corticospinal tract: diffusion magnetic resonance tractography with intraoperative correlation. J Neurosurg 2001;95(6):1082

24. Wu JS, Zhou LF, Hong XN, Mao Y, Du GH. [Role of diffusion tensor imaging in neuronavigation surgery of brain tumors involving pyramidal tracts]. Zhonghua Wai Ke Za Zhi 2003;41(9):662–666

25. Talos I, O'Donnell L, Westin CF, et al. Diffusion tensor and functional MRI fusion with anatomical MRI for image-guided neurosurgery. In: Ellis R, Peters T, eds. Medical Image Computing and Computer-Assisted Intervention - MICCAI 2003. Berlin/Heidelberg: Springer-Verlag; 2003: 407–415

26. Kamada K, Sawamura Y, Takeuchi F, et al. Functional identification of the primary motor area by corticospinal tractography. Neurosurgery 2005; 56(1, Suppl)98–109, discussion 98–109

27. Kinoshita M, Yamada K, Hashimoto N, et al. Fiber-tracking does not accurately estimate size of fiber bundle in pathological condition: initial neurosurgical experience using neuronavigation and subcortical white matter stimulation. Neuroimage 2005;25(2):424–429

28. Enders F, Iserhardt-Bauer S, Hastreiter P, Nimsky C, Ertl T. Hardware-accelerated glyph based visualization of major white matter tracts for analysis of brain tumors. In: Galloway RJ, Cleary K. eds. Medical Imaging 2005: Visualization, Image-Guided Procedures, and Display: Proceedings of SPIE Vol. 5744. Bellingham, WA:SPIE; 2005: 504–511

29. Merhof D, Hastreiter P, Nimsky C, Fahlbusch R, Greiner G. Directional volume growing for the extraction of white matter tracts from diffusion tensor data. In: Galloway RJ, Cleary K, eds. Medical Imaging 2005: Visualization, Image-Guided Procedures, and Display: Proceedings of SPIE Vol. 5744. Bellingham, WA:SPIE; 2005: 165–172

30. Nimsky C, Grummich P, Sorensen AG, Fahlbusch R, Ganslandt O. Visualization of the pyramidal tract in glioma surgery by integrating diffusion tensor imaging in functional neuronavigation. Zentralbl Neurochir 2005;66(3):133–141

31. Nimsky C, Ganslandt O, Fahlbusch R. Implementation of fiber tract navigation. Neurosurgery 2006; 58(4, Suppl 2)ONS-292–ONS-304

32. Nimsky C, Ganslandt O, Weigel D, et al. Intraoperative tractography and neuronavigation of the pyramidal tract. Jpn J Neurosurg 2008; 17:21–26

33. Duffau H, Capelle L, Denvil D, et al. Usefulness of intraoperative electrical subcortical mapping during surgery for low-grade gliomas located within eloquent brain regions: functional results in a consecutive series of 103 patients. J Neurosurg 2003;98(4):764–778

34. Yingling CD, Ojemann S, Dodson B, Harrington MJ, Berger MS. Identification of motor pathways during tumor surgery facilitated by multichannel electromyographic recording. J Neurosurg 1999;91(6): 922–927

35. Wu JS, Zhou LF, Tang WJ, et al. Clinical evaluation and follow-up outcome of diffusion tensor imaging-based functional neuronavigation: a prospective, controlled study in patients with gliomas involving pyramidal tracts. Neurosurgery 2007;61(5):935–948, discussion 948–949

36. Ganslandt O, Buchfelder M, Hastreiter P, Grummich P, Fahlbusch R, Nimsky C. Magnetic source imaging supports clinical decision making in glioma patients. Clin Neurol Neurosurg 2004;107(1):20–26

37. Krishnan R, Raabe A, Hattingen E, et al. Functional magnetic resonance imaging-integrated neuronavigation: correlation between lesion-to-motor cortex distance and outcome. Neurosurgery 2004;55(4): 904–914, 914–915

38. Goebell E, Fiehler J, Ding XQ, et al. Disarrangement of fiber tracts and decline of neuronal density correlate in glioma patients—a combined diffusion tensor imaging and 1H-MR spectroscopy study. AJNR Am J Neuroradiol 2006;27(7):1426–1431

39. Kinoshita M, Hashimoto N, Goto T, et al. Fractional anisotropy and tumor cell density of the tumor core show positive correlation in diffusion tensor magnetic resonance imaging of malignant brain tumors. Neuroimage 2008; 43(1)29–35

40. Stadlbauer A, Ganslandt O, Buslei R, et al. Gliomas: histopathologic evaluation of changes in directionality and magnitude of water diffusion at diffusion-tensor MR imaging. Radiology 2006;240(3):803–810

41. Stadlbauer A, Nimsky C, Buslei R, et al. Diffusion tensor imaging and optimized fiber tracking in glioma patients: histopathologic evaluation of tumor-invaded white matter structures. Neuroimage 2007; 34(3):949–956

42. Stadlbauer A, Nimsky C, Gruber S, et al. Changes in fiber integrity, diffusivity, and metabolism of the pyramidal tract adjacent to gliomas: a quantitative diffusion tensor fiber tracking and MR spectroscopic imaging study. AJNR Am J Neuroradiol 2007;28(3):462–469

43. Price SJ, Jena R, Burnet NG, Carpenter TA, Pickard JD, Gillard JH. Predicting patterns of glioma recurrence using diffusion tensor imaging. Eur Radiol 2007;17(7):1675–1684

44. Kamada K, Todo T, Masutani Y, et al. Visualization of the frontotemporal language fibers by tractography combined with functional magnetic resonance imaging and magnetoencephalography. J Neurosurg 2007;106(1):90–98

45. Catani M, Jones DK, ffytche DH. Perisylvian language networks of the human brain. Ann Neurol 2005;57(1):8–16

46. Parker GJ, Luzzi S, Alexander DC, Wheeler-Kingshott CA, Ciccarelli O, Lambon Ralph MA. Lateralization of ventral and dorsal auditory-language pathways in the human brain. Neuroimage 2005;24(3): 656–666

47. Powell HW, Parker GJ, Alexander DC, et al. Hemispheric asymmetries in language-related pathways: a combined functional MRI and tractography study. Neuroimage 2006;32(1):388–399

48. Vernooij MW, Smits M, Wielopolski PA, Houston GC, Krestin GP, van der Lugt A. Fiber density asymmetry of the arcuate fasciculus in relation to functional hemispheric language lateralization in both right- and left-handed healthy subjects: a combined fMRI and DTI study. Neuroimage 2007;35(3):1064–1076

49. Chen X, Weigel D, Ganslandt O, Buchfelder M, Nimsky C. Diffusion tensor imaging and white matter tractography in patients with brainstem lesions. Acta Neurochir (Wien) 2007;149(11):1117–1131, discussion 1131

50. Nimsky C, Ganslandt O, Hastreiter P, et al. Intraoperative diffusion-tensor MR imaging: shifting of white matter tracts during neurosurgical procedures—initial experience. Radiology 2005;234(1):218–225

51. Nimsky C, Ganslandt O, Hastreiter P, et al. Preoperative and intraoperative diffusion tensor imaging-based fiber tracking in glioma surgery. Neurosurgery 2005;56(1):130–137, discussion 138

52. Nimsky C, Ganslandt O, Von Keller B, Romstöck J, Fahlbusch R. Intraoperative high-field-strength MR imaging: implementation and experience in 200 patients. Radiology 2004;233(1):67–78

53. Nimsky C, Ganslandt O, Merhof D, Sorensen AG, Fahlbusch R. Intraoperative visualization of the pyramidal tract by diffusion-tensor-imaging-based fiber tracking. Neuroimage 2006;30(4):1219–1229

54. Nimsky C, Ganslandt O, Cerny S, Hastreiter P, Greiner G, Fahlbusch R. Quantification of, visualization of, and compensation for brain shift using intraoperative magnetic resonance imaging. Neurosurgery 2000;47(5):1070–1079, discussion 1079–1080

55. Dorward NL, Alberti O, Velani B, et al. Postimaging brain distortion: magnitude, correlates, and impact on neuronavigation. J Neurosurg 1998;88(4):656–662

56. Keles GE, Lamborn KR, Berger MS. Coregistration accuracy and detection of brain shift using intraoperative sononavigation during resection of hemispheric tumors. Neurosurgery 2003;53(3):556–562, discussion 562–564

57. Nabavi A, Black PM, Gering DT, et al. Serial intraoperative magnetic resonance imaging of brain shift. Neurosurgery 2001;48(4):787–797, discussion 797–798

58. Kamada K, Todo T, Masutani Y, et al. Combined use of tractography-integrated functional neuronavigation and direct fiber stimulation. J Neurosurg 2005;102(4):664–672

59. Merhof D, Soza G, Stadlbauer A, Greiner G, Nimsky C. Correction of susceptibility artifacts in diffusion tensor data using non-linear registration. Med Image Anal 2007;11(6):588–603

60. Kybic J, Thévenaz P, Nirkko A, Unser M. Unwarping of unidirectionally distorted EPI images. IEEE Trans Med Imaging 2000;19(2):80–93

61. Hellier P, Barillot C. Multimodal non-rigid warping for correction of distortions in functional MRI. In: Delp S, DiGioia A, Jaramaz B, eds. Proceedings of the Medical Image Computing and Computer-Assisted Intervention (MICCAI), 3rd International Conference: Lecture Notes in Computer Science. Berlin/Heidelberg: Springer-Verlag; 2000: 512–520

62. Merhof D, Hastreiter P, Soza G, Stamminger M, Nimsky C. Non-linear integration of DTI-based fiber tracts into standard 3D MR data. In: Girod B, Magnor M, Seidel H-P, eds. Vision, Modeling and Visualization 2004. Berlin: Akademische Verlagsgesellschaft Aka; 2004: 371–377

63. Tuch DS, Reese TG, Wiegell MR, Wedeen VJ. Diffusion MRI of complex neural architecture. Neuron 2003;40(5):885–895

64. Merhof D, Enders F, Hastreiter P, et al. Neuronal fiber connections based on A*-pathfinding. In: Manduca A, Amini A, eds. Proceedings of Medical Imaging 2006: Physiology, Function, and Structure from Medical Images. Bellingham, WA: SPIE; 2006: 1–8

65. Merhof D, Richter M, Enders F, et al. Fast and accurate connectivity analysis between functional regions based on DT-MRI. In: Larsen R, Nielsen M, Sporring J, eds. Proceedings of the Medical Image Computing and Computer-Assisted Intervention - MICCAI 2006. Berlin/Heidelberg: Springer-Verlag; 2006: 225–233

IV

Nonneoplastic Surgical Indications

16

Intraoperative Magnetic Resonance Imaging for Epilepsy Surgery

Michael Buchfelder, Christopher Nimsky, and Daniel Weigel

The basis of epilepsy surgery is a hypothetical focus, which is considered the origin of abnormal electrical activity within the brain that may or may not be associated with morphologic abnormalities. However, in many cases a lesion can be depicted by sophisticated imaging. Usually, pharmacoresistancy of seizures is required before an operation is considered and preoperative investigations are performed, which are hoped to reveal the origin and propagation of seizure activity.[1] With the availability of morphologic (such as computerized tomography [CT] and magnetic resonance imaging [MRI]) and functional (such as interictal and ictal single photon emission tomography, positron emission tomography [PET], and magnetoencephalography [MEG]) imaging, epilepsy surgery underwent another enormous evolution. To date, a variety of operative procedures are designed to resect or disconnect an epileptogenic focus in the brain, so that no more seizures are generated or the abnormal electrical activity can no longer spread across the brain.[2] Video electroencephalography (EEG) monitoring is usually the first step. It documents whether the patient actually suffers from epilepsy because it correlates the clinical manifestations of seizures to abnormal cortical discharges. Thereafter, a battery of structural and functional imaging methods are available that can reveal connatal or acquired lesions in the brain and areas of functional hyperactivity during convulsions or interictally. Based on these examinations a hypothesis is established as to where the abnormal discharges originate and how they spread throughout the brain. The aim of epilepsy surgery is either to resect this focus or to interrupt the propagation of abnormal electrical activity by disconnective operations. The cooperation of neurologists, neurosurgeons, psychologists, neuroradiologists, nuclear medicine specialists, and psychiatrists is very useful in this context. In any case, interdisciplinary cooperation should result in a well-structured treatment plan. With modern precise localization technologies being available, in many patients, foci such as unilateral mesial temporal sclerosis, slowly growing tumors typically associated with epilepsy, vascular anomalies, or cortical dysplasias are well defined in distinct areas of the brain. Recent developments in surgical techniques are targeted resections of what is believed to be epileptogenic tissues rather than the previously practiced standard resections of cerebral lobes. Whether a resection or disconnection actually accomplished the treatment plan was usually confirmed when postoperative MR images were obtained. Early attempts to utilize intraoperative MRI (iMRI) in epilepsy surgery to assess whether a tailored resection or disconnection procedure morphologically fulfills the individual needs of a patient were reported in 1998[3] and 1999[4] with the description of the systems and set-ups. The recently proposed concept of "as much as possible" limited tissue removal would support a more conservative resection than initially advocated by many centers to preserve tissue that is not necessarily epileptogenic or involved in propagation of the seizures. Its aim is mainly to reduce adverse neuropsychologic sequelae of brain tissue resection. Because a sophisticated MRI is one of the mainstays of a preoperative workup of an epilepsy patient who is prepared for surgery, it makes sense to depict the result of the operation also by MRI. Despite recent advances in epilepsy surgery[5] that encompass the evolution of more-refined investigative techniques for the preoperative evaluation of patients with pharmacoresistant seizures and sophisticated operative procedures, further progress contributing to better delineation and definition of the epileptogenic process and its potential responsiveness to surgical resection is still eagerly awaited. In general, the extent of a resection is estimated by the surgeon at the time of the operation. However, a radiologic documentation of the amount and precise localization of resected brain was until recently only available several weeks after surgery. In this chapter, we review the experience gained with iMRI during surgery for epilepsy in patients with pharmacoresistant seizures.

◆ Systems and Set-ups

In 2000, we initially reported on the first 61 epilepsy surgery procedures with intraoperative low-field MRI utilizing a 0.2 tesla (T) MR (Siemens Magnetom; Siemens AG, Erlangen, Germany) system installed in our operating theater between 1996 and 2001.[3] This had a shifting operating table on which the patient's head could be brought just outside of the 5 gauss (G) line where it was unrestrictedly accessible and use of standard surgical instruments was possible. We initially even used a "twin operating theater" with patient transport on an air-cushioned system so that we could perform intraoperative electrocorticography (ECoG) in a standard shielded operating theater. Mean scanning time was 15 minutes.[6] Nimsky et al[7] implemented a navigation microscope within the fringe field of this MRI scanner, so that an update of navigation was possible utilizing intraoperative MRI data. A similar system with the same 0.2 T magnet, but with a tiltable surgical table was described by Lewin et al.[8] They performed 21 operations for the treatment of seizures. Mean time required for their imaging sessions was 15.4 minutes for the intraoperative and 11 minutes for postoperative imaging sessions. The mean patient who had surgery for seizures underwent 1.67 imaging sessions. The Neurological Institute of New Jersey describe the use of their PoleStar N10 system (0.12 T; Medtronic Navigation, Inc., Louisville, CO) for assessing the extent of mesial temporal lobe resections in five patients.[9] Likewise, Levivier et al[27] provide a few pictorial examples of temporal lobe operations and excision of a left frontal cortical dysplasia with the PoleStar Medtronic system, in which the navigation tool of the equipment was also utilized. Walker et al[10] reported on the Boston experience with the 0.5 T GE Signa system (General Electric Medical Systems, Waukesha, WI). There were 13 patients with benign intraaxial lesions presenting with seizures. The intraoperative set-up in the GE system, where the patient is lying in the MRI scanner during the whole operation, allowed the use of the MR imager as an online navigation device, but had the drawback that intraoperative electrophysiologic examinations (such as ECoG and hippocampal recordings) could not be performed in the vicinity of the system due to the high strength of the magnetic field. The ceiling mounted, mobile 1.5 T IMRIS system (IMRIS, Winnipeg, Manitoba, Canada) installed in Calgary in 1997 was also used for epilepsy surgery procedures. Kaibara et al[11] reported on 14 patients with temporal lobe resections for pharmacoresistant seizures. They performed surgical planning and interdissection MRI in all 14 patients. Eight of the patients additionally had quality-assurance MR investigations. A set of coronal and axial images added 20 to 30 minutes to the operative procedure. Because this magnet can be moved away from the patient, ECoG can be performed in the same operating theater. A further analysis of the Calgary series experience with epilepsy surgery and iMRI comprising 70 patients by utilizing the 1.5 T high-field system was reported by Kelly et al.[12] Neuronavigation was registered based on the preoperative planning images in 38 of the 70 patients (55%). Interdissection images were obtained in all but one patient (98.6%). They confirm that interdissection images led to further tissue resections in 26% of the patients. The currently used set-up in Erlangen was described by Nimsky et al.[13] The "Brain Suite" consists of a 1.5 T MR imager equipped with a rotating operating table and located in a radiofrequency- (RF-) shielded operating theater. A navigation microscope placed inside the 0.5 millitesla (mT) zone and used with a ceiling-mounted navigation system enables integrated microscope-based neuronavigation. In this system, the patient moves. Draping the patient and rotating the operating table for scanning takes some 2 minutes. We have shown that intraoperative ECoG for epilepsy surgery is possible within the RF-shielded operating theater; in close vicinity to the MRI scanner (**Fig. 16.1**). During the 7.5 years between April 2002 and August 2009, 1424 operative cranial neurosurgical procedures were performed in this system and 170 of these were operations for epilepsy other than tumor resections. There were 12 implantations of electrodes, 156 resections, and two multiple subpial transections performed with 1.5 T MRI intraoperatively. One-hundred thirty temporal lobe resections and 25 extratemporal resections were performed. In 124 of the procedures, navigation was used based on intraoperatively acquired datasets. The improvements in workflow, image quality, and efficiency between the low- and high-field systems in the same department were analyzed by Nimsky et al.[14]

◆ Intraoperative Recordings and Positioning of Electrodes

Despite the considerable advances in imaging technology and sophisticated functional investigations, there remain a substantial number of patients in whom the noninvasive evaluations fail to precisely localize the focus. Further information is frequently gathered by the implantation of subdural or intracerebral electrodes for a few days or by intraoperative ECoG. Although attempts have been made to reduce invasive diagnosis to a minimum, its availability in difficult cases characterizes a universal epilepsy surgery program. It is a general custom to implant subdural electrodes through burr holes under radiofluoroscopic control. Their position is thus only estimated in relation to bony landmarks of the skull because the x-ray does not depict the brain.[5] Only grids are implanted via craniotomies and the position of electrodes is then directly visible on the brain surface. Direct cortical stimulation using these electrodes may reveal further information on functionally important regions. The intraoperative low-field MRI beautifully depicted the position of hippocampal and depth electrodes.[6] We thus confirmed in the operating theater that the electrodes were placed where we wanted to record. If required, repositioning could easily be achieved and the positions rechecked. The high-field system is advantageous, particularly concerning the quality of the images. **Figure 16.2** shows the

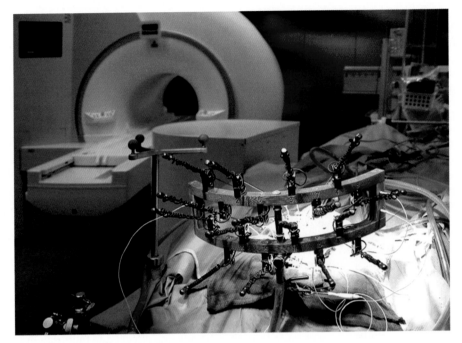

Fig. 16.1 Set-up for epilepsy surgery with intraoperative magnetic resonance imaging (MRI): electrocorticography with the Montreal system and reference star for neuronavigation (BrainLab VectorVision; BrainLab, Feldkirchen Germany) in the front; 1.5 T MRI scanner (Siemens Sonata, Maestro Class; Siemens AG, Erlangen, Germany) in the back.

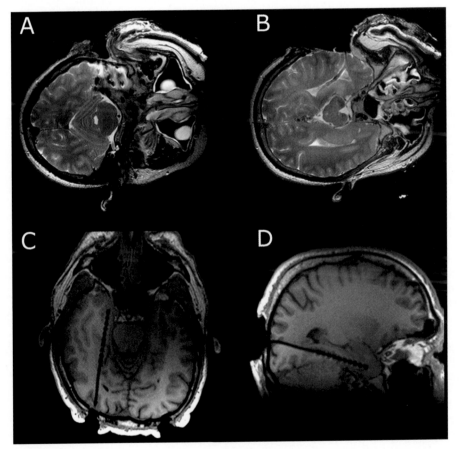

Fig. 16.2 Intraoperative localization of electrodes. **(A)** The subdural strips were placed for intraoperative electrocorticography. Their exact localization detected by intraoperative magnetic resonance imaging (iMRI) can be used for functional neuronavigation during surgery. **(B)** The hippocampal electrode was placed transcortically into the ventricle for intraoperative electrocorticography. The iMRI documents the correct placement and the anatomic relation to the hippocampus. **(C,D)** The deep brain electrode was placed with use of neuronavigation ("frameless stereotaxy") into the hippocampus for chronic recordings. The iMRI documents the correct placement.

basal subdural and hippocampal electrodes for intraoperative corticography, which allow for correlation between the neurophysiologic recordings and the topography of the brain. The figure also shows a depth electrode that records through the axis of the hippocampus. Mehta et al[15] describe the advantages of frameless stereotactic placement of depth electrodes with a commercially available navigation system in epilepsy surgery. Implementation of a navigation tool that uses the MR data registration within the same operating theater and patient position in which the operation is performed seems to be advantageous because it avoids potential inconsistencies and thus improves the accuracy of electrode placement. Ideally, the resulting electrode localization can be immediately visualized, which is also possible with an iMRI. Depiction of subdural and intracerebral electrodes by MRI is of no safety concern.[16]

◆ Temporal Lobe Resections

Temporal lobe resections are the most frequently performed neurosurgical operations for the treatment of pharmacoresistant epilepsy. A major advantage of these procedures is that most of these can be undertaken without causing a neurologic deficit at least in most patients and particularly in the nondominant hemisphere. The concept of standard resections of the anterior temporal lobe survived for decades. One of the ongoing controversies is that of structure–function relationship, which was more recently approached by systematic sophisticated assessment of the extent of tissue resection in relation to the pre- and postoperative loss of cognition and to the efficacy of the procedure with respect to seizure control. The background of tailored anterior or posterior temporal lobe resections is an attempt to achieve more precise resection, thus maximizing preservation of normal brain. Various suggestions as to how to achieve this goal have been made in the past and a variety of different surgical procedures have been devised.[5] We utilized intraoperative ECoG in addition to the preoperative investigations for tailoring the resections to the needs of the individual patient. As already mentioned, iMRI beautifully depicts the position of hippocampal and depth electrodes and allows for the establishment of some functional–anatomic relationship because of its ability to correlate anatomic structures and lesions within the brain and their relative location with respect to the electrodes. The individualized temporal lobe resections vary to date considerably from selective amygdalohippocampectomies to lesionectomies, usually with resection of some perilesional tissue. In all these different types of resections, the extent of mesial and neocortical resections should be documented. Moran et al[17] have suggested using a technique based on volumetric analysis based on the delayed postoperative MRI. They intended to determine a relationship between seizure and neuropsychologic outcome and the extent of resection. Some authors find a correlation between the radicality of resection of the mesial temporal lobe and seizure outcome.[18–21] Although such a correlation is difficult to significantly establish, analysis of surgical failures after an initial temporal lobe resection also found incomplete resection of the amygdala, hippocampus, and parahippocampal gyrus performed during the initial surgery. In many of these patients the outcome could be improved by extending the mesial temporal lobe resection.[22–24] One would now assume that generally neurosurgeons have learned from these observations and attack the mesial temporal lobe more aggressively. After all, there are anatomic landmarks that can help during temporal lobe resections. Undoubtedly, however, an iMRI would reveal what might be hidden to the surgeon because of its deep location medial to the temporal horn of the lateral ventricle and beneath the choroid plexus. We showed that the entire temporal lobe could be excellently imaged by iMRI using a magnetic field strength as low as 0.2 T during the operative procedure, depicting whether there was a lesion or not.[6,25] At that time, we classified hippocampal sclerosis as nonlesional, even when there was a clearly visible medial lobe atrophy. In 49 of the 58 cases reported in detail in another article, the intraoperative findings corresponded exactly to those obtained during follow-up MRI several months after surgery in different institutions.[26] The outcome in respect to seizure control was quite favorable. No adverse effects due to intraoperative imaging and intraoperative patient transportation, which was necessary in our setting to allow the combination of intraoperative neurophysiologic recordings with MRI were encountered. Neuronavigation, even functional navigation, was integrated in 11 patients. Extension of resection was performed in two lesional cases and one nonlesional case. Twenty-two of the 29 lesional patients and 17 of the 29 nonlesional patients became absolutely seizure-free. The overall complication rate was low. Specifically, there was only one instance of wound infection that necessitated removal of the infected bone flap and subsequent closure of the bony defect by a cranioplasty. This adverse event, however, cannot necessarily be attributed to intraoperative imaging. There was no symptomatic rebleeding. However, the true incidence of asymptomatic postoperative hematoma could only be estimated because the patients were not routinely scanned a few days after surgery. Kaibara et al[11] report on 14 patients: 10 patients underwent anterior temporal lobectomy and four patients who underwent selective amygdalohippocampectomy for seizures using the 1.5 T system. The interdissection images revealed residual unresected amygdala or hippocampus in seven patients. One unexpected acute hematoma was found by intraoperative imaging. Apart from one patient, all became seizure-free. In a later report from the Calgary group with 51 patients operated upon with temporal lobe resections, the initial findings were confirmed. Schwarz et al[7] used the PoleStar 0.12 T magnet to standardize amygdalohippocampectomy and found the image quality sufficient to improve the initial surgical result, just as Levivier et al[27] depict some examples of temporal lobe procedures in their article. Others also recognized that (apart from the total resection of lesions in lesional cases) the extent and completeness of mesial temporal lobe resection is important. Van Roost et al[28] recognized the importance of the problem and attempted to use neuronavigation to improve the standardization of

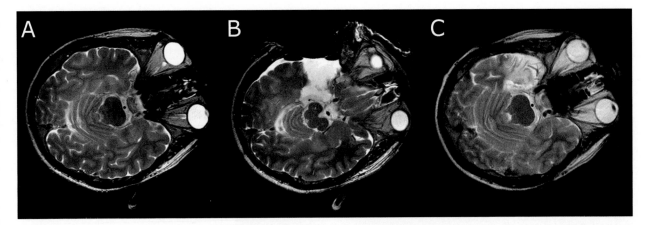

Fig. 16.3 A 37-year-old male patient with hippocampal sclerosis. **(A)** Preoperative magnetic resonance imaging (MRI). **(B)** A tailored neocortical and temporomesial resection was performed according to the findings of intraoperative electrocorticography. The intraoperative MRI documents the extent of the resection. **(C)** The follow-up MRI 6 months postoperatively shows normal postoperative findings. However, some shift of adjacent brain has occurred so that the extent of resection is less well reflected as in the intraoperative MRI.

amygdalohippocampectomy, but had the disadvantage of relying on preoperative data. The intraoperative use of a high-field MRI scanner allows an even better resolution of intraoperative images, which might be valuable even in nontumor cases. The actual extent of a resection is exactly depicted in the intraoperative 1.5 T MRI, while brain displacement into the resection cavity sometimes leads to underestimation of resection volume in the delayed postoperative MRI (**Fig. 16.3**). The delayed postoperative images were, however, in the past considered as the gold standard for assessing the amount of neocortical and mesial temporal lobe resection. These measures seem to be crucial in studies that would like to support a more conservative surgery in temporal lobe resections while sparing tissue not necessarily involved in epileptogenesis. Thus iMRI is a useful tool in such investigations. Many patients with seizures originating in one temporal lobe harbor lesions. Benign tumors that do not pose an onco-logic problem are typical examples. Because their complete resection correlates with seizure outcome, it should be unequivocally documented (**Fig. 16.4**). The desired resection pays tribute to the findings of preoperative investigations: electrophysiology and functional imaging. It is not desired to carry out a most elegant selective resection of the lesion. Essentially, at least within the temporal lobe, low-grade gliomas may be epileptogenic lesions. Thus, in our initial reports with the low-field system, there were a high proportion of lesions operated on for pharmacoresis-tant seizures, which turned out to be gliomas. The Erlangen policy of tailored resection resulted in different combinations of neocortical and mesial resections, albeit mostly there was some mesial resection performed. We found that postresection imaging necessitates a more objective documentation of the actual extent of resection than a subjective surgical description. The early postresection intraoperative MR images, just as routine postoperative imaging, could be utilized to precisely classify the type of temporal lobe resection.

◆ Extratemporal Resections

Much less-resective procedures in the field of epilepsy surgery concern regions outside the temporal lobe. Frequently, conclusive localization of the focus is very difficult in these cases, particularly if the MRI does not depict any abnormality.[29] Furthermore, in many such cases, the proximity to eloquent cortical regions poses a significant operative hazard. Implantation of subdural electrodes, functional navigation, and awake craniotomy are attempts to reduce neurologic deficit. Only the nondominant frontal lobe is less critical. Intraoperative ECoG is more frequently utilized and more generally accepted in extratemporal resections than in surgery of the temporal lobe. There are only very limited examples in the medical literature. Walker et al[10] present five lesional cases outside of the temporal lobe, where they accomplished total resection with confirmation by their 0.2 T scanner. Three of them were occipital and two were frontal. In addition, they describe resection of a hypothalamic hamartoma. Taniguchi et al[30] present two patients with vascular lesions presenting with epilepsy. They localized and resected the lesions with the support of an AIRIS 0.3 T MRI scanner (Hitachi Medical Corp., Tokyo, Japan) for which they devised a radiofrequency coil integrated with a stereotactic fame. Levivier et al[27] depict a frontal cortical dysplasia. Surprisingly, there is also a lack of reports on the use of other intraoperative imaging modalities, such as CT as referred to their specific application in epilepsy surgery. Only the usefulness of intraoperative ultrasound imaging, which is more frequently applied to resection control in glioma surgery, has been found useful during the tailoring of functional hemispherectomies.[31]

◆ Lesionectomies

If there is good evidence that a structural lesion in the brain is epileptogenic a lesionectomy might be an appropriate operation. Resection of the lesion is termed lesionectomy when

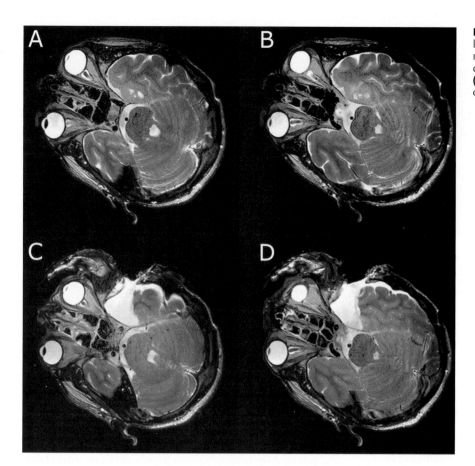

Fig. 16.4 A 22-year-old male patient with lesional epilepsy. **(A,B)** The preoperative magnetic resonance imaging (MRI) scans depict a temporomesial cystic ganglioglioma. **(C,D)** The intraoperative MRI scans document complete resection.

the dominating clinical symptoms are seizures and oncologic considerations do not press for surgical intervention. Caution, however, is necessary because lesions and concomitant nonlesional foci may be present. A lesion depicted in the MRI such as a cavernous hemangioma is frequently, but not necessarily always the focus of an epileptic disorder. Moreover, gliotic changes and tissue alterations in the close neighborhood of the vascular or tumorous lesion may be responsible for the abnormal discharges. Thus, the most brilliant minimal invasive and selective microsurgical resection might not be the ultimate solution for the patient. It seemed advantageous to also apply the principles of epilepsy surgery to lesions that produce seizures. Because the total resection of lesions seems to offer the best chance for improvement of epilepsy, the use of MR imaging to intraoperatively document the completed excision was reported by Walker et al.[10] They assessed the amount of resection of benign intracerebral tumors, such as dysembryoplastic neuroepithelial tumors (DNET) and gangliogliomas, but also cortical dysplasias and a hypothalamic hamartoma with the GE Signa SP scanner and used the intraoperative images also as an online navigational tool. Clinically, there was improvement of seizures in all patients, but the follow-up was relatively short. With their set-up, they could not use ECoG, the usefulness of which they question anyway. Apart from a deep venous thrombosis and one hemianopsia in a patient with an occipital cortical dysplasia there were no complications

reported. They concluded that intraoperative imaging could assure the completeness of resections in this cohort of patients as it did with gliomas, which were operated for oncologic indications.[32] Likewise, but not providing data from a series, Levivier et al[27] provide an example of a left frontal cortical dysplasia in which they used navigation and the comparison of pre- and postresection intraoperative images. Particularly with cortical dysplasias, which are difficult to depict, the application of high-field systems is advantageous (**Fig. 16.5**). The definition of a lesion within the surgical field is sometimes a problem. Although it offers much worse tissue contrast and also provides worse resolution, Miller et al,[33] in the lack of availability of iMRI, used intraoperative ultrasound to localize cortical dysplasias in their patients. Kelly et al[12] resected nine benign lesions and seven cortical dysplasias in their epilepsy patients with high-field MRI guidance. The tumors were gangliogliomas, gangliocytomas, and DNETs. Stefan et al[34] report on resection of a periventricular nodular heterotopia in a girl who harbored several lesions. Coregistration of several functional imaging data with the intraoperative 1.5 T MRI was crucial in identifying the lesion, documenting resection, and avoiding a distortion of visual pathways. Even benign tumors are tumors. Their resection may be selective if electrophysiology permits (**Fig. 16.6**). However, the completeness of resection must be assured. Apart from the benign tumors, in our opinion hypothalamic hamartoma is a specific lesion in which surgical

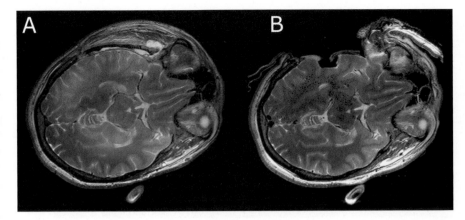

Fig. 16.5 A 20-year-old female patient with nonlesional epilepsy. **(A)** The preoperative magnetic resonance imaging (MRI) scan depicts no pathologic findings. **(B)** The intraoperative MRI scan documents the resection according to findings from presurgical invasive diagnostic. Histologically, in the resected cortex focal cortical dysplasia (type IIb) was found.

treatment with the use of intraoperative resection control is extremely useful. The clinical manifestations of hypothalamic hamartomas are precocious puberty and gelastic epilepsy. These nontumorous lesions are localized in the lower portion of the 3rd ventricle and may be intrinsic, embedded in the hypothalamus or more exophytic, protruding into the optico-chiasmatic cisterns, but still connected with the confines of the 3rd ventricle. The exophytic ones are easier to deal with. One of the characteristics of the intrinsic ones, however, is that their delineation appears much better in the MRI than in the surgical field. Walker et al[10] describe how they used their low-field system to assure total resection of a hypothalamic hamartoma, which they reoperated because at the first operation, the surgeon had missed a portion of the lesion. Although we had used our 0.2 T Magnetom open system for the surgery of hypothalamic hamartomas[25] we found 1.5 T high-field iMRI much better for the depiction and delineation of these lesions (**Fig. 16.7**). In several instances, even in good quality MR images the hypothalamic hamartomas are difficult to detect. Subtle signs, such as asymmetry of the 3rd ventricle or a minor bulging of tissue into the optico-chiasmatic cistern are the only radiological signs, which are difficult to detect on low-field MR images. One major advantage of intraoperative imaging is undoubtedly that a conservative resection may be performed, and in the case of residual hamartoma, the resection may be

extended. Intraoperatively, the lesions are ill defined and difficult to distinguish from the hypothalamus: lesions in the hypothalamus should be strictly avoided. In doubtful situations, updating navigation based on intraoperative images documenting residual hamartoma, just in tumor cases, may be particularly helpful in this pathologic entity.[35]

◆ Corpus Callosum Transsection

In patients who suffer from generalized multifocal seizures or drop seizures and are not considered suitable candidates for attacking a focus, transsection of the corpus callosum is an option. This palliative operative procedure is considered particularly useful for patients with drop seizures. With careful patient selection, some 70% of such patients will have a reduction in the magnitude and/or frequency of their seizures following the procedure which is performed through a paramedian craniotomy and interhemispheric dissection.[36,37] In the past, complete transsection of the corpus callosum was attempted. This is rarely performed to date and generally replaced by a two-third to three-quarter transsection, at least at the primary intervention. Corpus callosotomy is a good example for nonlesional, entirely functional epilepsy surgery because the corpus callosum as the target of surgery, usually shows no abnormality. Only a

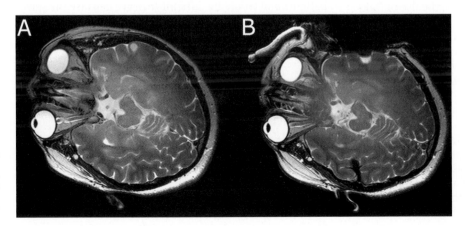

Fig. 16.6 A 25-year-old female patient with lesional epilepsy. **(A)** The preoperative magnetic resonance imaging (MRI) scan depicts a temporal ganglioglioma in the middle temporal gyrus. **(B)** The intraoperative MRI scan documents complete resection.

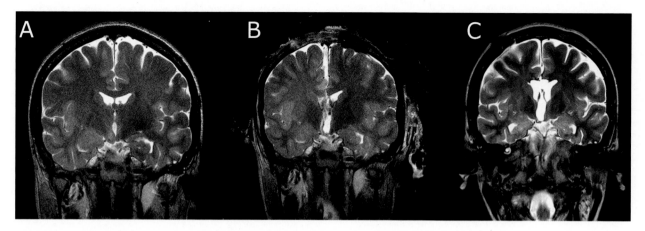

Fig. 16.7 A 33-year-old female patient with hypothalamic hamartoma. **(A)** The preoperative magnetic resonance imaging (MRI) scan detects the hypothalamic hamartoma in the 3rd ventricle. **(B)** The intraoperative MRI scan documents the complete resection via a transcallosal approach. **(C)** The follow-up MRI scan 6 months postoperatively shows normal postoperative findings.

few patients who underwent this operation with intraoperative imaging are to date reported in the medical literature. We described four patients, who underwent callosal sectioning for drop seizures studied intraoperatively with the 0.2 T system. The resolution of iMRI was not only sufficient to depict the exact extent of the callosotomy, but also revealed the crucial relation to the fornix[6] in all four patients assessed. Two more patients were added in a more recent publication including one extensive disconnection of the entire corpus callosum.[25] Similarly, Kelly et al comment that the intraoperative 1.5 T MR images obtained in their patient revealed the shape and extent of the callosotomy very well. Landmarks are rare along the corpus callosum;[38,39] thus usually the exact extent of the transection is only visible on the sagittal projection of a postoperative MRI.[37] With intraoperative imaging, the result of the transection can be immediately visualized and if necessary corrected before the patient leaves the operating theater.

◆ Conclusions

Just as in the surgery of intrinsic brain tumors or pituitary adenomas, in epilepsy surgery operations, the use of iMRI offers the best quality control that we presently have available. In contrast to the latter two entities, however, experience is still limited and the data that are available are still preliminary. Except for hemispherectomy, examples for the use of iMRI are meanwhile available for all intracranial epilepsy surgery procedures. It is easily conceivable that it is a major advantage to have the positioning of electrodes ascertained in relation to brain structures, to assure that the amount of tissue resection meets the treatment plan that has been made after considering morphologic and functional data and to detect hemorrhages as early as possible. This depiction of the reality offers the chance of intraoperative correction, so that at least when the patient goes to the intensive care unit, one knows that the resection or

disconnection looks as it is desired. The available data from the literature and our own experience suggest that, in general, the iMRI depicted the localization and extent of a resection with a good correlation to the routine postoperative images obtained 2 to 3 months after surgery. Discrepancies in this comparison of intra- and postoperative MRI resulted from changes that occurred during the postoperative period, such as a variation in ventricular size. The actual situation as created by the neurosurgeon within the brain is certainly better reflected during intraoperative imaging. This, on the other hand, does not reveal postoperative secondary changes, such as infarctions occurring with some delay, which undoubtedly, apart from the type of resection performed, also have an effect on the neuropsychologic outcome of the patient. The results of epilepsy surgery in relation to the seizure outcome in the few patients or small series reported to date are comparable with those reported in larger series without intraoperative imaging by expert centers. There is hitherto no evidence that the use of intraoperative imaging in epilepsy surgery causes specific complications. It has not yet been shown that the use of iMRI in the surgery for seizures improves the surgical results or reduces adverse effects. This would require higher numbers of patients and would be difficult to prove because the selection of patients who are recruited for operative treatment seems to determine the outcome rather than the expertise with which the surgical procedure is performed.[5]

References

1. Chang BS, Lowenstein DH. Epilepsy. N Engl J Med 2003;349(13):1257–1266
2. Engel J Jr. Surgery for seizures. N Engl J Med 1996;334(10):647–652
3. Steinmeier R, Fahlbusch R, Ganslandt O, et al. Intraoperative magnetic resonance imaging with the Magnetom open scanner: concepts, neurosurgical indications, and procedures: a preliminary report. Neurosurgery 1998;43(4):739–747, discussion 747–748
4. Sutherland GR, Kaibara T, Louw D, Hoult DI, Tomanek B, Saunders J. A mobile high-field magnetic resonance system for neurosurgery. J Neurosurg 1999;91(5):804–813

5. Buchfelder M, Stefan H. Neurosurgical treatment of epilepsy. Neurol Psychiatry Brain Res 1999;7:131–136
6. Buchfelder M, Ganslandt O, Fahlbusch R, Nimsky C. Intraoperative magnetic resonance imaging in epilepsy surgery. J Magn Reson Imaging 2000;12(4):547–555
7. Nimsky C, Ganslandt O, Kober H, Buchfelder M, Fahlbusch R. Intraoperative magnetic resonance imaging combined with neuronavigation: a new concept. Neurosurgery 2001;48(5):1082–1089, discussion 1089–1091
8. Lewin JS, Nour SG, Meyers ML, et al. Intraoperative MRI with a rotating, tiltable surgical table: a time use study and clinical results in 122 patients. AJR Am J Roentgenol 2007;189(5):1096–1103
9. Schwartz TH, Marks D, Pak J, et al. Standardization of amygdalohippocampectomy with intraoperative magnetic resonance imaging: preliminary experience. Epilepsia 2002;43(4):430–436
10. Walker DG, Talos F, Bromfield EB, Black PM. Intraoperative magnetic resonance for the surgical treatment of lesions producing seizures. J Clin Neurosci 2002;9(5):515–520
11. Kaibara T, Myles ST, Lee MA, Sutherland GR. Optimizing epilepsy surgery with intraoperative MR imaging. Epilepsia 2002;43(4):425–429
12. Kelly JJ, Hader WJ, Myles ST, Sutherland GR. Epilepsy surgery with intraoperative MRI at 1.5 T. Neurosurg Clin N Am 2005;16(1):173–183
13. Nimsky C, Ganslandt O, Von Keller B, Romstöck J, Fahlbusch R. Intraoperative high-field-strength MR imaging: implementation and experience in 200 patients. Radiology 2004;233(1):67–78
14. Nimsky C, Ganslandt O, Fahlbusch R. Comparing 0.2 tesla with 1.5 tesla intraoperative magnetic resonance imaging analysis of setup, workflow, and efficiency. Acad Radiol 2005;12(9):1065–1079
15. Mehta AD, Labar D, Dean A, et al. Frameless stereotactic placement of depth electrodes in epilepsy surgery. J Neurosurg 2005;102(6):1040–1045
16. Davis LM, Spencer DD, Spencer SS, Bronen RA. MR imaging of implanted depth and subdural electrodes: is it safe? Epilepsy Res 1999;35(2):95–98
17. Moran NF, Lemieux L, Maudgil D, Kitchen ND, Fish DR, Shorvon SD. Analysis of temporal lobe resections in MR images. Epilepsia 1999;40(8):1077–1084
18. Jooma R, Yeh HS, Privitera MD, Rigrish D, Gartner M. Seizure control and extent of mesial temporal resection. Acta Neurochir (Wien) 1995;133(1-2):44–49
19. Kanner AM, Kaydanova Y, deToledo-Morrell L, et al. Tailored anterior temporal lobectomy. Relation between extent of resection of mesial structures and postsurgical seizure outcome. Arch Neurol 1995;52(2):173–178
20. Nayel MH, Awad IA, Lüders H. Extent of mesiobasal resection determines outcome after temporal lobectomy for intractable complex partial seizures. Neurosurgery 1991;29(1):55–60, discussion 60–61
21. Wyler AR, Hermann BP, Somes G. Extent of medial temporal resection on outcome from anterior temporal lobectomy: a randomized prospective study. Neurosurgery 1995;37(5):982–990, discussion 990–991
22. Awad IA, Nayel MH, Lüders H. Second operation after the failure of previous resection for epilepsy. Neurosurgery 1991;28(4):510–518
23. Germano IM, Poulin N, Olivier A. Reoperation for recurrent temporal lobe epilepsy. J Neurosurg 1994;81(1):31–36
24. Wyler AR, Hermann BP, Richey ET. Results of reoperation for failed epilepsy surgery. J Neurosurg 1989;71(6):815–819
25. Buchfelder M, Nimsky C. Intraoperative low-field MR imaging in epilepsy surgery. Arq Neuropsiquiatr 2003;61(Suppl 1):115–122
26. Buchfelder M, Fahlbusch R, Ganslandt O, Stefan H, Nimsky C. Use of intraoperative magnetic resonance imaging in tailored temporal lobe surgeries for epilepsy. Epilepsia 2002;43(8):864–873
27. Levivier M, Wikler D, Massager N, Legros B, Van Bogaert P, Brotchi J. [Intraoperative MRI and epilepsy surgery]. Neurochirurgie 2008;54(3):448–452
28. Van Roost D, Schaller C, Meyer B, Schramm J. Can neuronavigation contribute to standardization of selective amygdalohippocampectomy? Stereotact Funct Neurosurg 1997;69(1-4 Pt 2):239–242
29. Ossenblok P, de Munck JC, Colon A, Drolsbach W, Boon P. Magnetoencephalography is more successful for screening and localizing frontal lobe epilepsy than electroencephalography. Epilepsia 2007;48(11):2139–2149
30. Taniguchi H, Muragaki Y, Iseki H, Nakamura R, Taira T. New radiofrequency coil integrated with a stereotactic frame for intraoperative MRI-controlled stereotactically guided brain surgery. Stereotact Funct Neurosurg 2006;84(4):136–141
31. Kanev PM, Foley CM, Miles D. Ultrasound-tailored functional hemispherectomy for surgical control of seizures in children. J Neurosurg 1997;86(5):762–767
32. Oh DS, Black PM. A low-field intraoperative MRI system for glioma surgery: is it worthwhile? Neurosurg Clin N Am 2005;16(1):135–141
33. Miller D, Knake S, Bauer S, et al. Intraoperative ultrasound to define focal cortical dysplasia in epilepsy surgery. Epilepsia 2008;49(1):156–158
34. Stefan H, Nimsky C, Scheler G, et al. Periventricular nodular heterotopia: a challenge for epilepsy surgery. Seizure 2007;16(1):81–86
35. Nimsky C, von Keller B, Schlaffer S, et al. Updating navigation with intraoperative image data. Top Magn Reson Imaging 2009;19(4):197–204
36. Maehara T, Shimizu H. Surgical outcome of corpus callosotomy in patients with drop attacks. Epilepsia 2001;42(1):67–71
37. Sorenson JM, Wheless JW, Baumgartner JE, et al. Corpus callosotomy for medically intractable seizures. Pediatr Neurosurg 1997;27(5):260–267
38. Awad IA, Wyllie E, Lüders H, Ahl J. Intraoperative determination of the extent of corpus callosotomy for epilepsy: two simple techniques. Neurosurgery 1990;26(1):102–105, discussion 105–106
39. Gonçalves Ferreira AJ, Farias JP, Carvalho MH, Melancia J, Miguéns J. Corpus callosotomy: some aspects of its microsurgical anatomy. Stereotact Funct Neurosurg 1995;65(1-4):90–96

17

Awake Craniotomy and Intraoperative MRI for the Resection of Gliomas

Arya Nabavi, Simone Goebel, Lutz Dörner, Nils Warneke, Stephan Ulmer, and Hubertus Maximillian Mehdorn

Throughout the development and implementation of intraoperative magnetic resonance imaging (iMRI), the goal has been to combine surgery and MRI[1-6] such that MRI provides surgical guidance without impeding the use of state-of-the-art microneurosurgical techniques. The results of various groups have shown that iMRI provides the basis for more extensive glioma resection.[1,4,7-11]

We installed our customized integrated MRI operating room (MRI-OR) with a 1.5 tesla MRI scanner (Intera; Philips Healthcare, Andover, MA) in 2005. Our primary indications involve primary and recurrent gliomas (see Chapter 12).

However, although most gliomas are situated in predominantly quiescent localizations and are thus potentially amenable to gross total volumetric resection, some lesions affect eloquent areas, in particular speech and motor cortex.

These areas may be merely displaced by the lesion, but also infiltrated.[12,13] Under the latter condition, gross total volumetric resection of the tumor is certain to cause unacceptable deficits affecting the patient's quality of life. Although biopsy might be an option to define pathology, surgical resection and volume reduction remains the first step in the subsequent multimodal therapy. The challenge in these cases rests in the balance between the most complete surgical excision and conserving or preferably improving function, and hence quality of life.

A thorough evaluation of such lesions has to combine structural as well as functional characteristics. Functional MRI (fMRI) is of great value in localizing areas at risk, either in the approach trajectory or the potential resection area. However, it does not yield certainty. It is well known that language production, comprehension, and association encompass multiple areas. Comprehensive investigation by imaging remains a challenge.[14-16] Even for motor skills, which often show a good overlap of functional and anatomic representation on preoperative evaluation,[17] direct motor responses may be elicited beyond the structural identifiable precentral gyrus.[18]

Acknowledging the incomplete representation of functional areas on preoperative imaging, we chose to gain additional information for surgical decision making. Therefore, we use direct cortical stimulation for electrophysiologic testing during "awake craniotomies"[19-21] for patients with lesions in eloquent areas. This allows testing and monitoring of function, specifically speech and motor skills,[22] and if necessary modification of surgical tactics. Since 1996, we have been acquiring experience with cortical stimulation during awake craniotomies. Building on this familiarity we transferred this technique to the setting of iMRI.

In this chapter we describe our practice of combining iMRI and awake craniotomy.

◆ Preparation and Procedure

Intraoperative MRI-Operating Theater Set-up

We installed a fully integrated iMRI-OR in our institution in 2005. At the core of this operating room is the short-bore 1.5 tesla MRI scanner (Intera; Philips Healthcare).[4,7] The sequences are the same as in conventional MRI. We use flexible surface coils. Usually, we position one coil below the patient's head, and for scanning the second coil is positioned on top of the head, opposite to the first one.

Conventional microneurosurgery is performed outside of the 5 gauss (G) line, using ferromagnetic tools and equipment (such as the microscope, ultrasonic aspirator, bipolar coagulation, and cortical stimulation), as well as a ceiling-mounted navigation system (BrainLab VectorVision; BrainLab, Heimstetten, Germany). The patient is transferred from the microneurosurgical operation site to the scanner using a pivoting angiography table, which connects to the MRI. For this transfer the surgical site is covered with adhesive sterile draping. According to the MR characteristics of the lesion (e.g., enhancing or nonenhancing, T2 hyperintense, fluid attenuation inversion recovery [FLAIR] abnormality) the appropriate sequences are chosen. The imaging time is kept as concise as possible. Usually one neurosurgeon remains with the patient during scanning, which most patients consider very reassuring. The images are directly transferred to our navigation system via Ethernet. The patient is returned to the microneurosurgical operation site. For updated navigation we reattach the dynamic reference frame if further resection is necessary.

Patients and Preoperative Evaluation

Between September 2005 and October 2008, 348 surgeries were performed in this integrated MRI-OR suite. The main pathologies were gliomas (227) and pituitary lesions (52). In all, 209 glioma cases were limited to either hemisphere (117 left, 92 right). Thirty-four patients were operated on with cortical stimulation; four underwent repeat surgery for recurrent disease. Therefore, 38 awake craniotomy procedures were performed. Thirty-two cases had left-sided lesions, of which 14 were tested primarily for motor skills, and 18 for speech. Six patients with right-sided pathology underwent intraoperative monitoring, testing motor skills. Age ranged from 23 to 69 years (median age of 42 years).

Initial patient selection was based on their neurologic symptoms and on the structural MRI. Patients harboring lesions within or abutting eloquent areas were considered for awake craniotomy. Mandatory workup included fMRI and neuropsychologic investigation.

Awake craniotomy was considered, if the patient's lesion extended into or infiltrated speech-associated areas: the left frontal operculum (for left dominant hemisphere) and the left dorsotemporal lobe. With regard to motor skill-associated areas, those lesions abutting or infiltrating the primary motor cortex, the left-sided supplementary motor area, and also the subcortical pathways were considered for awake craniotomy. Tumors within the right supplementary region, if the patient is clearly left dominant, are operated on under general anesthesia.

Major neurologic deficits, which preclude intraoperative testing, are contraindications, such as pronounced aphasia, which would prevent speech testing. As for motor areas, unless the patient is unable to move at all, awake craniotomy should not be ruled out. After debulking and reduction of mass effect, the paresis might improve. However, if infiltration predominates, this might not happen, but worsening can be potentially avoided by discontinuing the operation.

Subsequently, patients were evaluated by a neuropsychologist. Specific emphasis was given to potential compliance, anxiety, and intellectual capacity. Patients were excluded with a score below 23 points in the Mini Mental State Examination, and less than 50% in the examined language tests. Furthermore, inhibited, apathic, and disorganized behavior patterns were grounds to exclude patients because noncompliant behavior was likely (Goebel S, Nabavi A, Schubert S, et al. Patient perception of combined awake brain tumor surgery and intraoperative MRI. Accepted for publication in Neurosurgery). Naturally, claustrophobic patients cannot be considered for awake craniotomy in an iMRI.

Having explained the rationale for potential awake craniotomy before testing the patients, we then discuss the test results and the surgical technique with the patients. We have found most patients to be motivated and compliant following this preoperative procedure. Only one patient declined due to psychological problems. We ascribe the high rate of acceptance of this technique to the thorough assessment prior to recommending the procedure.

Overview of Procedure

The anesthesiologist provides cardiovascular and pulmonary monitoring during surgery. Nerve blockades and local anesthesia of the prospective surgical area are done by the anesthesiologist and the neurosurgeon. The patient is positioned for surgery in a specially adapted MRI-compatible Mayfield clamp, rigidly attached to the MRI-table. Initial microneurosurgical tumor removal is guided by neuronavigation using preoperative imaging and cortical stimulation during neurophysiologic testing. On demand MRI is acquired and used for updated navigation. Throughout the procedure, low doses of analgesics are given. After resection and final testing, sedating medication is begun. The distinct steps are discussed in detail below.

Initial Arrangement, Positioning, and Commencing Surgery

The anesthesiologist prepares the patient with intravenous (IV) and arterial lines, central venous catheter, and urethral catheter in a separate area for patient preparation. The occipital, temporal, and supraorbital nerves are blocked with depots of 2.5% Naropin (ropivacaine hydrochloride; AstraZeneca UK Ltd., London, UK). Then the patient is transferred to the iMRI-OR and placed on the table docked to the MRI.

Positioning awake patients in an iMRI unit is even more of a challenge than in a conventional OR. Special care has to be taken to ascertain comfortable arrangements as well as access to the patient for intraoperative testing. In the iMRI, the mentioned goals have to be achieved, while having the further restraints of the MRI tunnel. Thus we position in the immediate vicinity of the MRI, to ensure the free passage into the bore for imaging. Although the head is rigidly fixed in the MRI-compatible Mayfield clamp, we place cushions beneath the neck. Patients have been observed to relax their neck muscles subsequently. It is important to ensure that the patient is as comfortable as possible. Small discomforts at the onset of surgery may result in total noncompliance toward the end of the resection.

In addition, it should be noted that the table's mount permits only raising and lowering of the head, tilting along the table axis is not possible.

The patient's head is rigidly fixed to the table with a specially modified carbon-fiber Mayfield clamp (Promedics GmbH, Düsseldorf, Germany). The projected pin insertion sites were infiltrated with 2 to 4 milliliters of 7.5% Naropin. More Naropin is injected as needed. One coil is permanently positioned below the patient's head, within the Mayfield clamp, while the other surface coil is placed on top. This coil is removed during surgery, and repositioned for scanning (on top of the draping).

After positioning we acquire a T2-weighted image (T2WI), to rule out artifacts. The patient is transferred to the surgical

position; the navigation system is registered. The point of entry is defined using the navigation system, setting the best approach to the tumor. The flap is fashioned to provide enough space to perform cortical mapping and potentially use alternate routes to circumvent functional areas should they be encountered. The planned skin incision is infiltrated with 7.5% Naropin. If a straight incision is used, only the planned incision is infiltrated. For a skin flap, which is most frequently indicated, its base has to be infiltrated as well.

The drapes are arranged in a tent-like fashion (**Fig. 17.1**) allowing access to the patient as well as visual contact, to allow testing (e.g., naming of drawn objects).

Standard microneurosurgical techniques are employed. After placing the burr hole, additional Naropin-immersed cottonoids are placed on the dura. Throughout the opening additional doses of Ultiva (Remifentanil; Abbott Laboratories,

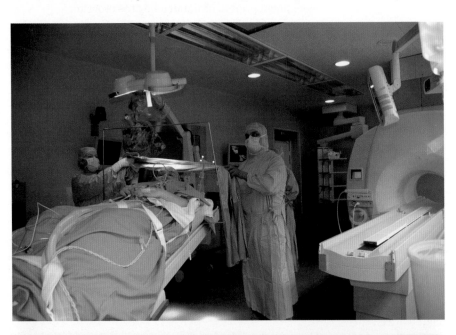

A

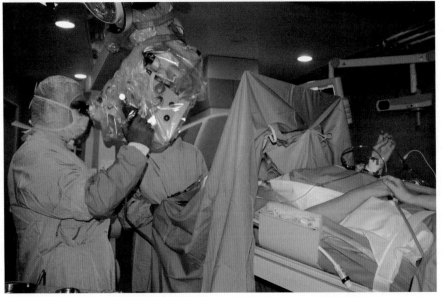

B

Fig. 17.1 **(A)** Patient positioned for surgery in the intraoperative magnetic resonance imaging- operating room (iMRI-OR) suite. Drapes are arranged to allow access to the patient and visual contact. The pivoting angiography table is disconnected from the MRI scanner, and turned, to place the patient's head into the "surgical area." The monitor of the ceiling-mounted navigation system is visible on the right side. Draped microscope on the left in the background. **(B)** Position after draping. View from the other table side. MRI in the background. Motor testing during resection of a recurrent malignant glioma, extending from the right postcentral gyrus anteriorly into the pyramidal tract. The contrast-enhancing lesion was removed completely, the resection cavity lined with Gliadel wafers (MGI Pharma, Bloomington, MN). The patient had no motor deficit, perception of a "heavy leg," as complained about prior to surgery, receded after tumor debulking.

Abbott Park, IL) are infused. Once the bone flap is turned, Naropin-immersed cottonoids are placed on the dura for local anesthesia. The dura is opened under the microscope. The brain itself is not pain-sensitive. However, the basal dura and larger vessels may elicit pain, when manipulated. Additional Naropin-immersed cottonoids are placed on the painful structures. Care must be taken that the anesthetic agent does not reach the cortical areas in question because that may hamper cortical stimulation. Employing neuronavigation, the best approach to the tumor is defined and its borders identified, respectively.

Various groups use propofol during craniotomy, and discontinue the drug before cortical stimulation. They have reported good results without adverse effect on cortical stimulation after the discontinuation of propofol.[23,24]

Intraoperative Testing

The neuropsychologist, typically the one who performed the preoperative evaluation, remains with the patient throughout the procedure. Testing is performed regularly as well as on the surgeon's request (**Fig. 17.1B**). Throughout the surgery, the neuropsychologist and the surgeon speak with the patient.

Cortical stimulation is established as a technique to identify functional cortical areas; subcortical stimulation helps to identify connective fiber tracts.

It uses electrical current which, depending on the examined area, may elicit or impede responses. We use a bipolar cortical stimulator to investigate the cortex in the planned trajectory and for superficial lesions around the tumor. The cortex is touched in various areas (**Fig. 17.2A, B,C**), while the neuropsychologist tests the functions associated with that specific area – either speech or motor tasks. The basic elements of the tests were rehearsed prior to surgery. Speech monitoring is the most complex, ranging from naming to association and free narration. If functional areas are touched with the probe, disruption of the cortical electrical activity results in functional deficits. These are reversible with removal of the probe.

If cortical stimulation results in reversible deficits, these areas may not be resected, even if obvious tumor infiltration is present.

If cortical stimulation does not produce deficits, but approaching through the tested area results in neurologic

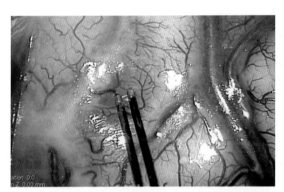

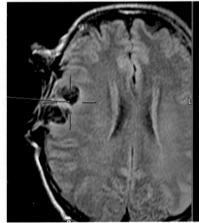 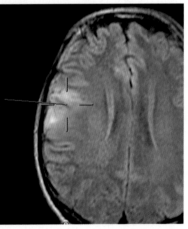

Fig. 17.2 Patient with focal seizures, beginning in the tongue was diagnosed with diffusely contrast-enhancing cortical lesion at the lateral portion of the right precentral gyrus. Fluid attenuation inversion recovery (FLAIR) and T2-weighted magnetic resonance imaging showed diffuse signal abnormality around the contrast-enhancing areas. For navigation FLAIR imaging was chosen. **(A)** Bipolar stimulator. No motor deficit was induced with stimulation of either side of the visible vein, corresponding to the sulcus, dividing two pathologic gyri. **(B)** Screen shot of the neuronavigation system after intraoperative update. *Left:* Intraoperative MR image after resection (acquired with flexible coils), showing the division of the two resection areas, and the resection cavities separated by the sulcal arachnoid and vessels. The adjacent sulci were reached at the bottom of the resection cavity. The pointer is depicted by the green crosshair in the axial FLAIR slices. *Right:* Corresponding image used for initial navigation, acquired with a conventional head coil before surgery.
(C) Postresection microscope image. Dividing vein was preserved. Frozen section had confirmed the diagnosis of malignant glioma. The cavity displayed on the intraoperative image is being lined with Gliadel wafers (MGI Pharma, Bloomington, MN). Throughout the surgery, the patient had performed well, and had no motor deficit. Around the third day after surgery she experienced speech difficulties, which we could contribute to the perifocal swelling. Transient neurologic deterioration with subsequent recovery is not rare following surgery adjacent to eloquent areas. This can be accredited to surgically induced edema or Gliadel-induced inflammatory reaction in the adjacent brain.

changes, this is mostly due to propagated pressure. These changes should disappear once the pressure is lifted. If such deficits persist, it may be necessary to use another approach. However, occasionally, in particular with larger lesions, swift debulking may relieve intrinsic pressure and subsequently resolve this transient neurologic impairment.

Contrary to these undulating changes, vascular compromise of cortical areas results in sudden onset of irreversible loss of function. When working in the supplementary motor area and in close vicinity to the subcortical pathways sudden onset paresis might also occur without vascular injury. Clinically indistinguishable from each other, DWI imaging allows a differentiation. These deficits without vascular lesion have a better prognosis.

If the patient experiences progressive loss of function, or the intervals needed for recuperation become progressively longer without regaining the previous functional level, surgery may have to be discontinued, unless the remaining tumor is in quiescent areas. Because repeated testing may tire the patient, we try to commence surgery in the most crucial areas, to ensure the best results in the critical regions.

Seizures may occur spontaneously, but may also be induced by the cortical testing. However, these events seldomly occur. We discontinued the routine recording of an electrocardiogram (ECG) previously, which facilitated the transfer to the MRI environment. Although cortical stimulation is unimpeded outside the 5 G line, an ECG would be more susceptible.

In our series there were no generalized seizures. Focal seizures were managed by cold irrigation of the cortex,[25] without the need for IV medication. Three of our patients had focal seizures during cortical stimulation. All of these events were overcome irrigating the cortex with cold saline.

However, particularly with motor function, postictal paresis might impede the progress of surgery. With repeated seizures, the restoration may take progressively longer, rendering the continuation of surgery impracticable.

One patient with a tumor within the precentral gyrus extending into the supplementary motor cortex experienced repeated focal seizures unrelated to cortical stimulation. Finally, a postictal paresis of the right arm developed, which precluded further electrophysiologic testing. The surgery was discontinued. The paresis resolved over the following days. There were no seizures during imaging. There were no complications due to the combination of cortical stimulation in the awake patient with intraoperative MRI.

Imaging

The imaging parameters are the same as conventionally used for iMRI (see Chapter 12). However, because the patient's cooperation and concentration are of major importance to ensure proper results on cortical stimulation and neuropsychologic evaluation, the time spent on imaging must be well planned. Depending on the lesion's imaging characteristics, 20 to 60 minutes were necessary per case. A member of the neurosurgical team stays with the patient throughout the scanning. Furthermore, the confined space within the bore adds to the discomfort. Therefore, the initial

resection has to be carried as far as possible, preferably until gross total tumor removal is accomplished, to limit repetitive scans. For nonenhancing lesions we acquire axial T2 and FLAIR imaging. If necessary, orthogonal images are acquired as well. For enhancing lesions, we employ routine T1 before and after contrast administration in the orthogonal planes. The patient receives ear plugs for scanning.

None of our patients demanded termination of the scanning. All T1WIs and T2WIs yielded diagnostic image quality, whereas FLAIR imaging seemed to be more variable.

Scanning is initiated on the surgeon's demand. Preparation and transfer to the "imaging" site takes 3 to 5 minutes. For the transfer the operating site is carefully covered. Special care has to be taken to arrange the drapes in such a way that the patient's face is not covered during scanning. Oxygen is administered through a nasal tube. It is helpful to place this slightly in front of the face with a high flow causing an air current.

The images are transferred to our ceiling-mounted neuronavigation system, if updated navigation is indicated. The dynamic reference frame (drf) is connected to the Mayfield-clamp. For scanning the drf is disconnected. A specific joint enables repositioning after scanning, reconstituting the previous geometry of the clamp–drf system. Thus navigation can be continued with updated information/images.

◆ Discussion

Our experience shows the feasibility of implementing intraoperative high-field MRI and the technique of awake craniotomy for lesions within eloquent regions. Patient selection according to a systematic process is crucial to ascertain patients' motivation and eventual cooperation. This is even more important because scanning adds time to the awake procedure. Still, 32 of 34 patients said they would undergo a second awake surgery in the MRI if necessary. Eventually four patients had second awake procedures for recurrent tumors. Only two had asked for discontinuation of the procedure due to fatigue and discomfort, which was less accorded to the MRI, but to the awake procedure itself. The appropriateness of our selection process is reflected by the constrained indication for 38 awake craniotomies in 3 years, as well as the high acceptance rate. The data on patients' acceptance as reported by other groups for conventional awake craniotomies are similar to our experience with the combined approach.[26,27] Albeit well received, awake craniotomy remains a strenuous experience for the patient, as well as for the OR team.[26,27]

The rationale for operating on patients with cortical stimulation while awake is based on the heterogeneity of functional areas.

Speech in particular involves multiple centers for its generation, comprehension, and association.[21] This complexity is underlined by the separated, nonoverlapping centers, performing similar tasks in bilingual patients.[28,29]

Although the motor cortex has structural and imaging features,[17] which often allow identification, it has been demonstrated that during direct stimulation almost one third of the responses were elicited from areas beyond the precentral gyrus.[18]

The presurgical depiction of functional areas with fMRI has been extensively investigated and yields a sufficient basis for initial risk assessment. Motor responses lead to reproducible information, correlating to the MRI anatomy of the given region. Furthermore, the Broca area can be identified regularly.[16,30] However, other areas with crucial contribution may be obscured if the tasks set for fMRI do not specifically involve their input.[15] Although there is a multitude of articles of various aspects of fMRI[31] the inherent limitations of this technology have to be conceded,[32] irrespective of the instructive quality of the three-dimensional (3D) fMRI representations.

Pragmatically, we use fMRI to verify the speech dominant hemisphere (which for our patients can be corroborated by neuropsychologic evaluation), as well as dominant motor areas, as for the hand and the leg. The sophistication of preoperative imaging and in particular its integrated representation in 3D[33] suggests a high level of security that functional centers and their connections can be sufficiently identified and preserved. The multimodal information certainly facilitates surgical planning and risk assessment. However, with aforementioned restraints in regard to the methodology as well as the incomplete representation of complex cognitive and neurophysiological processes, we decided to acquire additional information.

This is underscored by an additional difficulty. Although integration of fMRI into conventional navigation systems facilitates planning and guiding the craniotomy as well as the initial approach, these navigation systems lose their accuracy during the course of resection. They are unable to compensate intraoperative brain deformation, so-called brain-shift."[34] This brain shift invalidates preoperative functional and structural imaging[34,35] because of tissue displacement and deformation due to volume changes (resection, cerebrospinal fluid [CSF] drainage, etc.).

In regard to the structural data, intraoperative MRI circumvents this limitation.[35] On-demand new intraoperative images are acquired, which depict the residual lesion and the displacement of the surrounding tissue. Thus the structural data can be renewed intraoperatively and used for updated navigation, assisting surgical decision making.

To simulate the displacement of functional centers, elastic registration algorithms have been investigated.[34,36–39] Although these algorithms for elastic registration can describe the phenomenon of brain-shift, their predictive value of where a certain cortical area has shifted to remains very limited.

Another feature of contemporary MRI work-up involves the portrayal of connective fiber tracts. Together with fMRI this DTI can be extracted from specific imaging and integrated for neuronavigation. In contrast to fMRI data, DTI can be directly extracted from intraoperative MRI[40] and used for updated navigation (see Chapter 15). Depending on the extraction and postprocessing algorithms the depicted fiber tracts may differ considerably.[41]

Although functional imaging integrated into neuronavigation provides a very good basis for initial risk assessment,

there are a variety of parameters, which limit its validity during surgery, both methodologic[32] and practical (e.g., imaging time, brain-shift).

Nevertheless, violation of functional centers as well as their connecting fibers will lead to neurologic deficits. Testing and cortical stimulation in the awake patient permits more thorough intraoperative evaluation and provides more flexibility (e.g., bilingual testing, mathematics, comprehension, narration). The fiber connections can also be tested in the awake patient, using the fairly recent technique of subcortical stimulation,[42–45] which employs lower current and different probes, but adheres to the same principles as depicted for cortical stimulation. Subsequently, it provides online electrophysiologic confirmation of the fiber connections with technique-inherent safety margins (current modification).

iMRI may be limited in regard to updating fMRI and partially fiber tracts (which may consume additional time), but allows a comprehensive depiction of structural features, such as residual tumor.

Data from MRI-guided surgeries showed promising results in regard to achieving gross total tumor resection in high-grade gliomas.[1,4,7,8,10,11,46,47]

There are also encouraging results for low-grade lesions.[8,48] However the long natural course has to be taken into account,[49] and further follow-up of the patient populations operated on with iMRI guidance since 1996 is needed.[8,48]

That residual tumor presents a clear and present predicament was recently underscored, almost as a side-effect, of the study on the resection of high-grade gliomas with 5-aminolevulinic acid (5ALA) fluorescence-guidance.[50] In this randomized multicenter study the control group was operated on using standard microneurosurgical tools and techniques without 5ALA as a surgical adjunct. Standard postoperative MRI showed residual tumor in 62% of cases. This is even more astounding because the study design explicitly excluded lesions located within or close to eloquent areas and included only those tumors that were deemed "totally" resectable.

With the extent of resection being a determining factor for length of survival in primary brain tumors,[8,20,48,49,51] a more complete resection by MRI-guidance provides an important advantage and underscores the potential value of iMRI, where imaging can be used to identify residual tumor while it can still be resected.

◆ Conclusion

Gliomas within or in the vicinity of eloquent areas represent a special challenge.

Preoperative data integration into neuronavigation systems facilitates planning and approaching tumors in eloquent areas.[22] Residual uncertainty due to intraoperative displacement and deformation,[34,52] but also in regard to technical issues of fMRI[32] and DTI[53] remain, rendering their value for intraoperative surgical decision making ambiguous.

Although the capacity to detect structural changes, specifically residual tumor, in MRI is undisputed, the infiltration by visible and MRI-verified tumor may involve eloquent areas. Resecting these areas solely on imaging criteria could

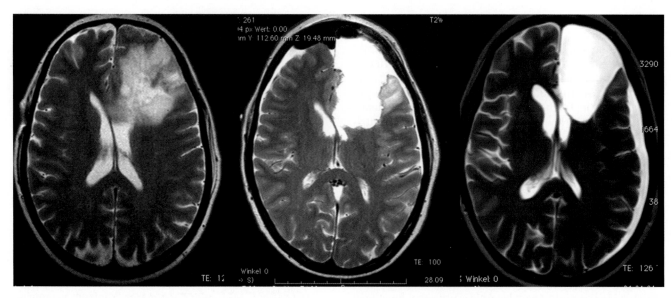

Fig. 17.3 Imaging and function. Image series of corresponding slice before (left), during (middle), and 9-month postoperative after radiotherapy. Case presentation: A 43-year-old right-handed woman with one seizure was diagnosed with a left frontal tumor (left image; preoperative). Functional magnetic resonance imaging (fMRI) had proven the left hemispheric dominance. Speech-associated areas were diagnosed to be at the dorsal border of the tumor in the frontal operculum. The resection was started with central debulking, eventually removing the anterior portion of the frontal lobe. Cortical stimulation revealed speech arrest while testing in macroscopically obvious tumor infiltrated and enlarged gyrus. Imaging confirmed tumor (middle image; intraoperative MRI, craniotomy is above image area). This area was not resected. The patient showed unimpaired speech during surgery. After

the initial days, she developed pronounced speech deficits. On her 3-month visit she had improved, on the 6-month visit she had recovered almost completely, revealing difficulties only on specific tasks. After 9 months she had begun to work part-time and has extended her working hours since then. Histopathology was an oligodendroglioma III. She received adjuvant radiation therapy, but rejected chemotherapy. T2 signal abnormality has almost disappeared after adjuvant radiotherapy. On her 9-month follow-up visit imaging showed a recurrence apical to the shown slice, without clinical symptoms. Chemotherapy was started. Her neurologic status has remained stable. Imaging shows diffuse infiltration reaching into motor pathways, but almost stable since the 15-month follow-up (at present 30 months after surgery).

yield satisfactory imaging at the unacceptable price of neurologic deficits (**Fig. 17.3**).

Thus we see the necessity to obtain further information to make our surgical assessment. In addition to preoperative functional and structural imaging, as well as updated iMRI and neuronavigation, we use cortical stimulation during awake craniotomies. This approach is demanding, but well tolerated by patients. Careful preoperative evaluation is essential to ensure compliance. There is no adverse effect from iMRI or from the results of cortical stimulation on the awake patient.[54]

Furthermore, surgical strategy has to be evaluated in light of multimodal tumor therapy. Particularly with malignant gliomas adjuvant therapy in continuation of surgery represents the standard of care. Although iMRI can show the necessary extent of a resection, conserving functional capacities is paramount (**Fig. 17.3**). We consider the implementation of direct iMRI visualization of tumor and online investigation of function with awake craniotomy an important tool in the multimodal treatment of cerebral gliomas in the vicinity of eloquent areas.

References

1. Black PM, Alexander E III, Martin C, et al. Craniotomy for tumor treatment in an intraoperative magnetic resonance imaging unit. Neurosurgery 1999;45(3):423–431, discussion 431–433
2. Tronnier VM, Wirtz CR, Knauth M, et al. Intraoperative diagnostic and interventional magnetic resonance imaging in neurosurgery. Neurosurgery 1997;40(5):891–900, discussion 900–902
3. Steinmeier R, Fahlbusch R, Ganslandt O, et al. Intraoperative magnetic resonance imaging with the Magnetom open scanner: concepts, neurosurgical indications, and procedures: a preliminary report. Neurosurgery 1998;43(4):739–747, discussion 747–748
4. Hall WA, Martin AJ, Liu H, et al. High-field strength interventional magnetic resonance imaging for pediatric neurosurgery. Pediatr Neurosurg 1998;29(5):253–259
5. Jolesz FA, Morrison PR, Koran SJ, et al. Compatible instrumentation for intraoperative MRI: expanding resources. J Magn Reson Imaging 1998;8(1):8–11
6. Sutherland GR, Louw DF. Intraoperative MRI: a moving magnet. CMAJ 1999;161(10):1293
7. Hall WA, Liu H, Martin AJ, Truwit CL. Intraoperative magnetic resonance imaging. Top Magn Reson Imaging 2000;11(3):203–212
8. Claus EB, Horlacher A, Hsu L, et al. Survival rates in patients with low-grade glioma after intraoperative magnetic resonance image guidance. Cancer 2005;103(6):1227–1233
9. Nimsky C, Fujita A, Ganslandt O, Von Keller B, Fahlbusch R. Volumetric assessment of glioma removal by intraoperative high-field magnetic resonance imaging. Neurosurgery 2004;55(2):358–370, discussion 370–371
10. Schneider JP, Trantakis C, Rubach M, et al. Intraoperative MRI to guide the resection of primary supratentorial glioblastoma multiforme—a quantitative radiological analysis. Neuroradiology 2005;47(7):489–500
11. Trantakis C, Winkler D, Lindner D, et al. Clinical results in MR-guided therapy for malignant gliomas. Acta Neurochir Suppl (Wien) 2003;85:65–71
12. Skirboll SS, Ojemann GA, Berger MS, Lettich E, Winn HR. Functional cortex and subcortical white matter located within gliomas. Neurosurgery 1996;38(4):678–684, discussion 684–685

13. Schiffbauer H, Berger MS, Ferrari P, Freudenstein D, Rowley HA, Roberts TP. Preoperative magnetic source imaging for brain tumor surgery: a quantitative comparison with intraoperative sensory and motor mapping. Neurosurg Focus 2003;15(1):E7

14. Petrovich Brennan NM, Whalen S, de Morales Branco D, O'shea JP, Norton IH, Golby AJ. Object naming is a more sensitive measure of speech localization than number counting: converging evidence from direct cortical stimulation and fMRI. Neuroimage 2007;37(Suppl 1):S100–S108

15. Petrovich N, Holodny AI, Tabar V, et al. Discordance between functional magnetic resonance imaging during silent speech tasks and intraoperative speech arrest. J Neurosurg 2005;103(2):267–274

16. Quiñones-Hinojosa A, Ojemann SG, Sanai N, Dillon WP, Berger MS. Preoperative correlation of intraoperative cortical mapping with magnetic resonance imaging landmarks to predict localization of the Broca area. J Neurosurg 2003;99(2):311–318

17. Naidich TP, Hof PR, Yousry TA, Yousry I. The motor cortex: anatomic substrates of function. Neuroimaging Clin N Am 2001;11(2):171–193, vii–viii vii–viii

18. Uematsu S, Lesser R, Fisher RS, et al. Motor and sensory cortex in humans: topography studied with chronic subdural stimulation. Neurosurgery 1992;31(1):59–71, discussion 71–72

19. Black PM, Ronner SF. Cortical mapping for defining the limits of tumor resection. Neurosurgery 1987;20(6):914–919

20. Berger MS, Rostomily RC. Low grade gliomas: functional mapping resection strategies, extent of resection, and outcome. J Neurooncol 1997;34(1):85–101

21. Ojemann GA. The neurobiology of language and verbal memory: observations from awake neurosurgery. Int J Psychophysiol 2003;48(2):141–146

22. Pinsker MO, Nabavi A, Mehdorn HM. Neuronavigation and resection of lesions located in eloquent brain areas under local anesthesia and neuropsychological-neurophysiological monitoring. Minim Invasive Neurosurg 2007;50(5):281–284

23. Olsen KS. The asleep-awake technique using propofol-remifentanil anaesthesia for awake craniotomy for cerebral tumours. Eur J Anaesthesiol 2008;25(8):662–669

24. Huncke K, Van de Wiele B, Fried I, Rubinstein EH. The asleep-awake-asleep anesthetic technique for intraoperative language mapping. Neurosurgery 1998;42(6):1312–1316, discussion 1316–1317

25. Sartorius CJ, Berger MS. Rapid termination of intraoperative stimulation-evoked seizures with application of cold Ringer's lactate to the cortex. Technical note. J Neurosurg 1998;88(2):349–351

26. Danks RA, Rogers M, Aglio LS, Gugino LD, Black PM. Patient tolerance of craniotomy performed with the patient under local anesthesia and monitored conscious sedation. Neurosurgery 1998;42(1):28–34, discussion 34–36

27. Palese A, Skrap M, Fachin M, Visioli S, Zannini L. The experience of patients undergoing awake craniotomy: in the patients' own words. A qualitative study. Cancer Nurs 2008;31(2):166–172

28. Bello L, Acerbi F, Giussani C, et al. Intraoperative language localization in multilingual patients with gliomas. Neurosurgery 2006;59(1):115–125, discussion 115–125

29. Walker JA, Quiñones-Hinojosa A, Berger MS. Intraoperative speech mapping in 17 bilingual patients undergoing resection of a mass lesion. Neurosurgery 2004;54(1):113–117, discussion 118

30. Brannen JH, Badie B, Moritz CH, Quigley M, Meyerand ME, Haughton VM. Reliability of functional MR imaging with word-generation tasks for mapping Broca's area. AJNR Am J Neuroradiol 2001;22(9):1711–1718

31. Connecting the dots. Nat Neurosci 2009;12(2):99

32. Logothetis NK. What we can do and what we cannot do with fMRI. Nature 2008;453(7197):869–878

33. Nimsky C, Ganslandt O, Fahlbusch R. Functional neuronavigation and intraoperative MRI. Adv Tech Stand Neurosurg 2004;29:229–263

34. Nabavi A, Black PM, Gering DT, et al. Serial intraoperative magnetic resonance imaging of brain shift. Neurosurgery 2001;48(4):787–797, discussion 797–798

35. Nimsky C, Ganslandt O, Cerny S, Hastreiter P, Greiner G, Fahlbusch R. Quantification of, visualization of, and compensation for brain shift using intraoperative magnetic resonance imaging. Neurosurgery 2000;47(5):1070–1079, discussion 1079–1080

36. Wittek A, Kikinis R, Warfield SK, Miller K. Brain shift computation using a fully nonlinear biomechanical model. Med Image Comput Comput Assist Interv 2005;8(Pt 2):583–590

37. Clatz O, Delingette H, Talos IF, et al. Robust nonrigid registration to capture brain shift from intraoperative MRI. IEEE Trans Med Imaging 2005;24(11):1417–1427

38. Ferrant M, Nabavi A, Macq B, et al. Serial registration of intraoperative MR images of the brain. Med Image Anal 2002;6(4):337–359

39. Ferrant M, Nabavi A, Macq B, Jolesz FA, Kikinis R, Warfield SK. Registration of 3-D intraoperative MR images of the brain using a finite-element biomechanical model. IEEE Trans Med Imaging 2001;20(12):1384–1397

40. Nimsky C, Ganslandt O, Fahlbusch R. Implementation of fiber tract navigation. Neurosurgery 2007; 61(1, Suppl)306–317, discussion 317–318

41. Bürgel U, Mädler B, Honey CR, Thron A, Gilsbach J, Coenen VA. Fiber tracking with distinct software tools results in a clear diversity in anatomical fiber tract portrayal. Cen Eur Neurosurg 2009;70(1):27–35

42. Duffau H. Contribution of cortical and subcortical electrostimulation in brain glioma surgery: methodological and functional considerations. Neurophysiol Clin 2007;37(6):373–382

43. Bello L, Gallucci M, Fava M, et al. Intraoperative subcortical language tract mapping guides surgical removal of gliomas involving speech areas. Neurosurgery 2007;60(1):67–80, discussion 80–82

44. Duffau H. Intraoperative cortico-subcortical stimulations in surgery of low-grade gliomas. Expert Rev Neurother 2005;5(4):473–485

45. Duffau H, Capelle L, Denvil D, et al. Usefulness of intraoperative electrical subcortical mapping during surgery for low-grade gliomas located within eloquent brain regions: functional results in a consecutive series of 103 patients. J Neurosurg 2003;98(4):764–778

46. Tummala RP, Chu RM, Liu H, Truwit CL, Hall WA. Optimizing brain tumor resection. High-field interventional MR imaging. Neuroimaging Clin N Am 2001;11(4):673–683

47. Nimsky C, Ganslandt O, Buchfelder M, Fahlbusch R. Intraoperative visualization for resection of gliomas: the role of functional neuronavigation and intraoperative 1.5 T MRI. Neurol Res 2006;28(5):482–487

48. Claus EB, Black PM. Survival rates and patterns of care for patients diagnosed with supratentorial low-grade gliomas: data from the SEER program, 1973-2001. Cancer 2006;106(6):1358–1363

49. Sanai N, Berger MS. Glioma extent of resection and its impact on patient outcome. Neurosurgery 2008;62(4):753–764, discussion 264–266

50. Stummer W, Pichlmeier U, Meinel T, Wiestler OD, Zanella F, Reulen HJ; ALA-Glioma Study Group. Fluorescence-guided surgery with 5-aminolevulinic acid for resection of malignant glioma: a randomised controlled multicentre phase III trial. Lancet Oncol 2006; 7(5):392–401

51. Laws ER, Parney IF, Huang W, et al; Glioma Outcomes Investigators. Survival following surgery and prognostic factors for recently diagnosed malignant glioma: data from the Glioma Outcomes Project. J Neurosurg 2003;99(3):467–473

52. Nimsky C, Ganslandt O, Hastreiter P, Fahlbusch R. Intraoperative compensation for brain shift. Surg Neurol 2001;56(6):357–364, discussion 364–365

53. Berman JI, Berger MS, Chung SW, Nagarajan SS, Henry RG. Accuracy of diffusion tensor magnetic resonance imaging tractography assessed using intraoperative subcortical stimulation mapping and magnetic source imaging. J Neurosurg 2007;107(3):488–494

54. Nabavi A, Goebel S, Doerner L, Warneke N, Ulmer S, Mehdorn M. Awake craniotomy and intraoperative magnetic resonance imaging: patient selection, preparation, and technique. Top Magn Reson Imaging 2009; 19(4):191–196

18

Intraoperative Magnetic Resonance Imaging and Cerebrovascular Surgery

Taro Kaibara, Robert F. Spetzler, and Garnette R. Sutherland

Since the initial development of intraoperative magnetic resonance imaging (iMRI) technology in the mid-1990s, a variety of MRI systems have evolved for use during neurosurgical procedures. The systems have ranged from low-field (0.12 tesla) to high-field (3.0 tesla) imaging magnets and have involved either operating within the magnetic field or outside the magnetic field.[1–8] In general, the field strength of the iMRI system determines image quality and imaging sequences or software applications available to the neurosurgeon. A broad spectrum of neurosurgical disease has been monitored with iMRI, in particular neoplastic pathology; however, there is a distinct paucity of literature regarding the use of iMRI in the surgical treatment of cerebrovascular disease.

The treatment of cerebrovascular disease has changed tremendously, relying heavily on advances in surgical technique, technology, and neuroimaging. Rigid cranial fixation without limiting head position is essential to allow maximal brain relaxation and to minimize brain retraction. A surgical microscope is a necessity and a microscope-interfaced surgical chair with mouth and foot controls is utilized by many cerebrovascular surgeons. High-resolution imaging modalities such as digital subtraction angiography (DSA), MRI/MR angiography (MRA), and more recently, rapid computed tomographic angiography (CTA) have tremendously improved the evaluation and treatment of cerebrovascular disease. Convergence of imaging modalities in the operating room (OR) is the natural next step toward refining and optimizing surgical treatment. Intraoperative technologies such as angiography, CT, ultrasound Doppler flow probes, neuronavigation, and near-infrared indocyanine green videoangiography (ICG) are among the techniques now available to the cerebrovascular surgeon. With the advent of MR systems in the OR, the utility of iMRI in treating vascular disease has been examined. Specific MR capabilities, such as MRA, diffusion weighted imaging (DWI), and diffusion tensor imaging

(DTI), represent potentially powerful tools to aid intraoperative management of cerebrovascular disease.

◆ Clinical Experience

Intraoperative MRI Systems

The cerebrovascular operations discussed in this chapter were performed at Barrow Neurologic Institute (BNI) in Phoenix, Arizona, or at the University of Calgary (UC), in Calgary, Alberta, Canada.

The iMRI system at BNI utilizes a General Electric (General Electric Medical Systems, Waukesha, WI) Signa HD 3.0 tesla (T) imaging magnet, based on the principle of moving the patient to a stationary magnet for imaging. The system is located in a separate radiofrequency- (RF-) shielded room within the main neurosurgical operating theater area, which houses 11 neurosurgical ORs. It is directly accessible from two adjacent ORs and indirectly from the remaining nine operating theaters. The operating tables in the adjacent two rooms are equipped with a translating table top, which slides onto the mobile MR gantry. A Mayfield-type MRI-compatible skull fixation system is incorporated into the table top. For intraoperative imaging, the intubated patient is transferred, with or without the surgical site open, onto the mobile MRI gantry by sliding the table top onto the docked gantry. The gantry is then transferred to the MRI suite and docks to the MRI system for imaging. An MRI-compatible ventilator is utilized in the imaging suite. Following completion of imaging, the patient is returned to the operating table in a similar fashion.

The GE HD 3.0 T system is equipped with high-power 23 to 50 mT/m gradients. Slew rate is 80 to 150 mT/m per millisecond. The magnet is 2.4 m tall, 2.2 m wide, and 2 m in length. It possesses a working bore of 60 cm and weighs

12,000 kg. The 5 gauss (G) fringe field is 2.8 × 5.0 m. The electronic OR table is custom made by Maquet (Rastatt, Germany), and possesses all of the positional capabilities of a standard OR table as well as standard head fixation attachments.

The iMRI system at The University of Calgary was initially based on a movable prototype 1.5 T magnet[4,9] and now a movable IMRIS 3.0 T magnet. The magnet (Siemens Verio 3.0 T, Erlangen, Germany) measures 1.73 m in length, with an internal diameter of 90 cm and a weight of 8,000 kg, compared with the prototype 5,100 kg 1.5 T system. The working aperture is 70 cm with shielded gradients in place. The 5 G fringe field measures only 4 m × 3.5 m. The system provides a large homogeneous field of view measuring 50 × 50 × 50 cm at the isocenter, maximum gradient strength of 45 mT/m, and a slew rate of 200 mT/m per millisecond. When not needed for surgery, the magnet is housed in an alcove adjacent to the OR. For imaging, the magnet is moved into the OR and over the OR table with the aid of an electric motor and ceiling I-beam rails. The OR table and patient enter the magnet bore with the head of the table located in the center of the magnet. Once imaging is completed, the magnet is returned to the alcove.

Frameless stereotaxy is utilized routinely at both sites. The Stealth Treon (Medtronic Navigation, Inc., Louisville, CO) stereotactic neuronavigation system is utilized in all BNI ORs and is integrated with the surgical microscope. In Calgary, a prototype ceiling-mounted BrainLab (BrainLab, Heimstetten, Germany) neuronavigation system was used. Intraoperative MR images at each site can be easily transferred to either the Stealth or BrainLab systems, and are utilized to update the navigation system to correct for brain and lesion deformation and shift as a result of surgery.

Vascular Lesions

All surgeries were performed with standard patient-positioning, skull fixation, microsurgical tools, techniques, and microscopes. Standard neuroanesthetic management was utilized. Aneurysm clipping was performed with commercially available standard titanium aneurysm clips (Spetzler, Yasargil, or Sugita). Controlled hypotension and temporary clipping was applied as required in the standard fashion.

In this series, 20 patients harboring 23 aneurysms have had aneurysm clipping monitored with iMR imaging. All except two aneurysms were unruptured and were located throughout the cerebral circulation, 20 aneurysms involved the anterior circulation and three involved the posterior circulation (**Table 18.1**). In general, surgical planning iMRI showed the aneurysm and its relationship to conventional

Table 18.1 Total Number of Cerebrovascular Surgeries Performed Utilizing iMRI Monitoring

Pathology	Number	Gender	Age
Cavernous angioma	74	M:33, F:41	Mean: 33+17, Range: 0.25–69
Aneurysm	20	M:6 F:14	Mean: 51+19, Range: 13–76
AVM	33	M:20 F:13	Mean: 30+16, Range: 1–56
EC-IC bypass	5	M:4 F:1	Mean: 55+19, Range: 36–74
Carotid Endarterectomy	4	M:2 F:2	Mean: 76+4, Range: 72–79
MVD	1	M:1 F:0	n/a, Range: 37

Aneurysm Location	Number	AVM Location	Number
Anterior Communicating	4	Sylvian fissure	3
Anterior cerebral (A1)	1	Frontal	4
Carotid	6	Parietal	13
MCA	6	Temporal	9
Posterior circulation	3	Cerebellar	2
		Occipital	1

Cavernous Angiomas Location	Number
Frontal	15
Parietal	3
Temporal	18
Occipital	6
Cerebellar	3

(Continued on page 172)

Brainstem	26
Corpus callosum	1
Orbital	1
Cervical spine	1

Abbreviations: iMRI, intraoperative magnetic resonance imaging; AVM, arteriovenous malformation; EC-IC, extracranial to intercranial; MVD, microvascular decompression; MCA, middle cerebral artery; M, male; F, female.

surgical corridors. Interdissection and quality-assurance MRA showed susceptibility artifact that prevented accurate assessment of the aneurysm neck. The desire to negate this observation has resulted in the development of MR invisible clips based on ceramic materials.[10] In certain cases, aneurysm clipping was also immediately evaluated with ICG angiography, which demonstrated patency of daughter and parent vessels, and obliteration of the aneurysm. Quality-assurance iMRA obtained on these patients confirmed these findings.

A superficial temporal artery to middle cerebral artery (STA-MCA) bypass was performed along with supraclinoid carotid ligation in a patient with a giant cavernous carotid aneurysm (**Fig. 18.1**). All vessels, including the bypass, were visualized, except the proximal internal carotid artery, which demonstrated the expected occlusion. All iMRA studies demonstrated significant susceptibility artifact at the clip site (**Fig. 18.2**). In another case, a ruptured anterior communicating artery aneurysm underwent clipping. At surgery a prominent perforator adherent to the dome and neck of the aneurysm could not be preserved. Diffusion weighted imaging did not demonstrate any significant ischemic deficit in this patient (**Fig. 18.3**). Hemorrhage was excluded in all patients prior to extubation.

Seventy-one patients have had their cavernous malformation (CM) resection monitored with iMRI. Of these patients, 26 were located in the brainstem or diencephalon and the remainder were hemispheric, except for one orbital and one cervical cord lesion (**Table 18.1**). Surgical planning iMRI with or without surgical navigation was often utilized to accurately localize the CM, thereby optimizing craniotomy placement and surgical trajectory. Among the brainstem patients, interdissection MRI was used when needed to accurately localize the lesion in relationship to the planned brainstem entry site. Complete resection of the CM and absence of a postoperative hematoma was confirmed by the iMRI quality assurance imaging in all cases (**Fig. 18.4**). More recently, diffusion tensor tractography has been applied to patients with CM (**Fig. 18.5**). Fiber tracking demonstrates well the relationship of white matter tracts to both the surgical corridor and the cavernoma. This intraoperatively acquired knowledge makes the surgeon aware of the location of important structures to be avoided during the resection of these vascular malformations.

Thirty-two patients with an arteriovenous malformation (AVM) of the brain were monitored with iMRI. These AVMs were distributed in a typical fashion throughout the cerebral hemispheres and cerebellum. In general, surgical planning iMRI with or without surgical navigation optimized craniotomy placement, whereas quality-assurance iMRI confirmed complete resection of the lesion and excluded acute surgical complications such as hemorrhage or cerebral edema.

Five patients underwent extracranial to intercranial (EC-IC) bypass for occlusive cerebrovascular disease. Perfusion deficit defined on either preoperative or surgical planning iMRI studies, was immediately reversed following

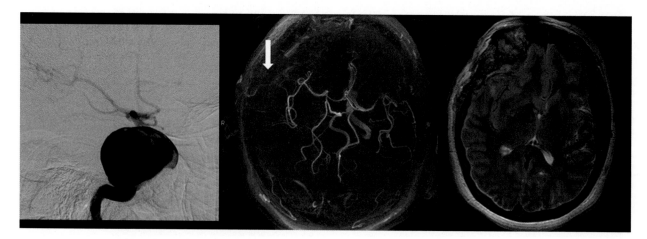

Fig. 18.1   A 61-year-old woman with a giant right cavernous sinus aneurysm. She underwent a craniotomy for superficial temporal artery to middle cerebral artery; an extracranial to intercranial (EC-IC) bypass was performed as well as Hunterian ligation of the aneurysm/internal carotid artery. Left: preoperative right internal carotid artery angiogram demonstrating the giant aneurysm. Middle: Intraoperative magnetic resonance angiography (iMRA) demonstrating patent bypass (*white arrow*) and occluded intracranial internal carotid artery. Right: T2-weighted axial intraoperative magnetic resonance imaging (iMRI) obtained prior to extubation demonstrating the absence of immediate complications.

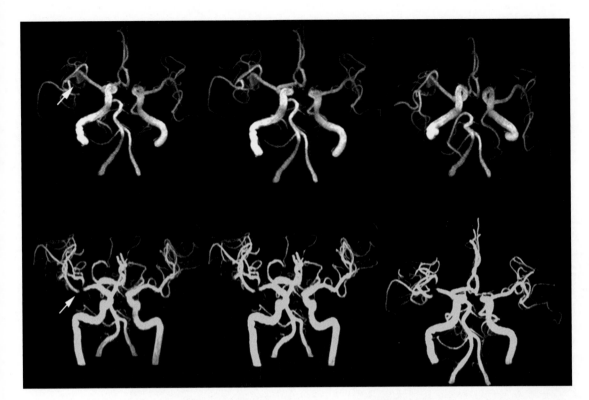

Fig. 18.2 This 59-year-old man was involved in a motor vehicle accident in which he sustained a minor closed head injury. Diagnostic computed tomography (CT) brain imaging showed a 10 × 7 × 7 mm right middle cerebral artery bifurcation aneurysm. The patient was brought to the operating room where surgical planning intraoperative magnetic resonance imaging (iMRI) including MR angiography (MRA; top row) showed well the aneurysm (white arrow) and its relationship to the middle cerebral artery bifurcation. Quality assurance iMRA studies (bottom row) showed susceptibility artifact related to the MR-compatible titanium clip (*arrow*), illustrating the need for an MR-invisible aneurysm clip.

bypass. For the four carotid endarterectomies reported, quality-assurance iMRI showed patency of the carotid and the absence of cerebral ischemia. One patient with trigeminal neuralgia was positioned laterally on the operating table. Intraoperatively acquired images showed the vascular compression defined on diagnostic studies.

◆ Discussion

The number of installed iMRI systems worldwide continues to increase annually. As more neurosurgeons gain experience with iMRI, it is becoming increasingly evident that certain pathologies are more likely to benefit from the monitoring of their surgery with iMRI. Likely due in part to the complexity of surgical treatment for these disorders, and the high quality of presently available intraoperative imaging modalities, the application of iMRI to cerebrovascular surgery has been somewhat limited.[11,12]

Aneurysms

Intraoperative angiography (IA)[13–19] demonstrates that incomplete aneurysm clipping or vessel occlusion requiring clip repositioning can be as high as 12%. Despite this, IA can be cumbersome and time consuming, utilizing potentially harmful ionizing radiation. With the availability of rapid and dependable intraoperative vascular evaluation with ICG[20–22] and microdoppler flow probes,[23,24] IA is generally reserved for the evaluation of more complex lesions.

Effective high-resolution MRA, DWI, or DTI all require high-field MR systems coupled with high-power gradients to maximize signal-to-noise ratio (SNR). This is necessary for both image quality and shorter imaging time. Particularly relevant is overall time spent in acquiring the images, as the duration of ischemia is inversely correlated to tissue recovery upon reperfusion.[25,26] Imaging time includes not only the actual image acquisition duration, but also time required for patient draping, surgical equipment storage, and travel time of the patient to and from the MR system, or vice versa. If imaging time is protracted, clip readjustment or reexploration will likely be of limited clinical benefit.

Although high-resolution MRA has been successfully obtained to evaluate the vasculature surrounding a clipped aneurysm, it is arguable whether it is of sufficient resolution. At present, the intraluminal direction of flow cannot be determined, although this may become possible with newer techniques. Image distortion and signal loss related to the titanium aneurysm clips renders detailed evaluation of the neck of the aneurysm impossible. This problem may

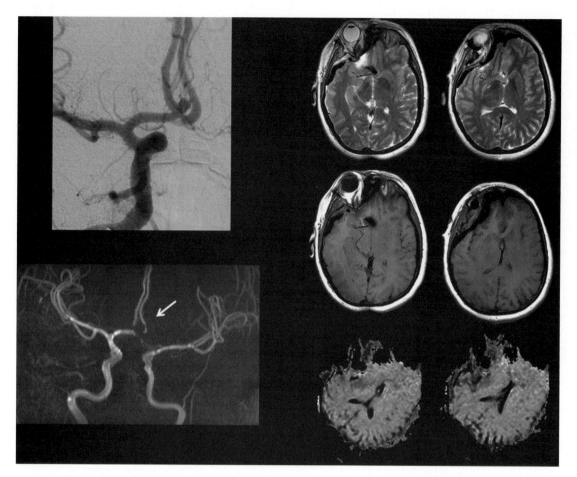

Fig. 18.3 A 49-year-old woman with a subarachnoid hemorrhage from a ruptured anterior communicating aneurysm (top left: preoperative contrast angiogram). Bottom left: following craniotomy for aneurysm clipping intraoperative magnetic resonance angiography (iMRA) demonstrating clearly the patent A1 and A2 vessels, but also again the significant susceptibility artifact related to the MR-compatible titanium clip (*arrow*). Right column: Quality assurance intraoperative T2-weighted magnetic resonance imaging (top), T2-weighted (middle), and diffusion-weighted imaging (DWI; bottom) demonstrating the lack of surgical complications including ischemic change.

be resolved as clips manufactured with other materials, such as ceramic, become available.[10]

Diffusion-weighted imaging (DWI) has been utilized to evaluate ischemic deficits in the surrounding brain parenchyma related to inadvertent vessel compromise, which may not be visualized on IA or ICG. In all cases presented in this study, rapid, high-quality DWI demonstrated no diffusion abnormality related to the surgical procedure or aneurysm clipping. This was particularly noteworthy in a case in which a large perforator was necessarily sacrificed during aneurysm clipping. Susceptibility artifact at the air–brain interface has not created any significant image distortion or caused image interpretation difficulties.

Vascular Malformations

The surgical resection of CMs, particularly given their typical size and subcortical location, has been particularly enhanced by the advent of intraoperative neuronavigation. Smaller, localized craniotomies directly over the lesion,

with limited corticectomies are typical for resection of these lesions. Navigation also allows for safer targeting of deep, less-accessible lesions such as those located in the brainstem. Intraoperative MRI in these cases has confirmed the complete resection of the lesion as well the absence of any significant postresection hemorrhage, which is of particular importance for brainstem CM.

Well known for demonstrating variable signal characteristics, iMR images of CM can be confounded by the surgical manipulation of the surrounding brain, postoperative fluid in the cavity, brain-shifts, and residual hemosiderin staining. Postoperative blood and fluid may have variable appearances on iMRI. The placement of hemostatic materials in the resection cavity is also common and should also be recognized when interpreting the images. The presence and location of any associated venous anomalies, malformations, or draining structures must also be noted intraoperatively for interpretation of iMR images. These structures may become more apparent following resection of the cavernous malformation and decompression of the veins. Thus it is essential that the surgeon correlate the iMR

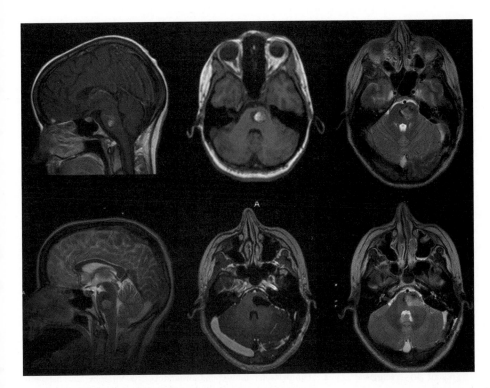

Fig. 18.4 A 28-year-old woman with a symptomatic left pontine cavernous malformation. Top row: preoperative sagittal and axial magnetic resonance MR images demonstrating the brainstem cavernous malformation. Bottom row: Quality assurance intraoperative magnetic resonance imaging (iMRI) demonstrating complete resection of the lesion and the absence of immediate complications.

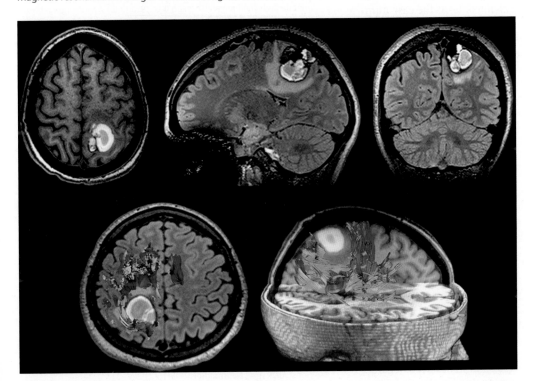

Fig. 18.5 A 23-year-old right-handed woman presented with acute headache and right-sided paresthesia secondary to a cavernous malformation. She was brought to the operating room, and surgical planning intraoperative magnetic resonance imaging (iMRI), including fiber tract diffusion tensor imaging, showed well the lesion and its relationship to predicted motor and sensory tracts (top row: the paracentral lesion in standard diagnostic format; bottom row: relationship of the lesion to adjacent fiber tracts as positioned for surgical approach). The lesion was resected through a small craniectomy. Quality assurance iMRI showed complete resection of the cavernoma with preservation of the fiber tracts (not shown). The patient made a full recovery.

images with the intraoperative findings, to verify the completeness of resection.

Craniotomy placement and size for patients undergoing AVM surgery are more accurate with the use of both iMRI and stereotactic navigation. Intraoperative MRA and MRI have demonstrated completeness of resection and the absence of significant hematoma. However, iMRA and the prominence of normal peri-AVM vasculature postresection must be interpreted with caution and correlated to intraoperative findings. The hemodynamic instability associated with AVM is well recognized, as are the risks of postresection hemorrhage and hyperperfusion.[27,28] Evaluation and interpretation of immediate postresection iMRI/DWI may provide a better understanding of this phenomenon. Identification of iMRI markers that predict a higher risk of perfusion-related complications will certainly enhance peri-operative AVM resection management.

In the treatment of vascular malformations in deep locations or adjacent to eloquent structures and neuronal tracts advanced in MR techniques afforded by high-field MR may be useful. As diffusion tensor imaging (DTI) and tractography become more readily available, their routine incorporation into surgical planning, resection, and iMRI monitoring may aid in minimizing surgical morbidity and in helping to identify those patients at risk of postresection complication.

Although iMRI has been applied to patients with vascular occlusive disease, its value is limited, other than for the immediate assessment of surgical outcome. As the case numbers of EC-IC bypass and carotid endarterectomy are limited, it is not possible to quantify this potential benefit, or compare it to other techniques used to monitor blood flow. The microvascular decompression for a trigeminal neuralgia case was included as a demonstration of the ability of iMRI to localize the craniectomy in relationship to the transverse sinus. Given this anecdotal case, it is not possible to comment on potential benefit.

◆ Conclusions

The neurosurgical management of cerebrovascular pathology is constantly undergoing evolution. Endovascular techniques are now commonplace and endosaccular coils, endoluminal stents, and embolic materials are constantly being refined. Similar to standard surgical approaches, access to rapid, high-field iMRI may be helpful in monitoring endovascular procedures to demonstrate early procedure-related changes in iMRI or DWI and allowing optimized therapy. This concept has already been developed by Matsumae et al, who have equipped an operating theater with fluoroscopy, angiography, CT, and iMRI, in addition to standard open surgery capability.[29]

The implication of DWI changes on iMRI has been debated. Although these changes are known to develop shortly following the onset of ischemia, the reversal of DWI changes following flow restoration reflects both time and degree of ischemia, and does not necessarily correlate with tissue survival.[30] In the setting of immediate postaneurysm clipping or AVM

resection, these changes may be misleading should temporary clipping or hypotension be utilized intraoperatively. Time of acquisition of iMR images after ischemia will also further confound interpretation of DWI changes.

Monitoring cerebrovascular surgery with iMRI is an exciting field with significant potential. Efficacy and success will depend upon maximization of the basic, essential criteria of iMRI: fast, high-resolution imaging with minimal disruption of standard surgical techniques and understanding and correlating imaging findings to surgical observations and techniques. Information regarding cerebral ischemia, blood flow, perilesional metabolism, neuronal tracts, and more are possible, and the refinement of MRI sequences and protocols to gain useful data beyond that which is currently available must be demonstrated.

References

1. Black PM, Moriarty T, Alexander E III, et al. Development and implementation of intraoperative magnetic resonance imaging and its neurosurgical applications. Neurosurgery 1997;41(4):831–842, discussion 842–845

2. Tronnier VM, Wirtz CR, Knauth M, et al. Intraoperative diagnostic and interventional magnetic resonance imaging in neurosurgery. Neurosurgery 1997;40(5):891–900, discussion 900–902

3. Steinmeier R, Fahlbusch R, Ganslandt O, et al. Intraoperative magnetic resonance imaging with the Magnetom open scanner: concepts, neurosurgical indications, and procedures: a preliminary report. Neurosurgery 1998;43(4):739–747, discussion 747–748

4. Sutherland GR, Kaibara T, Louw D, Hoult DI, Tomanek B, Saunders J. A mobile high-field magnetic resonance system for neurosurgery. J Neurosurg 1999;91(5):804–813

5. Hall WA, Liu H, Martin AJ, Pozza CH, Maxwell RE, Truwit CL. Safety, efficacy, and functionality of high-field strength interventional magnetic resonance imaging for neurosurgery. Neurosurgery 2000;46(3):632–641, discussion 641–642

6. Bohinski RJ, Kokkino AK, Warnick RE, et al. Glioma resection in a shared-resource magnetic resonance operating room after optimal image-guided frameless stereotactic resection. Neurosurgery 2001;48(4):731–742, discussion 742–744

7. Hadani M, Spiegelman R, Feldman Z, Berkenstadt H, Ram Z. Novel, compact, intraoperative magnetic resonance imaging-guided system for conventional neurosurgical operating rooms. Neurosurgery 2001;48(4):799–807, discussion 807–809

8. Hall WA, Galicich W, Bergman T, Truwit CL. 3-Tesla intraoperative MR imaging for neurosurgery. J Neurooncol 2006;77(3):297–303

9. Kaibara T, Saunders JK, Sutherland GR. Advances in mobile intraoperative magnetic resonance imaging. Neurosurgery 2000;47(1):131–137, discussion 137–138

10. Sutherland GR, Kelly JP, Boehm DW, et al. Ceramic aneurysm clips for improved MR visualization. Neurosurgery 2008;62:400–406

11. Sutherland GR, Kaibara T, Wallace C, Tomanek B, Richter M. Intraoperative assessment of aneurysm clipping using magnetic resonance angiography and diffusion-weighted imaging: technical case report. Neurosurgery 2002;50(4):893–897, discussion 897–898

12. Sutherland GR, Kaibara T. Neurosurgical suite of the future. III. Neuroimaging Clin N Am 2001;11(4):593–609

13. Parkinson D, Legal J, Holloway AF, et al. A new combined neurosurgical headholder and cassette changer for intraoperative serial angiography. Technical note. J Neurosurg 1978;48(6):1038–1041

14. Derdeyn CP, Moran CJ, Cross DT, Grubb RL Jr, Dacey RG Jr. Intraoperative digital subtraction angiography: a review of 112 consecutive examinations. AJNR Am J Neuroradiol 1995;16(2):307–318

15. Chiang VL, Gailloud P, Murphy KJ, Rigamonti D, Tamargo RJ. Routine intraoperative angiography during aneurysm surgery. J Neurosurg 2002;96(6):988–992

16. Payner TD, Horner TG, Leipzig TJ, Scott JA, Gilmor RL, DeNardo AJ. Role of intraoperative angiography in the surgical treatment of cerebral aneurysms. J Neurosurg 1998;88(3):441–448

17. Tang G, Cawley CM, Dion JE, Barrow DL. Intraoperative angiography during aneurysm surgery: a prospective evaluation of efficacy. J Neurosurg 2002;96(6):993–999

18. Klopfenstein JD, Spetzler RF, Kim LJ, et al. Comparison of routine and selective use of intraoperative angiography during aneurysm surgery: a prospective assessment. J Neurosurg 2004;100(2):230–235

19. Alexander TD, Macdonald RL, Weir B, Kowalczuk A. Intraoperative angiography in cerebral aneurysm surgery: a prospective study of 100 craniotomies. Neurosurgery 1996;39(1):10–17, discussion 17–18

20. Raabe A, Beck J, Gerlach R, Zimmermann M, Seifert V. Near-infrared indocyanine green video angiography: a new method for intraoperative assessment of vascular flow. Neurosurgery 2003;52(1):132–139, discussion 139

21. Raabe A, Nakaji P, Beck J, et al. Prospective evaluation of surgical microscope-integrated intraoperative near-infrared indocyanine green videoangiography during aneurysm surgery. J Neurosurg 2005; 103(6):982–989

22. Dashti R, Laakso A, Niemelä M, Porras M, Hernesniemi J. Microscope-integrated near-infrared indocyanine green videoangiography during surgery of intracranial aneurysms: the Helsinki experience. Surg Neurol 2009;71(5):543–550, discussion 550

23. Charbel FT, Hoffman WE, Misra M, Hannigan K, Ausman JI. Role of a perivascular ultrasonic micro-flow probe in aneurysm surgery. Neurol Med Chir (Tokyo) 1998;38(Suppl):35–38

24. Akdemir H, Oktem IS, Tucer B, Menkü A, Ba_aslan K, Günaldi O. Intraoperative microvascular Doppler sonography in aneurysm surgery. Minim Invasive Neurosurg 2006;49(5):312–316

25. Christou I, Alexandrov AV, Burgin WS, et al. Timing of recanalization after tissue plasminogen activator therapy determined by transcranial doppler correlates with clinical recovery from ischemic stroke. Stroke 2000;31(8):1812–1816

26. Kaplan B, Brint S, Tanabe J, Jacewicz M, Wang XJ, Pulsinelli W. Temporal thresholds for neocortical infarction in rats subjected to reversible focal cerebral ischemia. Stroke 1991;22(8):1032–1039

27. Spetzler RF, Wilson CB, Weinstein P, Mehdorn M, Townsend J, Telles D. Normal perfusion pressure breakthrough theory. Clin Neurosurg 1978;25:651–672

28. Spetzler RF, Hargraves RW, McCormick PW, Zabramski JM, Flom RA, Zimmerman RS. Relationship of perfusion pressure and size to risk of hemorrhage from arteriovenous malformations. J Neurosurg 1992; 76(6):918–923

29. Matsumae M, Koizumi J, Fukuyama H, et al. World's first magnetic resonance imaging/x-ray/operating room suite: a significant milestone in the improvement of neurosurgical diagnosis and treatment. J Neurosurg 2007;107(2):266–273

30. Li F, Han SS, Tatlisumak T, et al. Reversal of acute apparent diffusion coefficient abnormalities and delayed neuronal death following transient focal cerebral ischemia in rats. Ann Neurol 1999;46(3): 333–342

19

Skull Base Surgery and Intraoperative Magnetic Resonance Imaging

Taro Kaibara and Robert F. Spetzler

The surgical treatment of lesions involving the cranial base has evolved significantly over the past several decades. As in other neurosurgical disciplines their surgical management has relied heavily upon advances in technology and imaging modalities. Surgical adjuncts such as high-powered microscopes, ultrasonic aspirators, and endoscopes have refined skull base surgery techniques. Nerve stimulation and motor and sensory evoked potential monitoring provide invaluable electrophysiologic information regarding anatomy as well as the progress and effects of surgery. High-resolution computerized tomographic imaging (CT), magnetic resonance imaging (MRI), and advanced angiographic systems and techniques have greatly refined the preoperative localization and anatomic understanding of many of these lesions, particularly with regard to bony, soft tissue and neurovascular relationships.

The development of computerized surgical navigation systems has had tremendous impact upon many aspects of skull base surgery.[1-3] Based upon preoperatively acquired imaging, these image guidance systems are used to plan more refined surgical approaches to lesions and craniotomies that are smaller and more directly over the target. Intraoperatively, real-time image-based guidance allows the surgeon to accurately approach the lesion and provides constant information on the progress of surgery as well as the anatomic relationships of the various surrounding structures. This is of particular importance in skull base lesions where eloquent structures such as brainstem and/or cranial nerves are often incorporated within or are in very close proximity to a lesion and normal anatomic relationships are frequently distorted or destroyed.

The development of intraoperative magnetic resonance imaging (iMRI) systems over the past two decades has provided a unique tool for the surgeon to evaluate and assess the effects and progress of a surgical procedure. A variety of iMRI systems have been developed by different vendors in conjunction with surgeons throughout the world.[4-11] These systems differ vastly from one another in several characteristics. The main differences are magnet field strength (ranging from 0.12 tesla [T] to 3.0 T), whether the surgery is performed within the magnetic field, and whether the patient is transported to the magnet or whether the magnet is transported to the patient for imaging. Despite this heterogeneity of iMRI systems, it has become evident that the acquisition of high-resolution MR imaging and advanced MRI techniques require higher-field systems,[9,12] which allow the MRI evaluation of the anatomic and when warranted, the physiologic effects of surgery. Furthermore, by updating image-guidance systems with iMRI data, the inaccuracies in stereotaxy induced through operation and surgical resection can be corrected and residual lesion precisely localized.[13,14] Skull base lesions, given their relationships to complex but relatively constant anatomic structures represent unique lesions with particular potential to benefit from iMRI.

◆ The Intraoperative MRI System

The operations on skull base lesions discussed in this report were performed at Barrow Neurologic Institute (BNI) in Phoenix, Arizona. The iMRI system at the BNI utilizes a GE Signa HDx (General Electric Medical Systems, Waukesha, WI) 3.0 T MRI unit. The magnet is identical to the commercially available diagnostic unit marketed by GE. The magnet has a working aperture of 60 cm and weighs 12,000 kg. It is equipped with high power 23 to 50 mT/m gradients. Slew rate is 80 to 150 mT/m per millisecond. The magnet is 2.4 m tall, 2.2 m wide, and 2 m in length. The 5 gauss (G) fringe field is 2.8 × 5.0m, well within the confines of the imaging suite. The electronic operating room (OR) table is a specially designed unit by Maquet (Maquet GmbH, Rastatt, Germany) and possesses all of the positional capabilities of a standard OR table as well as a specially designed MRI-compatible skull fixation attachment.

The iMRI system is located in a suite within the main neurosurgical operating room area and is directly accessible from two adjacent, connecting ORs (**Fig. 19.1**). For iMRI the patient is transported, anesthetized, and intubated into the MRI scanner. Only patients undergoing surgery in either of the two directly adjacent rooms can undergo iMRI while remaining in skull fixation and the surgical site open. Although patients in the remaining rooms must have their wound closed and be removed from skull fixation prior to being transported for imaging, all 11 neurosurgical ORs have access to the MRI scanner for intraoperative imaging.

For a variety reasons including patient positioning restrictions due to patient size, instrumentation and magnet working aperture, time restrictions, etc., the majority of iMRI performed is with the surgical wound closed and the patient removed from skull fixation. The OR equipment and room is always maintained sterile for potential return for further surgery following iMRI.

Frameless stereotaxy is utilized in all cases. The Stealth Treon (Medtronic Navigation, Inc., Louisville, CO) stereotactic neuronavigation system is available in all the ORs and is closely integrated with the surgical microscopes. iMR images can be readily transferred to the Stealth system and are utilized to update the navigation system to correct for brain and lesion deformation and/or shift as a result of surgery. Accuracy has been well maintained during this data transfer and re-registration with iMR images.

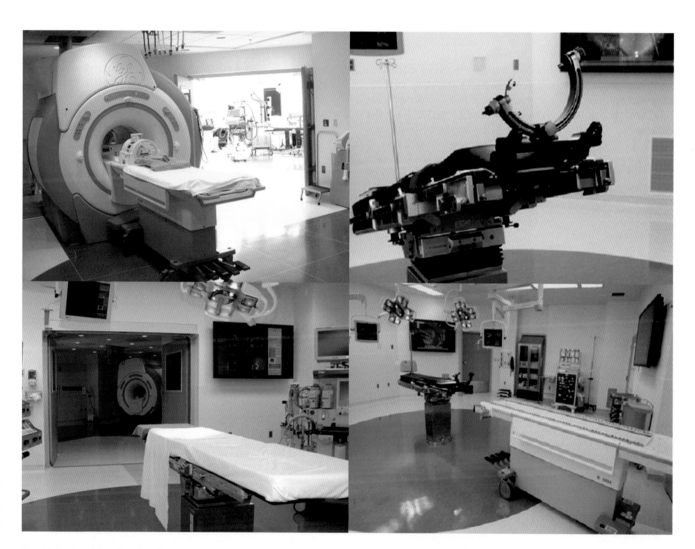

Fig. 19.1 Top left: GE 3.0 tesla intraoperative magnetic resonance imaging (iMRI) system (General Electric Medical Systems, Waukesha, WI) with one of directly accessible two adjacent operating rooms (ORs) in the background. Gantry is docked to magnet in imaging position. Bottom left: View from other OR with doors leading to iMRI suite open. Operating table in foreground. Top right: Maquet OR table (Maquet GmbH, Rastatt, Germany) with MRI-compatible head holder. Bottom right: The mobile MR gantry preparing to dock with OR table for transfer to iMRI suite.

◆ Clinical Experience

Surgical Technique

As the magnetic field within the operating room is negligible, all surgical procedures were performed using standard microneurosurgical instruments, equipment and techniques. This included use of ultrasonic aspiration, CO2 laser, endoscope, standard high-powered surgical microscope, etc., as needed. A Zeiss Pentero (Carl Zeiss AG, Oberkochen, Germany) microscope with surgical chair and foot and mouth controls was utilized for all operations. Electrophysiologic monitoring including somatosensory evoked potentials (SSEPs) and/or any other applicable modalities, such as brainstem auditory evoked potentials (BAERs) and cranial nerve monitoring, were utilized as deemed necessary by the surgeon. All monitoring leads were removed for iMRI.

Imaging Studies

All iMR images were obtained with the patient intubated and anesthetized. For transfer to the imaging suite ventilation was applied by the anesthesiologist by bag-mask. For iMRI with the patient remaining in skull fixation with the wound exposed ($n = 4$), all non-MR-compatible leads and instruments are removed and a draping protocol is utilized to maintain sterility of the surgical site. The patient is then transferred with the mobile tabletop on to the mobile MR gantry and transported to the iMR suite for MRI. In the MR suite an MR-compatible ventilator is utilized during imaging. Following MRI, the patient is transported back to the OR and the tabletop and patient are transferred back to the OR table. The sterile draping is unfolded and the surgery site reexposed, navigational data transferred to the Stealth system, and surgery resumed.

All standard MRI sequences were available and obtained as requested by the surgeon. These included T1-weighted, T2-weighted, fluid attenuation inversion recovery (FLAIR), gradient echo, gadolinium-enhanced, diffusion-weighted, and MR angiography. Average imaging time for this group of patients was 55 minutes.

Surgery of Skull Base Pathology

The surgical treatment of a broad range of skull base pathologies was monitored utilizing iMRI. Included in this series were any lesions involving the following regions: sellar/parasellar, cavernous sinus, orbit, clivus, nasopharynx, petrous bone, and posterior fossa ($n = 68$, see **Table 19.1**). The vast majority of these lesions were tumors with the most common pathologies

Table 19.1 Characteristics of Patients with Base Pathology Grouped by Diagnosis ($n = 68$)

Pathology	Location	Sex and Number Female	Male	Mean Age (Years)
Meningioma	Overall	13	5	57.2
	Petroclival	6	3	
	Cavernous sinus	3		
	Sphenoid wing	2	2	
	Foramen magnum	2		
Schwannoma	Overall	5	5	51.0
	Vestibular	5	3	
	Trigeminal		1	
	Jugular foramen		2	
Pituitary adenoma	Sellar	2	2	35.5
Cavernous Malformation	Brainstem	7	4	30.5
Chordoma	Clivus		1	57.0
Chondrosarcoma	Petrous		2	31.0
	Clival	1		40.0
Sinonasal carcinoma	Nasopharynx		1	49.0
Squamous cell carcinoma	Meckel cave	1	1	61.0
Teratoma	Head/neck/clivus	1		1.0
Craniopharyngioma	Suprasellar	1		4.0
Epidermoid	Cerebellopontine		2	54.0
Hemangioblastoma	Cerebellar	1	2	49.5
Choroid plexus papilloma	4th ventricle	1		1.0

Table 19.1 (*Continued*)   Characteristics of Patients with Base Pathology Grouped by Diagnosis (*n* = 68)

Ependymoma	4th Ventricle	1	2	37.3
Medulloblastoma	Cerebellum	1		32
Pilocytic astrocytoma	Pineal			32
	Sellar	1	1	1
	Brainstem	1		3
Metstatic breast carcinoma	Optic chiasm	1		64
Chiari malformation		1		1
Hemangioma	Orbit		1	59

being meningiomas (13 females, five males; mean age = 57.2 years), schwannomas (five females, five males; mean age = 51.0 years), pituitary adenomas (two females, two males; mean age = 35.5 years) and brainstem cavernous malformations (seven females, four males; mean age = 30.5 years). The remainder represented a broad spectrum of skull base pathologies including chondrosarcoma, clival chordoma, skull base carcinoma, hemangioblastoma, etc.

All patients underwent maximal resection prior to iMRI.

Meningioma

Eighteen patients harboring complex meningiomas had their tumor resection monitored with iMRI. Nine patients had large petroclival tumors; four involved the sphenoid wing, three involved the cavernous sinus, and two were located at the foramen magnum. Twelve patients were deemed to have gross total resection of the tumor while six patients underwent subtotal resection. Those undergoing subtotal resection included large petroclival tumors adherent to the brainstem and cranial nerves and those involving

the cavernous sinus. iMRI in this group of patients did not show any unanticipated residual tumor or hemorrhage and no patient returned to surgery based upon iMRI.

Schwannoma

Ten patients presented with complex schwannoma involving the skull base. Seven patients harbored large vestibular nerve lesions; one patient underwent two operations one year apart for an aggressive, recurrent jugular foramen schwannoma; and one patient harbored a trigeminal nerve schwannoma in the Meckel cave (**Fig. 19.2**). Of the tumors involving the vestibular nerve three were deemed to have gross total resection confirmed by iMRI while four patients were treated with subtotal resection due to adherence of tumor to brainstem and/or cranial nerves. The patient with the jugular foramen meningioma was initially treated with subtotal resection and remained without neurologic deficit. Following progression despite adjunctive treatment and development of significant tongue weakness, the patient underwent reresection with gross total removal of the tumor. The

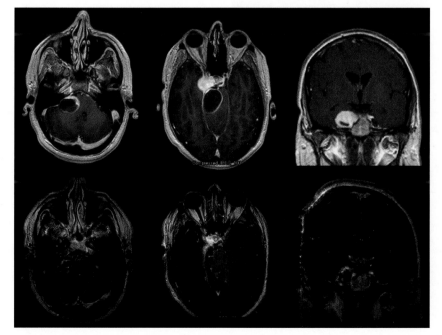

Fig. 19.2 Preoperative (top row) and intraoperative (bottom row) gadolinium-enhanced T1-weighted magnetic resonance (MR) images in a patient with a right-sided trigeminal schwannoma involving the cavernous sinus with a large posterior fossa cyst. Intraoperative MR images demonstrate excellent decompression of the brainstem and resection of the tumor.

trigeminal nerve schwannoma was completely resected. iMRI in these 10 patients did not demonstrate any unexpected residual tumor or hematoma in the surgical site.

Pituitary Adenoma

Four patients harboring a pituitary adenoma and undergoing transsphenoidal surgery were monitored with iMRI. Two patients underwent gross total resection and two had subtotal resection. In one patient unexpected residual tumor was encountered and in two patients further surgery was performed. One patient with subtotal resection of the tumor had residual tumor identified on iMRI over the planum sphenoidale. Navigation was updated with the iMRI and further surgery performed. However, on enlarging the craniotomy to resect this residual tumor, significant bleeding from the intercavernous sinus was encountered and surgery was halted in favor of a different approach. The other patient with subtotal resection had significant involvement of the cavernous sinus. In all patients, initial tumor resection was explored and evaluated with an endoscope.

Cavernous Malformation

Cavernous malformations of the brainstem are complex lesions whose treatment can be complicated with significant morbidity. Their management is dictated by their presentation to the surface of the brainstem and the optimal surgical approach may often require a creative skull base approach. Eleven patients with symptomatic brainstem cavernous malformations were monitored during surgery with iMRI. Imaging demonstrated complete resection in all of the patients and confirmed the absence of hemorrhage in the resection bed (**Fig. 19.3**; please see Chapter 18).

Miscellaneous Lesions

The surgeries for a broad variety of miscellaneous lesions were monitored using iMRI. This group included lesions such as pilocytic astrocytoma, hemangioblastoma, chondrosarcoma (**Fig. 19.4**), craniopharyngioma, choroid plexus papilloma, epidermoid cysts, as well as more malignant lesions such as medulloblastoma, sinonasal carcinoma, ependymoma, and chordoma. In eight of these 25 patients subtotal resection and the absence of surgical hematoma was confirmed with iMRI. This group of eight patients included a chondrosarcoma involving the petrous apex and cavernous sinus, a large 4th ventricular ependymoma resected through a midline craniotomy with significant tumor growth through the foramen of Lushka treated with a staged lateral craniotomy, and a large clival chondrosarcoma. Gross total resection and the absence of hematoma was confirmed with iMRI in the remainder of the patients. Demonstration of complete resection and the absence of complications was particularly useful in a patient undergoing a level III craniofacial resection of a sinonasal carcinoma.

In one patient harboring a recurrent hemangioblastoma, iMRI clearly demonstrated unexpected residual tumor high in the resection cavity (**Fig. 19.5**). The Stealth navigation system was updated with the iMR images and resection of the residual lesion performed. This was confirmed with a second iMRI. Interestingly, an unexpected residual lesion or a surgical complication requiring additional surgery was encountered in only one of the 25 patients in this group. In the remaining cases, either complete resection or expected residual tumor was demonstrated. Surgical complications such as hemorrhage or infarct were not observed on any of the iMRI studies.

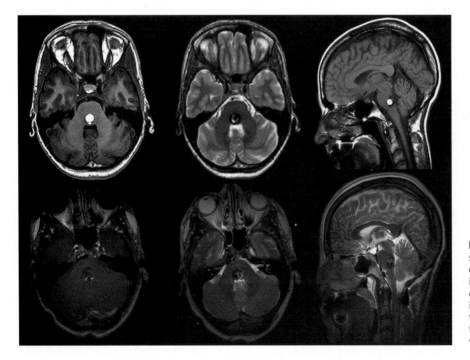

Fig. 19.3 T1- and T2-weighted axial and sagittal preoperative (top row) and intraoperative (bottom row) magnetic resonance images in a patient with a dorsal pontine cavernous malformation. Intraoperative MR images demonstrate complete resection of the lesion, the absence of acute complications, and the associated draining vein now visible in the resection cavity.

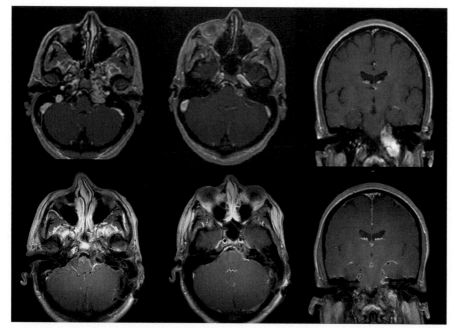

Fig. 19.4 T1-weighted gadolinium-enhanced axial and coronal preoperative (top row) and intraoperative (bottom row) magnetic resonance (MR) images in a patient with a large left petroclival chondrosarcoma. The intraoperative MR images demonstrate complete resection of the tumor with no acute complications.

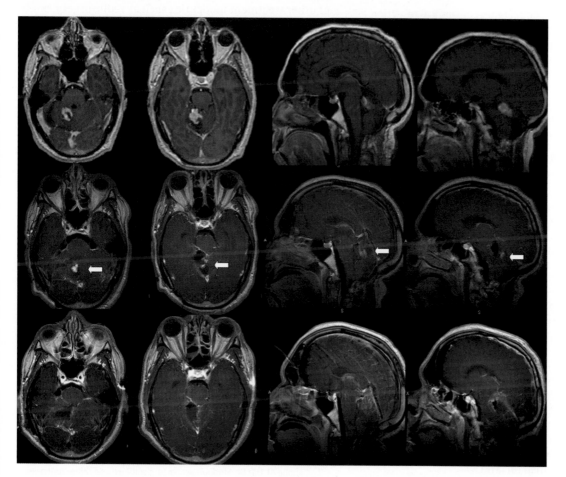

Fig. 19.5 T1-weighted gadolinium-enhanced axial and sagittal preoperative (top row) intraoperative (middle row) and second intraoperative (bottom row) magnetic resonance (MR) images in a patient with a recurrent cerebellar hemangioblastoma. Intraoperative MR (iMR) images demonstrated unexpected residual lesion (*white arrows*, middle row) which was then targeted with updated neuronavigation and resected, as demonstrated on second iMR images (bottom row).

◆ Discussion

The most significant advances that have affected neurosurgery over the past few decades have been those related to neuroimaging and its applications. Subsequently, MRI-based neuronavigation revolutionized the identification and classification, localization, and treatment of neurosurgical disease. Subsequently MRI and based neuronavigation, or frameless stereotaxy, has had tremendous impact upon the ease and safety of performing neurosurgery. This is achieved by providing simple, real time cranial localization for smaller, more accurate craniotomy placement. During surgery, real-time high-resolution microscope-integrated intraoperative navigation directs the surgeon to the lesion and its surrounding structures. Of the neurosurgical subspecialties, skull base surgery has likely experienced the greatest impact from the development of frameless stereotaxy. With the relatively fixed and rigid anatomy of most skull base lesions, they are relatively unaffected by the brain and lesion deformation and shift associated with craniotomy, cerebrospinal fluid egress, and surgical resection. The navigation system accuracy is maintained for longer periods during surgery and the need for updated MRI data are less.

The monitoring of the completeness of surgical resection – resection control – and the updating of surgical navigation systems to account for brain and tumor shifts are among the most commonly described benefits of iMRI. The clear demonstration of the absence of acute complication such as resection cavity hemorrhage, subdural hematoma, or cerebral infarct particularly following lengthy operations or in surgeries involving eloquent tissue such as the brainstem, is also a very important benefit of iMRI. In this series the iMR images very effectively demonstrated the absence of significant or worrisome complications such as hematoma or ischemia. This was very relevant given the frequently prolonged nature of these operations and the unforgiving characteristics of the surrounding structures, particularly so in the patients harboring cavernous malformations of the brainstem.

As is evident from the content of other chapters in this text, certain pathologies demonstrate a clear benefit from the iMRI monitoring of their surgery. Those lesions in which maximal resection is related closely to prognosis and survival certainly will likely benefit the most from surgical monitoring with iMRI. Pituitary adenoma resection has been shown by several authors to provide significant improvement in the completeness of resection.[15-19] Unexpected residual tumor identified on iMRI has been reported in up to 66% of patients undergoing transsphenoidal resection. The authors of these reports are uniformly impressed by the frequency of residual pituitary adenoma on iMRI. In our series, although the numbers of operations are small, pituitary adenoma resection patients clearly demonstrated the highest rate, 50% (two of four patients) of further surgery for residual lesion identified on iMRI.

In this series, patients harboring and undergoing surgery for skull base lesions, the number of patients in which unexpected residual lesion was identified on iMRI prompting unplanned further resection was very small: only 2 of the 68 patients. This low percentage is likely related to several factors. Although the OR and surgical instruments are always maintained sterile during iMRI for possible return to the OR, the patient transfer and imaging can be time-consuming. In this series, this took up to 55 minutes on average. The surgeon may thus be more apt to continue with maximal aggressive tumor debulking and resection, and completely close the craniotomy prior to iMRI. Patient positioning for skull base surgery is also often more demanding than for routine craniotomy and thus use of the iMRI system table is frequently not possible. This necessitates wound closure, removal from skull fixation, and return to a supine position for iMRI, again providing impetus for aggressive maximal resection prior to imaging. A small percentage of patients were also found to have residual lesion on iMRI, which was expected or felt to be not clinically significant to warrant the potential morbidity associated with further resection. These were primarily patients harboring benign lesions such as meningioma and schwannoma affecting the petroclival region that were large and/or densely adherent to brainstem and cranial nerves or in surgeries that were prolonged. This may reflect a general paradigm shift in skull base surgery toward the utilization of other treatment modalities such as radiosurgery, or observation for the management of residual disease rather than to incur morbidity from aggressive initial complete resection.

◆ Conclusions

Intraoperative MR systems demonstrate the versatility to accommodate the monitoring of complex skull base operations with high-resolution imaging during surgery. iMRI can enhance skull base surgery by allowing the surgeon to identify acute postoperative complications and unexpected residual lesion. Due to the inherent properties of basal lesions, the refinement of frameless stereotaxy has had tremendous impact on skull base surgery and the safety and maximization of lesion resection. iMRI, through the acquisition of high-resolution images, can update and augment the accuracy and effectiveness of these systems. Pituitary adenoma resection has been clearly shown to warrant monitoring with iMRI given the high rate of unsuspected residual lesion. Paradigm shifts in skull base surgery toward decreasing surgical morbidity and embracing adjuvant treatment modalities may decrease emphasis upon aggressive, maximal initial resection of certain lesions.

References

1. Hayashi N, Kurimoto M, Hirashima Y, et al. Efficacy of navigation in skull base surgery using composite computer graphics of magnetic resonance and computed tomography images. Neurol Med Chir (Tokyo) 2001;41(7):335–339
2. Gandhe AJ, Hill DL, Studholme C, et al. Combined and three-dimensional rendered multimodal data for planning cranial base surgery: a prospective evaluation. Neurosurgery 1994;35(3):463–470, discussion 471
3. McDermott MW, Gutin PH. Image-guided surgery for skull base neoplasms using the ISG viewing wand. Anatomic and technical considerations. Neurosurg Clin N Am 1996;7(2):285–295

4. Black PM, Moriarty T, Alexander E III, et al. Development and implementation of intraoperative magnetic resonance imaging and its neurosurgical applications. Neurosurgery 1997;41(4):831–842, discussion 842–845

5. Hadani M, Spiegelman R, Feldman Z, Berkenstadt H, Ram Z. Novel, compact, intraoperative magnetic resonance imaging-guided system for conventional neurosurgical operating rooms. Neurosurgery 2001;48(4):799–807, discussion 807–809 PubMed PMID: 11322440.

6. Steinmeier R, Fahlbusch R, Ganslandt O, et al. Intraoperative magnetic resonance imaging with the Magnetom open scanner: concepts, neurosurgical indications, and procedures: a preliminary report. Neurosurgery 1998;43(4):739–747, discussion 747–748

7. Tronnier VM, Wirtz CR, Knauth M, et al. Intraoperative diagnostic and interventional magnetic resonance imaging in neurosurgery. Neurosurgery 1997;40(5):891–900, discussion 900–902

8. Sutherland GR, Kaibara T, Louw D, Hoult DI, Tomanek B, Saunders J. A mobile high-field magnetic resonance system for neurosurgery. J Neurosurg 1999;91(5):804–813

9. Hall WA, Liu H, Martin AJ, Pozza CH, Maxwell RE, Truwit CL. Safety, efficacy, and functionality of high-field strength interventional magnetic resonance imaging for neurosurgery. Neurosurgery 2000;46(3):632–641, discussion 641–642

10. Bohinski RJ, Kokkino AK, Warnick RE, et al. Glioma resection in a shared-resource magnetic resonance operating room after optimal image-guided frameless stereotactic resection. Neurosurgery 2001;48(4):731–742, discussion 742–744

11. Hall WA, Galicich W, Bergman T, Truwit CL. 3-Tesla intraoperative MR imaging for neurosurgery. J Neurooncol 2006;77(3):297–303

12. Nimsky C, Ganslandt O, Von Keller B, Romstöck J, Fahlbusch R. Intraoperative high-field-strength MR imaging: implementation and experience in 200 patients. Radiology 2004;233(1):67–78

13. Samset E, Hirschberg H. Neuronavigation in intraoperative MRI. Comput Aided Surg 1999;4(4):200–207

14. Wirtz CR, Tronnier VM, Bonsanto MM, et al. Image-guided neurosurgery with intraoperative MRI: update of frameless stereotaxy and radicality control. Stereotact Funct Neurosurg 1997;68(1-4 Pt 1): 39–43

15. Nimsky C, von Keller B, Ganslandt O, Fahlbusch R. Intraoperative high-field magnetic resonance imaging in transsphenoidal surgery of hormonally inactive pituitary macroadenomas. Neurosurgery 2006;59(1):105–114, discussion 105–114

16. Gerlach R, du Mesnil de Rochemont R, Gasser T, et al. Feasibility of Polestar N20, an ultra-low-field intraoperative magnetic resonance imaging system in resection control of pituitary macroadenomas: lessons learned from the first 40 cases. Neurosurgery 2008;63(2):272–284, discussion 284–285

17. Fahlbusch R, Ganslandt O, Buchfelder M, Schott W, Nimsky C. Intraoperative magnetic resonance imaging during transsphenoidal surgery. J Neurosurg 2001;95(3):381–390

18. Bohinski RJ, Warnick RE, Gaskill-Shipley MF, et al. Intraoperative magnetic resonance imaging to determine the extent of resection of pituitary macroadenomas during transsphenoidal microsurgery. Neurosurgery 2001;49(5):1133–1143, discussion 1143–1144

19. Dort JC, Sutherland GR. Intraoperative magnetic resonance imaging for skull base surgery. Laryngoscope 2001;111(9):1570–1575

20

Treatment of Spinal Disorders

Carlo M. DeLuna

The growth of intraoperative magnetic resonance imaging (iMRI) technology has led to significant advances in the field of cranial neurosurgery. MRI's ability to visualize the surgical field in multiple planes and to combine physiologic data with near-real-time imaging has begun to change the way tumors are being resected.[1–4] In contrast, there are currently no iMRI systems that are in common use for the adult spine. There are also fewer published reports describing spinal applications for iMRIs. Part of the reason may be that, unlike cranial operations, spinal surgery does not easily fit inside a magnet. Another reason could be due to MRI's superior ability to visualize intracranial lesions and this has naturally led to a greater focus on these surgeries. Regardless of the reason, iMRI could potentially have more usefulness for diseases of the spine than the brain. If cranial neoplasms have traditionally been the most common indication for intraoperative imaging, neoplasms of the spinal cord and vertebral column are far more prevalent when metastatic disease is included.[5,6] Degenerative diseases causing spinal cord or nerve root compression are even more common and account for a greater proportion of operations than cranial or spinal neoplasms in most general neurosurgery practices. Finally, spine surgery already incorporates intraoperative imaging. This is most commonly seen in spinal stabilization procedures to check for correct positioning of implants. The added ability to intraoperatively assess the spinal cord during such procedures or to confirm the radiologic success of a decompression would be an easily recognizable advantage of MRI.

If the recent history of cranial surgery is a guide, iMRI for spine surgery will likely grow with technological advances. The direction of this growth will depend on which systems are adopted by the surgical community. Therefore, as this field is in its infancy, understanding the history and current state of the art can lead to a better understanding of where spinal intraoperative imaging will be in the future.

◆ History

MRI is the most recent imaging technology being adapted to the neurosurgical operating room (OR). The use of portable ultrasound for localizing intracranial tumors has a long history.[7] Intraoperative angiograms using portable fluoroscopy have already become standard additions to the neurosurgical armamentarium for clipping aneurysms.[8] Ultrasound is also being studied to assist spinal surgery.[9,10] The successful introduction of any imaging technology into the OR is subject to numerous factors. The above examples suggest that portability and convenience are key components.

Although a discussion of MRI technology is beyond the scope of this chapter, it is relatively apparent that traditional MR diagnostic systems are neither portable nor easy to use in an OR. The first systems developed in the late 1990s required modifications to the OR to accommodate intraoperative imaging.[11,12] Regardless, the initial experience of spinal surgeries using MRI were performed on these systems. In 1999, Verheyden et al described 16 thoracic and lumbar surgeries utilizing instrumentation that were performed within a GE Signa SP (General Electric Medical Systems, Waukesha, WI) double-donut MRI scanner.[13] Woodard et al in 2001, used a similar system to perform iMRI during nine cervical and three lumbar operations.[14] Hall et al, in a review of high-field iMRI procedures at the University of Minnesota in 2000, included one lumbar operation, three thoracic operations, and one sacral operation using a Philips Gyroscan (Philips Healthcare, Andover, MA).[15]

Each of these studies demonstrated the safety and feasibility of iMRI for spinal surgery in a magnetic environment. Otherwise, the number of cases performed was generally small and a search of the literature showed no other published reports for spine surgery in any of the major journals. The absence of additional observations appears to parallel the lack of acceptance that these systems received outside their respective centers.

More recently, several newer systems developed for neurosurgical applications, such as PoleStar (Medtronic Navigation, Inc., Louisville, CO),[16] Brainsuite (Laboratory of Neuro Imaging, UCLA),[17] and IMRIS (IMRIS, Winnipeg, Manitoba, Canada),[18] have adopted the strategy of having lower impact on the surgical environment. None of these newer systems, however, are designed to intraoperatively image the adult spine. These developments and the paucity of recent studies utilizing MRI for spinal surgery indicate that technologic advances have not yet been applied to this field. One way to illustrate what the future may hold is to review the experience using iMRI on a personal, unpublished series of recent cervical spine operations performed at Wilkes-Barre General Hospital in Pennsylvania.

◆ Penn State/Wilkes-Barre Experience

The IMRIS at Wilkes-Barre General Hospital was one of the first systems installed in the United States that utilized a large-bore, high-field magnet mounted on rails (**Fig. 20.1**). It allowed general neurosurgical procedures to be performed in a suite where the magnet was brought in as surgical circumstances warranted. This site had the additional advantage of being associated with a general neurosurgery practice. There was therefore an ample population of spinal surgeries which could be exposed to this technology.

During the early utilization of the system, it became apparent that a standard craniotomy position allowed the IMRIS to visualize the superior cervical spine. This property had been described before. Kaibara et al in 2001, reported on three transoral resections for odontoid pathology that used intraoperative imaging.[19] This demonstrated that a mobile magnet could image the cervicomedullary junction during surgery and that the information could alter surgical planning. At Wilkes-Barre, it was noticed that positioning the patient 10 to 20 cm superior on the OR table allowed imaging of the entire cervical spine (**Fig. 20.2**).

Given the relative ease of visualizing the cervical spine, a decision was made to use IMRIS in these operations. Clinical usefulness, however, was not the initial goal at Wilkes-Barre. Cervical surgeries were performed frequently enough that they could be used to make OR personnel proficient with MRI protocols. Otherwise, the preparation and imaging were similar to cranial operations and these were the surgeries that were expected to benefit from intraoperative imaging. As experience developed, these initial procedures revealed several distinct drawbacks that demonstrated how much more difficult cervical spine surgeries were when using iMRI.

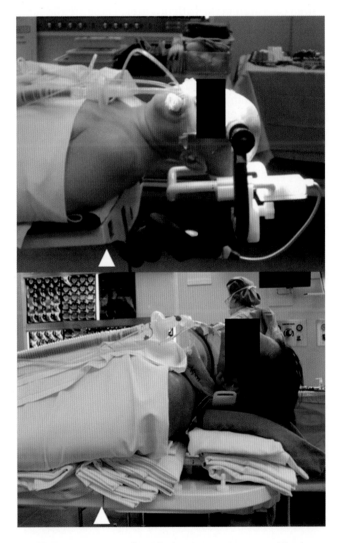

Fig. 20.2 Comparison of standard supine craniotomy position in pins (top) to supine anterior cervical diskectomy position on bolsters (bottom). In cervical diskectomy position, head is ~15 cm. superior. *White arrow* indicates table break.

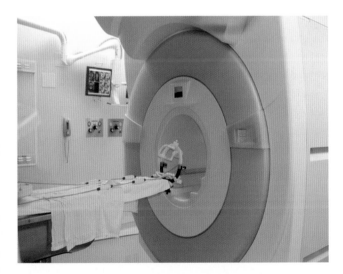

Fig. 20.1 The IMRIS (IMRIS, Winnipeg, Manitoba, Canada) suite at Wilkes-Barre General Hospital with Siemens Open Bore Espree 1.5 tesla magnetic resonance imaging (MRI) scanner positioned at the head of operating room table. Head holder is attached to the table with paired two channel coils in place.

The overall length of time to start the operation was prolonged. As in cranial magnet cases, care had to be taken to adequately pad the patient and avoid skin to conductive surface contact. This required the attention of both the anesthesiologist and the circulating nurse. Because IMRIS entered the room on rails, anesthesia equipment and the anesthesiologist were positioned at the patient's foot. Extension tubing was added to allow the anesthesia machine to sit outside the 5 gauss (G) line when the magnet was in the room. Adjusting to this distance was consistently labor intensive. Even though the magnet was in the operating suite for a fraction of the surgery, constant surveillance was enforced so that all metal instruments were accounted for. Finally, the OR table had a narrower axial profile to allow the patient to sit inside the bore. This required careful wrapping of the patient to ensure they were secured to the operating table and still compact enough to fit within the magnet.

Imaging the cervical spine in IMRIS requires positioning paired coils around the patient's neck. These are the same coils used for cranial MRIs. These rigid coils were designed to lie in close proximity to the patient's head. They are configured as paired half cylinders positioned superior and inferior to the surgical site. Positioning these coils to fit under the patient's neck would sometimes cause them to protrude into the base of the cervical spine. This happened most frequently in obese or broad-shouldered individuals and extra care was taken to pad these patients. In extreme cases, it was found that if the inferior paired coil could not fit, the

other coil could be placed on top of the surgical site. The images obtained were usually adequate enough to visualize the cervical spine.

Although these steps prolonged the preparation time for the surgery, they did not affect the operation. What had the greatest impact on the operation were those systems that were in physical contact with the patient. Physiologic monitoring became limited. Because of inherent constraints to electrocardiogram (EKG) monitoring during MR imaging, cardiac electrodes could not be dispersed in the standard montage. Axis deviation and changes in signal polarity could not be reliably measured. In addition, the copper wires and stainless steel needles for electrophysiologic monitoring can have potentially deleterious effects in a high-field magnet. Prior to imaging, all of these wires are removed. Therefore, no further monitoring can be performed after the first intraoperative image. Finally, the wrapping and padding of the patient restricts access to the prominence of the iliac crest. This severely limits how easily autologous bone graft can be harvested. In some cases cutting through the drapes can alleviate this, but it was occasionally difficult to obtain a sufficient amount of autologous bone graft.

Except for these preparations, the actual surgical procedure could be performed in a routine manner. Between May 2006 and April 2008, 32 cervical surgeries were performed. Case characteristics are summarized in **Table 20.1**. In every case, a standard approach using normal instrument trays was performed. Surgical time was prolonged due to the MR

Table 20.1 Cervical Spine Operations Performed at Penn State Neurosurgery/Wilkes-Barre General Hospital Utilizing Intraoperative Magnetic Resonance Imaging: Patient Characteristics and Outcomes, May 2006–April 2008

Case	Age	Sex	Diagnosis	Procedure	Outcome
1	54	M	Screw back-out	Removal of steel anterior cervical plate	Acquired MRI proficiency, newly diagnosed syrinx
2	46	F	R C6–7 HNP	ACDF with instrument and bone	Acquired MRI proficiency
3	38	F	C5–6 stenosis	ACDF with instrument and bone	Confirmed decompression
4	41	M	L C6–7 HNP	ACDF with instrument and bone	Confirmed decompression
5	42	M	R C5–6 HNP	ACDF with instrument and bone	Acquired MRI proficiency
6	48	M	L C5–6 HNP/osteophyte	ACDF with instrument and bone	Acquired MRI proficiency
7	45	M	R C5–6 HNP/osteophyte	ACDF with instrument and bone	Acquired MRI proficiency
8	39	M	R C6–7 osteophyte	Posterior C6–7, C7–T1 laminotomy and foraminotomy	Acquired MRI proficiency
9	43	F	R C6–7, C7–T1 HNPs	C6–7, C7–T1 ACDF with instrument/bone	Acquired MRI proficiency
10	44	M	C5–6, C6–7 stenosis	C5–6, 6–7 ACDF with instrument/bone	Acquired MRI proficiency
11	43	M	R C5–6 HNP	ACDF with instrument/bone	Acquired MRI proficiency, no change in cord compression
12	39	M	Bilateral C6–7 perched facets	C6–7 360 degree fusion with instrument/bone	No cord contusion, plate artifact
13	44	F	C5–6 stenosis	ACDF with instrument/bone	Acquired MRI proficiency
14	58	M	L C5–6 HNP/osteophyte	ACDF with instrument/bone	Confirmed decompression, plate artifact
15	44	M	L C5–6 HNP/osteophyte	ACDF with instrument/bone	Acquired MRI proficiency
16	56	M	C4–5, C5–6 stenosis/contusion	C4–5, 5–6 ACDF with instrument/bone	Confirmed decompression of cervical cord

Case	Age	Sex	Diagnosis	Procedure	Outcome
17	71	F	C4–5 stenosis/contusion	ACDF with instrument/bone	Confirmed decompression of cervical cord
18	52	F	C6–7 discitis/osteomyelitis	C6 corpectomy and C5–7 anterior fusion with bone	Confirmed decompression at C7
19	45	M	R C5–6 osteophyte	ACDF with instrument/bone	Confirmed decompression and allograft placement
20	44	F	R C6–7 osteophyte	ACDF with instrument/bone	Acquired MRI proficiency
21	72	F	C3–4 stenosis	C3, partial C4 laminectomy	Post positioning MRI shows no contusion, intraoperative MRI shows good decompression, limited bone removal
22	48	F	C4–5, C6–7 stenosis	Posterior C5–6 laminectomy	Confirmed decompression of cervical cord
23	44	M	R C6–7 HNP	R posterior C6–7 foraminotomy, discectomy	Confirmed decompression
24	62	F	C4 intramedullary tumor	Posterior C3–4 laminectomy and tumor biopsy	Confirmed biopsy
25	21	M	Chiari I malformation/syrinx	Suboccipital and C1 decompression, duraplasty	Confirmed decompression, syrinx unchanged
26	32	M	L C6–7 HNP	ACDF with bone	Confirmed decompression
27	58	M	C4–5, C5–6 stenosis, contusion	C4–5, 5–6 ACDF with instrument and bone	Confirmed decompression, increased T2 signal
28	66	F	C5–6 disk/osteophyte	ACDF with bone	Confirmed decompression and allograft placement
29	83	M	Central C5–6 HNP	ACDF with instrument/bone	Confirmed decompression and allograft placement
30	73	F	C3–4 stenosis, cord atrophy, subluxation	Partial C3 and C4 posterior laminectomy	Confirmed decompression of cervical cord, limited bone removal
31	37	F	L C5–6 HNP	ACDF with instrument/bone	Confirmed decompression
32	80	F	Unstable C2, type II fracture	C1–2 Harms fusion with autograft	C1–2 foramina patent

Abbreviations: M, male; F, female; L, left; R, right; HNP, herniated nucleus pulposus; ACDF, anterior cervical discectomy and fusion; MRI, magnetic resonance imaging.

imaging. In general, it would take at least 15 to 20 minutes to prepare the surgical field to bring in the magnet, another 20 minutes to acquire the images, and a final 15 to 20 minutes to resume the surgery. Interrupting this surgery was analogous to performing an intraoperative angiogram during aneurysm clipping.

Reviewing the 32 operations, there were no adverse effects from positioning, anesthesia, or MR imaging. There were also no complications from the prolonged preparation or surgical times. Isolated problems arose when imaging quality was poor. These occurred early in the program and were mostly attributed to radiofrequency interference from sources inside the OR. Several observations were made during these surgeries that underscored the advantage of intraoperative imaging.

◆ Anterior Cervical Discectomies

The majority of intraoperative imaging for cervical spine surgery was for anterior cervical discectomies with fusion. Seventeen single-level and four two-level discectomies were performed for degenerative spine disease. Most of the procedures performed in the first year were used for training purposes. Patients would be prepared for a magnet case, the surgical procedure was performed including instrumenting with an anterior plate, and then the MRI was obtained prior to removing the surgical drapes and transferring the patient. These images were therefore not clinically different than obtaining an outpatient MRI following surgery.

As proficiency improved, however, review of the images showed subjectively better detail than standard outpatient studies. It was unclear whether this was due to the proximity of the coil to the neck or the absence of movement with the patient under anesthesia. Metal artifact from the anterior plate and screws obscured some detail but overall, the initial cases proved the feasibility of intraoperative imaging for anterior cervical discectomies. More importantly, the information from the intraoperative images became useful for the cervical surgeries themselves. It provided immediate feedback that the herniated disk was removed or that the stenosis was relieved. This gave a subjective sense of certainty that the goal of surgery had been accomplished. It is

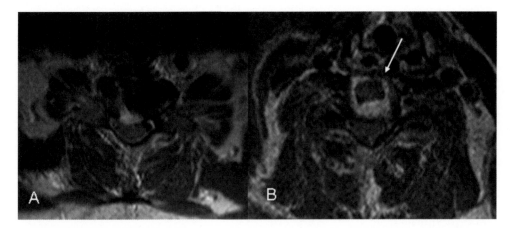

Fig. 20.3 Axial T2-weighted intraoperative magnetic resonance imaging scans of two different anterior cervical discectomy and fusion surgeries obtained **(A)** after and **(B)** prior to placement of instrumentation. Note the decreased artifact without instrumentation and the allograft bone spacer in the decompressed disk space (*white arrow*).

analogous to the objective confirmation that occurs after obtaining a plain x-ray to check the position of an anterior cervical plate.

As more discectomies were performed, greater comfort developed with using the magnet. It became obvious that an MRI taken after the decompression and before the instrumentation gave less-distorted images of the disk space (**Fig. 20.3**). This led to better resolution of the spinal cord without the artifact from cervical screws. It showed more clearly that an adequate decompression had been performed and allowed an improved assessment of the position of the bone graft. Another immediate advantage was the ability to utilize landmarks, such as the lateral margins of the bone graft or the location of the distracter pin hole, to better center the cervical plate. Intraoperative measurement of the rostrocaudal height between disk spaces helped select plates that did not overlap adjacent disk spaces. Vertebral depth measurements could accurately gauge the length needed for a vertebral body screw to avoid entering the central canal. None of this information is readily available on lateral radiographs and is only possible because of the MRI software.

iMRI had become a standard part of an anterior cervical fusion. As it became more commonplace to use the MRI after decompression, the clinical importance of this information also became apparent. This is best illustrated in the following example.

A 58-year-old man presented several days after a motor vehicle accident with long tract signs and worsening upper extremity weakness. His preoperative images (**Fig. 20.4A,B**) revealed posterior osteophytes at C4–5 and C5–6. There were signal changes suspicious for cervical cord edema over both levels. He underwent a two-level anterior cervical discectomy and fusion for critical central canal stenosis. The intraoperative image (**Fig. 20.4C,D**) showed a much larger area of T2 signal within the cervical cord. His central cord syndrome did not improve after surgery.

The information from the MRI did not alter this patient's surgical plan. With the potential liability associated from the mechanism of injury, the intraoperative image at least served as an objective snapshot of the spinal

cord immediately after decompression. The amount of cord edema after decompression was larger than what would have been anticipated from the preoperative images. The MRI confirmed that the underlying pathology was removed and the central canal was decompressed, but it also gave an early indication that this patient's central cord syndrome would probably not improve over time. As an aside, it was generally unpredictable what the contour of the cervical cord would be after decompression. In this last case, there was swelling into the disk space (**Fig. 20.4D**). In other cases, the cervical cord would remain deformed (**Fig. 20.3A**).

Posterior Decompression

As proficiency and timing improved further, other cervical surgeries were performed with intraoperative imaging. Five posterior decompressions were performed including three laminectomies and two foraminotomies. Unlike the anterior cervical approaches, intraoperative imaging had a greater potential to guide the extent of a posterior decompression. The following case serves as a useful illustration.

A 73-year-old woman with a history of osteoarthritis presented with worsening myelopathy. On workup, she was found to have central canal stenosis at C3–4 from spondylosis and a 3 to 4 mm anterolisthesis (**Fig. 20.5A**). She was taken to the OR for a planned C3–4 laminectomy. During her surgery, a minimally invasive approach was used to remove the C3–4 ligamentum flavum and the inferior lamina of C3. An intraoperative image (**Fig. 20.5B**) demonstrated a complete decompression and the surgery was concluded without further bone removal. The patient went on to improve following the operation.

As the above case illustrates, targeted removal of a focal constriction is possible with intraoperative imaging. There was a concern that a decompression in this patient could worsen her anterolisthesis. Her age would have put her at increased risk of posterior instrument failure if she underwent a stabilization procedure. She directly benefitted from

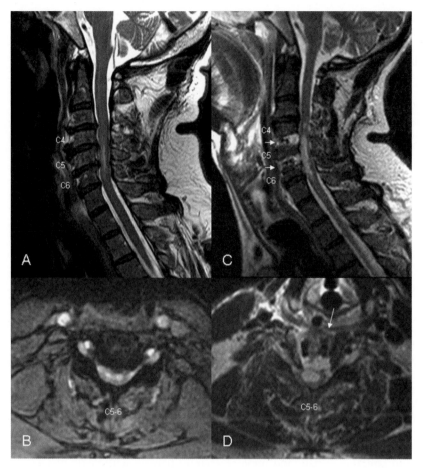

Fig. 20.4 **(A)** Sagittal and **(B)** C5–6 axial T2-weighted magnetic resonance images of the cervical spine from a patient presenting with upper extremity weakness. Visible on the sagittal views are C4–5 and C5–6 osteophytes causing central canal stenosis and cervical cord edema. **(C)** Sagittal and **(D)** axial T2-weighted intraoperative magnetic resonance images obtained after decompression and before instrumentation. Increased cervical cord edema can be seen overlying C5 and C6 vertebral bodies on sagittal views. *White arrows* indicate allograft bone spacers in C4–5 and C5–6.

the intraoperative imaging because the smaller laminectomy allowed most of her posterior elements to remain intact. Two of the three laminectomies in this series required less bone removal after the MRI showed a complete decompression.

Suboccipital Decompression

One suboccipital decompression for a symptomatic Chiari I malformation was performed with iMRI. Images were obtained after the duraplasty and this showed the patency of

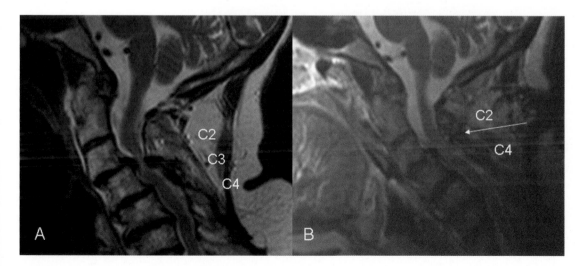

Fig. 20.5 **(A)** Sagittal T2-weighted magnetic resonance (MR) images of a 73-year-old patient presenting with myelopathy and showing C3–4 stenosis, anterior subluxation, and myelomalacia. C2 and C4 spinous processes are marked. **(B)** Intraoperative MR imaging showing decompression. *White arrow* indicates residual C3 lamina.

the decompression. A preexisting cervical syrinx was also visualized and it showed no change in size. Although cinegating to assess cerebrospinal fluid (CSF) flow was not done in this particular care, this would have been a relatively easy study. The surgical positioning and the site of the incision are particularly conducive to imaging with IMRIS. There are reports in the literature where decompressions are being performed without a duraplasty based on the preoperative absence of CSF flow on MRI.[20] Intraoperative imaging to assess CSF flow may have far-reaching applications for the surgical treatment of Chiari malformations. This could theoretically limit the amount of occipital bone removed or even avoid the need to perform a C1 laminectomy in select cases.

Cervical Trauma

The use of instrumentation to perform an arthrodesis is a common adjunct to the treatment of cervical fractures. Even though modern spine implants are made of MRI-compatible materials, there is significant image artifact in the area of surgery.[21] Based on the Wilkes-Barre experience with anterior cervical discectomies, which used cervical plates and screws, this artifact did not impair the ability to visualize the decompressed cervical cord. The quality of the image, however, was insufficient to assess proper placement of the instrumentation. In a case involving a type II odontoid fracture, the MRI coil was placed in close proximity to the operative site in an attempt to visualize the vertebral body screws. A posterior C1–2 fusion using Harms technique was performed, which involved inserting screws into the lateral mass of C1 and pedicles of C2. Despite using different imaging parameters, the screw placement in relation to the bone

could not be reliably imaged. The most useful clinical information obtained was that the C1–2 foramen on both sides and the central canal were patent.

Although complicated reconstructions are not a contraindication for intraoperative imaging, another cervical trauma further demonstrated this limitation of MRI. A patient underwent a combined anterior and posterior approach to treat an unstable subluxation of C6–7 with bilateral perched facets. An intraoperative image was obtained after spinous process wiring and anterior cervical plating. This confirmed that the spinal canal was patent, but because of metal artifact, even the alignment could not be properly assessed. In this particular case, C-arm fluoroscopy was used liberally to track the reduction and assess the instrumentation during the operation.

From these examples, it appears that iMRI is a useful addition, but an unlikely alternative to plain radiographs for treating cervical fractures that require instrumentation.

Tumor Surgery

Finally, this leads to what may be the most useful advantage of intraoperative imaging for cervical spine surgery: the ability to visualize soft tissue pathology. MRI is superior to other imaging modalities for visualizing osteolytic lesions.[22] When surgery involves decompression of the central canal, the ability to monitor the resection of these lesions can affect patient outcome. In the Wilkes-Barre series, the following case illustrates this concept.

A 52-year-old woman presented with worsening cervical pain and upper extremity paresis. Radiologic images revealed an osteolytic lesion involving the C5 and C6 vertebral bodies and destruction of the C5–6 disk space (**Fig. 20.6A**).

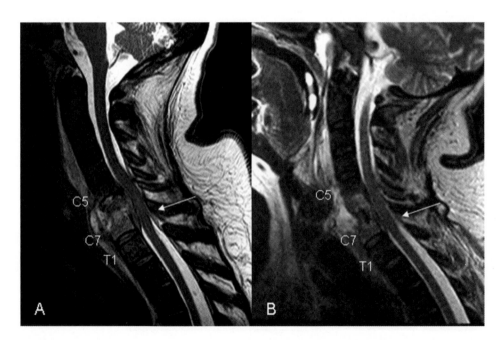

Fig. 20.6 Sagittal T2-weighted magnetic resonance (MR) images of a 52-year-old female with C5–6 discitis. **(A)** Preoperative MR imaging shows granulation tissue posterior to C7 (*white arrow*). **(B)** Intraoperative MR imaging shows central canal decompressed with inferior C7 vertebral body intact.

There was soft tissue in the central canal causing stenosis. A component of the soft tissue extended over the vertebral body of C7.

She underwent a corpectomy of C6 with debridement of the superior endplate of C7 and inferior endplate of C5. The pathology turned out to be an infectious discitis with osteomyelitis. During the decompression, it was unclear whether granulation tissue posterior to C7 was still causing stenosis. An iMRI showed no residual stenosis and no further bone was removed (**Fig. 20.6B**).

Although this case was diagnosed as an infection, the same general principles would have applied if this were a metastatic tumor. The ability to visualize anatomy beyond the surgical field had a demonstrated impact on surgical planning. Without imaging, the surgery probably would have required an additional corpectomy of C7 to ensure a complete decompression.

Another case illustrates this but also shows the advantage of high-field imaging in detecting smaller lesions.

A 62-year-old woman presented with signs of worsening myelopathy. Preoperative imaging showed a 2 to 3 mm enhancing intramedullary lesion in the dorsal cervical cord over the vertebral bodies of C3 and C4 (**Fig. 20.7A**). Following a laminectomy, no abnormality could be detected on the surface of the cervical cord. A midline myelotomy (**Fig. 20.7 B**) was performed and questionable gliotic tissue was encountered and debulked.

An iMRI showed that the myelotomy was in the tumor capsule (**Fig. 20.7C,D**). Because the lesion was densely adherent to normal tissue and there were no visible tumor

planes, it was decided not to proceed further knowing at least a biopsy was performed. The patient awoke without any new deficits and only a minor increase in her arm paresthesias.

In this situation, iMRI gave information that led to a reasonable judgment about avoiding further dissection. Because of the size of the lesion, it was unlikely that any other imaging modality short of a high-field MRI would have visualized it.

◆ Future Applications

The cervical spine experience at Wilkes-Barre was made possible by taking advantage of the configuration of the IMRIS system. Given the relatively small number of surgeries, any conclusions about the efficacy of this system are based at best on anecdotal experience. However, other centers with an iMRI have also used their system to visualize the cervical spine.[23] Therefore, the current state of intraoperative imaging for spinal disorders appears to be most promising for cervical pathology. The future of iMRI for the rest of the spine will ultimately depend on which technology can be adapted to body imaging. All current systems adequately address the needs of cranial neurosurgery, but some are more amenable to modification to suit extracranial surgery than others. Based on the IMRIS experience with cervical surgery and what is known about thoracic and lumbar surgery, there are several characteristics that would predict which systems will be successful.

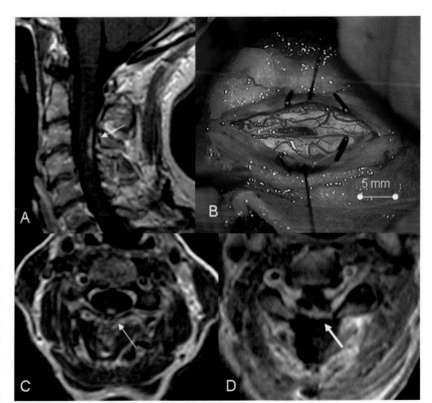

Fig. 20.7 Gadolinium-enhanced T1-weighted cervical spine magnetic resonance imaging (MRI) scan of a patient who presented with worsening myelopathy. **(A)** Sagittal images show an intramedullary enhancing lesion in the midline dorsal cervical cord over C3 and C4 (*white arrow*). **(B)** Intraoperative photomicrograph shows myelotomy after attempted debulking of lesion. Note absence of any visible pathology on surface of cervical cord. **(C)** Preoperative axial gadolinium-enhanced T1-weighted MRI showing enhancing lesion (*small white arrow*). **(D)** Intraoperative MRI showing myelotomy cleft (*large white arrow*) during surgery.

For most craniotomies, the OR table is of minimal importance. The table serves to ensure that the torso is well supported. In contrast, the OR table is of major importance in spine surgery. Unlike the head, the spine is generally not fixed to the OR table. Any movement of the patient could adversely affect the surgery. Patients in a lateral position or in a prone position with lumbar flexion are particularly prone to shifting even when the OR table is stationary. Therefore, any system that moves the patient must transition with minimal impact. The table itself must be able to perform multiple roles. It must be large enough to accommodate the different positions required for spine surgery. It must still be small enough to fit inside an MRI bore. It must adjust to different physiques but still be able to center the operative area within the MRI. Finally, it is necessary for the table to be both MRI compatible and radiolucent.

Similar to cranial neurosurgery, the most likely indication for intraoperative spine imaging is tumor resection. As most spinal tumors are extraaxial, future intraoperative systems will need to accommodate the possibility that surgical stabilization will be needed. Most spinal implants are nonferrous, but the instruments that insert them are stainless steel. It would be economically prohibitive to make all these instruments MRI compatible. Likewise, spinal operations will continue to rely on radiographs to visualize implanted hardware for the foreseeable future. Any new system should not preclude the use of fluoroscopy and portable x-ray during surgery.

All current iMRI systems take advantage of narrow, defined approaches used in cranial neurosurgery. Because the head can be positioned to accommodate the approach, the amount of "elbow room" for the surgeon and an assistant can be small. Spine cases on the other hand usually involve larger surgical fields. Approaches can vary significantly. A surgeon's line of sight varies by a much wider angle in spinal operations than craniotomies. Inherent in this is a greater need for freedom of movement around the surgical site. This is particularly the case when instrumenting for spinal stabilization. A new system should optimally have large areas of access to the surgical site.

Finally, one of the key elements that made IMRIS acceptable for cervical spine surgery was its easy integration into the OR. Despite the additional preparatory steps, the surgery was performed in a standard manner. Obtaining an image was a simple matter of moving away from the patient. The MRI, instead of becoming the focus of the operation, became another imaging modality in the room. This is probably the key component for any new iMRI system: it must be convenient for the surgeon.

Based on the above characteristics, there is no current system that addresses all these needs. Any intraoperative MRI that cannot perform body imaging would almost certainly be excluded from spinal operations. Systems that perform surgery in a dedicated, magnetic friendly environment or within the "fringe" borders of a magnetic field would probably require some modification of the surgical technique. The ultimate drawback for all current systems is the table. All existing systems would require extensive modifications to allow comfortable use for spine operations.

The most likely system that will be adopted for spinal imaging will either be a mobile magnet that is brought into the OR, or a mobile OR table that can seamlessly transport a patient into an MRI. Both of these solutions maintain an optimal environment from the surgeon's standpoint. From a practical standpoint, the ultimate solution for any given location will most likely depend on a compromise between neurosurgery and radiology.

◆ Conclusion

Intraoperative magnetic resonance imaging for spinal surgery is in its infancy. Like imaging for cranial surgery, more experience is needed to unequivocally determine whether these images are clinically useful or if they justify the expense of new technology. Extrapolating from the short history of intraoperative imaging for cranial neurosurgery, there is always a need for detailed images. MRI, however, is not the optimal imaging modality to visualize bone or the vertebral column. Spine surgery already has an array of less-expensive and well-documented radiographic tools. These include fluoroscopy, plain radiographs, and portable CT. It would seem that an additional imaging modality would only be useful in a small number of cases.

If there is any rationale for utilizing intraoperative MRI in the spine, one only needs to look at the current state of spine surgery. Newer technologies are evolving that not only repair or resect an underlying pathology, but augment and stabilize as well. This involves constant changes in the instrumentation and materials that are being used in the spine. All prostheses to some extent exhibit MR artifact.[24] Some of the newer prostheses already prevent accurate postoperative MRI images from being obtained.[25] Prior to inserting or applying these new constructs, there is a benefit to assessing the spinal cord and nerve roots. In these cases, MRI after the definitive surgical procedure and before insertion of artifact inducing constructs is the only way to accurately visualize this anatomy. Also, as in all other fields of surgery, there is a growing trend toward minimally invasive operations. As the Wilkes-Barre experience with laminectomies shows, iMRI can be a valuable tool to limit the extent, and ultimately the cost, of a surgical procedure.

The other, more important advantage of iMRI is obtaining immediate information. MRI has been known to be superior to other modalities when visualizing acute trauma to the spinal cord.[26] Prior studies have shown that there is clinical value in measuring signal changes over time in the injured spine.[27] More recent studies have suggested that signal changes observed during intraoperative imaging can have prognostic value, particularly in cervical myelopathy.[23] The ability to visualize these changes so soon after an operation has not been possible until now, but the Wilkes-Barre series has suggested that this information can have an impact on surgical planning.

It is probably inevitable that the technology for intraoperative spine imaging will advance as the success of cranial imaging becomes known. The systems to image the spine during surgery are closely linked to body imaging. Based on the number of applications alone, body imaging is a major incentive to the intraoperative MR industry. As more centers acquire the capacity to visualize the spinal cord during surgery, the value of this information will become apparent. Spine surgery will probably supplant cranial neurosurgery in both volume and need. iMRI is already beginning to revolutionize cranial neurosurgery and it is likely that newer technology will have a similar impact on the surgery of spinal disorders.

References

1. Sutherland GR, Kaibara T, Louw DF. Intraoperative MR at 1.5 Tesla—experience and future directions. Acta Neurochir Suppl (Wien) 2003;85:21–28
2. Jankovski A, Francotte F, Vaz G, et al. Intraoperative magnetic resonance imaging at 3-T using a dual independent operating room-magnetic resonance imaging suite: development, feasibility, safety, and preliminary experience. Neurosurgery 2008;63(3):412–424, discussion 424–426
3. Hall WA, Liu H, Martin AJ, Pozza CH, Maxwell RE, Truwit CL. Safety, efficacy, and functionality of high-field strength interventional magnetic resonance imaging for neurosurgery. Neurosurgery 2000;46(3):632–641, discussion 641–642
4. Nimsky C, Ganslandt O, von Keller B, Fahlbusch R. Preliminary experience in glioma surgery with intraoperative high-field MRI. Acta Neurochir Suppl (Wien) 2003;88:21–29
5. Frosch MP, Anthony DC, De Girolami U. The central nervous system. In: Kumar V, ed. Robbins and Cotran: Pathologic Basis of Disease. 7th Ed. Philadelphia, PA: Elsevier Saunders; 2005: 1401
6. Sundaresan N, Hughes JEO, DiGiacinto GV. Surgical management of primary and metastatic tumors of the spine. In: Schmidek HH, ed. Operative Neurosurgical Technique: Indications, Methods and Results. 3rd Ed. Philadelphia: WB Saunders Co.; 1995: 1981
7. Unsgaard G, Rygh OM, Selbekk T, et al. Intra-operative 3D ultrasound in neurosurgery. Acta Neurochir (Wien) 2006;148(3):235–253, discussion 253
8. Alexander TD, Macdonald RL, Weir B, Kowalczuk A. Intraoperative angiography in cerebral aneurysm surgery: a prospective study of 100 craniotomies. Neurosurgery 1996;39(1):10–17, discussion 17–18
9. Mirvis SE, Geisler FH. Intraoperative sonography of cervical spinal cord injury: results in 30 patients. AJR Am J Roentgenol 1990;155(3):603–609
10. Mihara H, Kondo S, Takeguchi H, Kohno M, Hachiya M. Spinal cord morphology and dynamics during cervical laminoplasty: evaluation with intraoperative sonography. Spine 2007;32(21):2306–2309
11. Black PM, Moriarty T, Alexander E III, et al. Development and implementation of intraoperative magnetic resonance imaging and its neurosurgical applications. Neurosurgery 1997;41(4):831–842, discussion 842–845
12. Hall WA, Martin AJ, Liu H, Nussbaum ES, Maxwell RE, Truwit CL. Brain biopsy using high-field strength interventional magnetic resonance imaging. Neurosurgery 1999;44(4):807–813, discussion 813–814
13. Verheyden P, Katscher S, Schulz T, Schmidt F, Josten C. Open MR imaging in spine surgery: experimental investigations and first clinical experiences. Eur Spine J 1999;8(5):346–353
14. Woodard EJ, Leon SP, Moriarty TM, Quinones A, Zamani AA, Jolesz FA. Initial experience with intraoperative magnetic resonance imaging in spine surgery. Spine (Phila Pa 1976) 2001;26(4):410–417
15. Hall WA, Liu H, Martin AJ, Pozza CH, Maxwell RE, Truwit CL. Safety, efficacy, and functionality of high-field strength interventional magnetic resonance imaging for neurosurgery. Neurosurgery 2000; 46(3):632–641, discussion 641–642
16. Hadani M, Spiegelman R, Feldman Z, Berkenstadt H, Ram Z. Novel, compact, intraoperative magnetic resonance imaging-guided system for conventional neurosurgical operating rooms. Neurosurgery 2001;48(4):799–807, discussion 807–809
17. Nimsky C, Ganslandt O, von Keller B, Fahlbusch R. Preliminary experience in glioma surgery with intraoperative high-field MRI. Acta Neurochir Suppl (Wien) 2003;88:21–29
18. Sutherland GR, Kaibara T, Louw DF. Intraoperative MR at 1.5 Tesla—experience and future directions. Acta Neurochir Suppl (Wien) 2003;85:21–28
19. Kaibara T, Hurlbert RJ, Sutherland GR. Intraoperative magnetic resonance imaging-augmented transoral resection of axial disease. Neurosurg Focus 2001;10(2):E4
20. Ventureyra EC, Aziz HA, Vassilyadi M. The role of cine flow MRI in children with Chiari I malformation. Childs Nerv Syst 2003;19(2):109–113
21. Rudisch A, Kremser C, Peer S, Kathrein A, Judmaier W, Daniaux H. Metallic artifacts in magnetic resonance imaging of patients with spinal fusion. A comparison of implant materials and imaging sequences. Spine (Phila Pa 1976) 1998;23(6):692–699
22. Ghanem N, Uhl M, Brink I, et al. Diagnostic value of MRI in comparison to scintigraphy, PET, MS-CT and PET/CT for the detection of metastases of bone. Eur J Radiol 2005;55(1):41–55
23. Mastronardi L, Elsawaf A, Roperto R, et al. Prognostic relevance of the postoperative evolution of intramedullary spinal cord changes in signal intensity on magnetic resonance imaging after anterior decompression for cervical spondylotic myelopathy. J Neurosurg Spine 2007;7(6):615–622
24. Ortiz O, Pait TG, McAllister P, Sauter K. Postoperative magnetic resonance imaging with titanium implants of the thoracic and lumbar spine. Neurosurgery 1996;38(4):741–745
25. Sekhon LH, Duggal N, Lynch JJ, et al. Magnetic resonance imaging clarity of the Bryan, Prodisc-C, Prestige LP, and PCM cervical arthroplasty devices. Spine (Phila Pa 1976) 2007;32(6):673–680
26. Mirvis SE, Geisler FH, Jelinek JJ, Joslyn JN, Gellad F. Acute cervical spine trauma: evaluation with 1.5-T MR imaging. Radiology 1988;166(3): 807–816
27. Morio Y, Teshima R, Nagashima H, Nawata K, Yamasaki D, Nanjo Y. Correlation between operative outcomes of cervical compression myelopathy and mri of the spinal cord. Spine (Phila Pa 1976) 2001;26(11):1238–1245

V
Design, Equipment, and Logistics

21

Promising Advances in Intraoperative MRI-Guided Neurosurgery

Ferenc A. Jolesz and Alexandra J. Golby

The concept of intraoperative magnetic resonance imaging (MRI) guidance was first envisioned in 1990 in the Image-Guided Therapy (IGT) Program at the Brigham and Women's Hospital, Harvard Medical School, Boston, MA.[1] This program, a collaboration with General Electric (General Electric Medical Systems, Waukesha, WI), introduced the Signa SP MRI with the nickname "double-doughnut" that refers to its special open configuration.[2] The first of its kind, this scanner was located in a fully functional operating room (OR) suitable for open neurosurgery. During interventional procedures and surgeries the patient stayed on the MRI table that also served as an OR table. This MRI configuration based on novel magnet design and technology complemented and augmented the neurosurgeons' vision, enabling them to see beyond and "under" the exposed surfaces and to discriminate tumors from normal tissue. MRI guidance not only improves localization and targeting of tumors, but also, within the limits of MRI's contrast and spatial resolution, identifies tumor margins—a critical step to ensure complete tumor removal.[3-5] Since then real-time or iterative intraoperative MR imaging (iMRI) at the Brigham has guided over 3,000 surgical and interventional procedures.[6] The procedures, among others, have included open brain surgeries, MRI-guided thermal ablations, and brain biopsies as well as nonneurosurgical procedures such as endoscopic sinus surgery and prostate brachytherapy.[7-11] Coupled with new therapy devices and surgical navigation, these procedures have become systems that have taken on a pivotal role in opening new directions in the surgical management of cancer in general and in neurosurgery of primary brain tumors in particular.[3] Within a short period, many new interventional and/or intraoperative MRI centers were established around the world, and iMRI became widely accepted in neurosurgery.[12-17]

The fundamental goal of neurosurgery is to target, access, and address the lesion without causing significant damage to normal brain tissue or vascular structures. The overall concern is the preservation of neurologic function, an outcome that requires precise delineation of functional anatomy and correct definition of the resection target volume. To improve outcomes and decrease invasiveness, neurosurgical treatment is increasingly taking advantage of rapid developments in imaging and data presentation. The combining of imaging and neurosurgery has a long history. In fact, neurosurgical progress parallels the developments of improved visualization. From early efforts with ventriculography and angiography to the introduction of the operating microscope to the development of cross-sectional imaging and the recent widespread adoption of neuronavigation, neurosurgeons have dramatically improved the precision, safety, and effectiveness of brain surgery for the treatment of many conditions. iMRI, for example, provides unprecedented intraoperative visualization capabilities. It has enhanced the surgeon's ability to accurately define margins and their relationship to critical structures during the resection of brain tumors. Over the past 20 years, specialized neuronavigational tools have been developed to assist the surgeon in these endeavors; the development of MRI-guided navigation systems, for instance, represents a significant improvement in the surgical treatment of various intracranial lesions. In recent years, several groups have proposed integrating functional data into the neuronavigation system.[18,19] Since its introduction in the early 1990s, the field of intraoperative and interventional MRI has grown and changed significantly. It has become increasingly obvious that *full access* open MRI, like the Signa SP, is not the only solution for guiding procedures. Indeed, numerous procedures require higher-field strength and more advanced image acquisition technology than can be accomplished with an open-magnet configuration. Several groups using iMRI for neurosurgery have moved to a higher-field strength using closed-bore 1.5 tesla (T) and even 3.0 T MRI systems.[20,21]

In terms of selecting an existing design or developing a new magnet for interventions or intraoperative guidance, tradeoffs exist with respect to magnet configuration, field strength, and gradient strength. Although the cylindrical configuration of conventional high-field MRI systems precludes direct access to the patient, the higher signal-to-noise ratio of higher field magnets improves spatial, temporal, and contrast resolution and can enable techniques such as temperature or flow-sensitive imaging, functional brain MRI, diffusion imaging, or MR spectroscopy (MRS). All of these techniques can be useful for surgical planning, image guidance, and treatment monitoring. The optimum configuration would have the openness and patient access of the Signa SP with high field 3.0 T; today, that points to a closed-bore unit.

Such a configuration does lack direct access, prohibiting real-time intraoperative imaging for open surgeries and certain minimally invasive procedures. Nevertheless, when the patient is moved in and out of the closed-bore magnet, image updates can be obtained during open procedures. In addition, within the closed bore of the high-field magnet, patients can be monitored in real-time during certain catheter-based applications and most thermal ablations. The trend in iMRI, especially in neurosurgery, is a move toward more widespread deployment of the high-field magnet as well as use of more advanced imaging techniques presently not feasible for less-expensive low- and midfield systems. Activities in the field of iMRI focus on moving most of the procedures (open surgeries, thermal ablations) to the advanced 3.0 T imaging platform to achieve faster and more flexible image acquisition that, in turn, will improve localization, targeting, monitoring, and therapy control for those procedures adapted to this new application environment.

The major goal of interventional or intraoperative MRI is to provide near real-time dynamic, interactive image guidance for surgical and percutaneous interventional procedures. Today, this type of image guidance is not available for open surgeries but can be provided for catheter-based or endoscopic procedures. In neurosurgery, iMRI has been successfully developed and implemented for multiple interventional and surgical procedures, including biopsies and the placement of electrodes, craniotomies for image-guided resection, or the treatment of various intracranial tumors and epileptogenic foci, intracranial cyst drainages, and thermal ablations for malignant and benign tumors.[3–5,7,16,22–33] In the future, potential applications will expand, and the use of iMRI guidance will be utilized for functional neurosurgery and for the treatment of benign brain tumors, especially those at the skull base as well as neurovascular abnormalities and various diseases of the spine. As far as the original use of iMRI for glioma surgery is concerned, that surgery's goal of obtaining as complete a resection as possible can only be accomplished with better techniques to detect the full extent of infiltrative tumor and more detailed information about the functional and structural anatomy of the brain tissue that surrounds the tumor.

As interventional MRI matures, its improved visualization opens doors to new treatment approaches. Once tools, tissue, and treatment effects can be monitored in near-real or real-time, numerous treatment approaches can be developed that do not require direct visualization and that represent a move away from open surgery. This major progress and expansion requires the development of new imaging methods, navigational techniques, surgical instruments, and interventional tools that will spawn other approaches to transform open surgeries into less-invasive procedures. One of the most promising, noninvasive thermal ablation using MRI-guided focused ultrasound (US), or MRgFUS as it has been named, has great potential to change neurosurgical practice.

The use of new molecular imaging techniques may improve the detection of tumor margins, but that development requires the use of modalities other than MRI. This multimodality environment suited to molecular imaging-guided surgeries should include nuclear and optical imaging modalities and/or navigation-assisted handheld probes that have higher sensitivity for tumor detection. The integration of functional (fMRI) and diffusion tensor imaging (DTI) into surgical planning and intraoperative guidance systems will further improve the preservation of neurologic functions and, ultimately, the completeness of resections.

◆ Intraoperative MRI-Guidance for Brain Tumor Surgery

Most open neurosurgery, whether using iMRI or not, aims to remove brain tumors. The original, and still compelling, reason for using intraoperative imaging during neurosurgery is to compensate for brain-shift. Navigational systems in the operating room acquire preoperatively a single three-dimensional (3D) image database, limiting the detection time window. As surgery progresses from craniotomy to resection, this preoperative information becomes less and less representative of the anatomy. An iMRI can update this preoperative dataset and provide more accurate guidance based on the actual anatomy. Although this improved navigation can be helpful for tumor removal, in some cases, intraoperative imaging may be restricted to the end of the surgery, when, before closing, a single imaging dataset is acquired to check the completeness of resection by looking for residual, MRI-visible tumor tissue. This so-called tumor control method is a practical and well-accepted use of iMRI. However, such a single imaging session at the completion of surgery cannot take full advantage of the information from iMRI that can provide more frequent correct brain-shift-compensated guidance for the safe removal of tumors.[33]

The early success of iMRI was due in large part to its ability to detect residual tumor prior to the end of surgery rather than postoperatively. At that time, most intraoperative sites did not have the computerized tools necessary to use the platform as a complex navigational system. In the future, iMRI will be extensively used as a de facto image-guidance and navigation system to capitalize on the benefits of image guidance to most tumor surgeries. Eventually, iMRI will fundamentally change the way surgery is performed by allowing the adoption of less-invasive surgical approaches that use novel technologies.

Intraoperative MRI Guidance for Primary Brain Tumors

Given its capabilities, iMRI can benefit patients who have cerebral gliomas for whom neurosurgical resection is the primary therapeutic intervention.[34] Gliomas are the most common types of primary malignant brain tumors; rarely circumscribed or well-defined, they grow diffusely within the brain. An interventional MRI scanner allows for the near-total removal of this type of tumor. That outcome can be achieved, although it is difficult due to the inherent uncertainty in visually distinguishing glial tumor tissue from adjacent brain tissue. The goal of minimizing the number of infiltrating glioma cells in the adjacent brain tissue is desirable for several reasons: prolonged survival, prolonged time to malignant progression, decreased risk of seizures, and eligibility for future oncologic therapies. Use of iMRI can achieve more complete tumor removal than surgery using just the human eye due to the higher sensitivity of the MRI in detecting and differentiating low-grade glial neoplasms from surrounding, often gliotic brain tissue.[3-5]

Maximizing the resection of glial tumor tissue while minimizing neurologic deficits is challenging in part because functional brain tissue may reside close to or even within gliomas, and the inadvertent removal of tumor-infiltrated, but functioning brain tissue can result in neurologic deficits.[35] iMRI increases the chances of preserving this functional brain tissue. Tissue that remains functional despite being edematous and infiltrated to an unspecified extent by glioma cells may be seen on nonenhancing T1-weighted images as hypointense areas and on T2-weighted images as hyperintense areas. Thus, even when resections are limited to within the MRI abnormality, postoperative neurologic deficits can result, suggesting that functioning white matter fiber tracts may exist within the tumor. Therefore, maximal resection, complicated by brain-shift, requires precise understanding of the anatomic features of the tumor and the individual functional organization of adjacent brain tissue.

The main predictor of an incomplete tumor resection was the proximity of the lesion to eloquent white matter tracts, such as the corticospinal tract or optic radiations.[36] In the absence of fiber tract visualization, the surgeon tends to perform a more conservative resection to avoid postoperative neurologic deficits. The effect of glial tumors on the architecture of hemispheric white matter is still largely unknown. Clearly, to achieve the goal of maximal resection while preserving neurologic function, knowledge of white matter tract location and its relationship to the glioma is as important as defining the tumor's relationship with the eloquent cortex. Information from multiple brain mapping modalities may provide optimal understanding of the complex structural and functional anatomy of glial tumors in eloquent brain areas, including fMRI and DTI and other preoperatively acquired brain mapping studies such as magnetoencephalography (MEG) or transcranial magnetic stimulation (TMS).[37] To be maximally useful, information derived from all imaging modalities must be accurately coregistered with the patient's brain during the operation and, importantly, updated to account for shifts in the brain shape as surgery proceeds.

Whenever possible, most neurosurgeons recommend a near total or gross total resection of all enhancing tumor volume and regionally infiltrated brain as defined on MRI (T2, fluid attenuation inversion recovery [FLAIR]). However, given the infiltrative nature of most gliomas, a gross total tumor resection is, in most cases, not possible, even though it has been shown to increase survival and time to progression.[34] To achieve the safest and most accurate resection of glial neoplasms, iMRI has become the method of choice because it allows the surgeon to more carefully delineate tumor margins as he or she performs a more aggressive and thorough tumor resection and to preserve surrounding regions of functioning normal brain. The development of techniques capable of accurately depicting tumor margins in vivo is important to determine the most appropriate surgical treatment for gliomas. To date, we at the Brigham and Women's Hospital have performed more than 1,000 craniotomies in the magnetic resonance therapy (MRT) suite.[5,6,26,38] In doing so, we assessed the main variables that affect the complete MRI-guided resection of low-grade gliomas.[19] The statistical analyses identified tumor characteristics to be predictive of incomplete tumor resection: diffuse margin on T2-weighted MRI, histopathologic type, tumor volume, and involvement of the corticospinal tract. More radical resections did not increase the risk of postoperative neurologic deficits.[28] An association between MRI-guidance and survival was also found.[34,39]

Statistical findings such as these underscore the importance of multiparametric imaging for surgical planning and guidance. Also, they evidence that a more complete, iMRI-guided resection can be obtained with high-field MRI and functional navigation. Then, if molecular imaging agents and/or methods are developed for the detection of tumor boundaries, even further improvements in glioma surgery can be expected. Such a step-up requires multimodality imaging in which MRI definition of tumor margins is complemented with optical or nuclear positron emission tomography (PET) or computed tomography (CT) imaging, molecular imaging, and more refined functional and anatomic mapping using fMRI and DTI. By integrating multimodality and multiparametric imaging, an even more complete resection without neurologic impairment can result. And although whether it is an independent predictor remains uncertain, a more complete resection offers a modest survival benefit even in high-grade glioma.[34,40] In addition, glioma excision under MRI guidance offers other clinical benefits including limiting surgical morbidity and substantially debulking the glioma to improve the effectiveness of adjuvant therapies such as chemo- and radiation therapy. Should a trial be ethically possible, which it is not, a randomized controlled trial would be the ideal way to resolve the issue of whether (and to what extent) surgical resection leads to improved patient outcomes and survival. Well-controlled retrospective studies may also provide valuable data for a multivariate analysis of all potential confounding factors.

Intraoperative MRI Guidance for Benign Brain Tumors

Experience using iMRI for benign brain tumors such as meningioma, acoustic neuroma, and pituitary tumors is limited. Conventional surgery with the help of navigational guidance in the operating room is usually successful in removing the tumor completely without complications. Nevertheless, situations arise when intraoperative imaging can help the surgeon to identify residual tumor or to provide essential intraoperative volumetric data, especially if the surgery is performed through a small craniotomy, a transsphenoidal approach, or through neuroendoscopy. In these situations, and when significant brain-shift is present, intraoperative imaging-based guidance can be extremely helpful.

An early success in iMRI was the image guidance for the transsphenoidal removal of pituitary tumors.[28] In addition to the suprasellar compartment, intra- and parasellar structures were also visualized intraoperatively in great detail. Such intraoperative imaging acts as an immediate "second look," allowing not only an increase in the resection, but also an increase in the percentage of complete removals. Neurosurgeons are frequently surprised by the extent of residual tumor after an initial resection attempt and find the intraoperative images useful for guiding further resection.[28] However, even high-field iMRI could not detect tumor remnants in every case. To identify localized tumor more precisely, dynamic contrasted-enhanced MRI can be used to distinguish residual tumor from normal gland and postoperative changes.[41] Gadolinium-soaked cotton pledgets have also been used to identify residual tumor at low-field strength.[42]

To further improve intraoperative visualization of intra- and parasellar anatomy, provide the best surgical guidance, and facilitate a complete resection, iMRI and endoscopic transsphenoidal surgery can be combined.[43] Each method provides complementary information to safely maximize the extent of resection. The evolution of the endoscopic endonasal transsphenoidal technique, which was exclusively used for sellar lesions through the sphenoid sinus, has opened a new access to large areas of the skull base from the nose. This path allows midline access and visibility without brain retraction to the suprasellar, retrosellar, and parasellar space as well as to the areas in the anterior and posterior cranial fossae to make possible the transsphenoidal treatment of a variety of skull base lesions that traditionally have been approached transcranially. Defining the future limits of these extended approaches that most likely require intraoperative image guidance using MRI is difficult. What is easier to predict? Real-time 3D information made available from iMRI may alter the way neurosurgeons approach skull base tumors.[44]

Intraoperative MRI Guidance for Vascular Neurosurgery

Intraoperative diffusion and/or perfusion MRI can also diagnose acutely developed vascular occlusion during surgeries and/or endovascular procedures.[45] In particular, MR venography (MRV), MR angiography (MRA), and diffusion-weighted imaging can identify vascular structures and functions that may prevent injury during surgery.

iMRI may also be used for microsurgical treatment of various vascular lesions. In particular, image guidance has been beneficial for the location of small vascular lesions like cavernomas and for control to ensure a complete resection.[46] A navigated approach to access deep-seated lesions is less accurate due to intraoperative brain-shift and brain retraction. During surgery, MRI can identify a patient's vascular anatomy, including the feeding arteries and draining veins of an intracranial arteriovenous malformation (AVM). However, MR-based imaging's usefulness as intraoperative angiography remains unknown. Any intraoperative assessment of technical results prior to wound closure does offer the neurosurgeon the opportunity to resect or obliterate a vascular malformation completely to obviate a second operation.

Real-time perfusion and diffusion imaging monitors the condition of the brain. Such anatomic and functional monitoring of vascular surgeries and endovascular interventions could significantly improve the safety of planned embolizations or occlusions and clip placements, particularly those in the vicinity of critical perforating vessels. During embolization, diffusion and perfusion intraprocedural imaging is necessary to recognize changes in anatomy (feeding and draining vessel flow and perfusion) and to detect impending infarction. Today, perfusion measurements can be obtained in less than 1 minute of scan time, making this approach a clinically feasible potential adjunct to catheter angiography.[47]

Intraoperative MRI Guidance for Spine Surgery

So far, only a small number of spinal surgical procedures have been performed with iMRI including lumbar discectomies, anterior cervical discectomies with/without fusion, cervical vertebrectomies with fusion, two cervical foraminotomies, and cervical laminectomy. iMRI provides rapid and accurate localization and assessment of the adequacy of decompression. Future applications of iMRI to spine surgery may include intraoperative guidance for resection of the spine and spinal cord tumors and trajectory planning for spinal endoscopy or screw fixation. Certain approaches, such as the transoral route to the cervicomedullary junction, are compromised by a tight surgical corridor and narrow angle of view, making the satisfactory decompression/resection difficult to determine. iMR images can help to determine the adequacy of surgical decompression. The acquisition of iMR images does not adversely affect operative time or neurosurgical techniques, including instrumentation procedures.[48] MRI temperature-sensitive imaging can also be used in laser discectomy and vertebroplasty to prevent thermal damage to nerve roots and the spinal cord and to make the procedure safer and better controlled.[49]

◆ Technical Challenges

MRI-Guided Neuroendoscopy

Because of the introduction of smaller endoscopes, neuroendoscopy has become an expanding field of neurosurgery. Neuroendoscopy is part of the trend in modern neurosurgery toward minimally invasive surgical procedures. These procedures can be accomplished by access and visualization through the narrowest entry and through maximum effective action at the target point with minimal disruption to normal tissue. The endoscopic removal of solid brain tumors from the intraventricular compartment would impose additional technical demands by requiring specialized instrumentation and image guidance preferably with iMRI.

The first MRI-guided endoscopic application was endoscopic sinus surgery.[9,10] The integration of endoscopy with optical tracking and intraoperative interactive imaging allows localization of anatomic landmarks during the procedure.

Since that beginning, the endoscope has been used for all types of neurosurgery, including transventricular neuroendoscopy, a procedure aimed at several intracerebral pathologies inside the ventricular system, for which the endoscope is used in real-time iMRI guidance and/or preoperative image-based navigation. Neuroendoscopy has also been expanding beyond just ventriculostomy procedures to those that treat intraventricular tumors, skull base tumors, degenerative spine disease, intracranial cysts, and hydrocephalus. Especially if image guidance is available, the use of the endoscope in neurosurgery has enormous potential.

Whereas neuroendoscopic images provide a direct high-resolution view of cavities and spaces in the intracranial compartment, they can be insufficient, without additional navigation capability, for the safe targeting of a lesion. More specifically, they cannot directly locate anatomic structures or pathologies that lie hidden beyond this surface and may only show the internal surface of a cavity. During endoscopic third ventriculostomy (ETV), neuroendoscopic imaging may not reveal the basilar artery that must be avoided to prevent life-threatening vascular damage. A navigation-enhanced neuroendoscope system can be developed that works in the MRI environment.[50] Such enhanced neuroendoscopy will be both faster and safer than conventional neuroendoscopy with an even greater ability to minimize possible complications. The developed method will significantly improve the surgeon's ability to navigate in the ventricles and access remote lesions with less tissue trauma. This new approach favors the use of a flexible endoscope as the use of a rigid endoscope is far from ideal. The rigid endoscope remains the standard due to the difficulties of orienting the flexible endoscope in the ventricle cavity, even though the flexible endoscope is superior to the rigid endoscope in accessibility and flexibility. The navigation-enhanced flexible endoscope should remove much of this difficulty as it will assist physicians in better comprehending the anatomic structures on an image. Once successfully developed, the MRI-guided endoscopic method will be applicable to the resection of intracerebral deep-seated tumors. For example, thalamic gliomas, that are difficult to access through open surgery or standard minimally invasive surgery, may be biopsied or even resected using MRI-guided endoscopes.

To introduce MRI-guided endoscopy, a strong need exists to develop MRI-compatible flexible endoscopes equipped with trackable coils. Tracking sensors can detect the position of the tip of the flexible endoscope in the cerebral cavity and show it on 3D MRI models. Then, even in cases of severe anatomic anomalies, flexible neuroendoscopy is safe and accurate. When the images from the MRI are overlaid on the real endoscopic view, previously invisible structures critical in flexible neuroendoscopy can be made visible. MRI-guided neuroendoscopy is particularly useful in the management of complex cystic lesions of the brain when the normal anatomic landmarks on which conventional neuroendoscopy are based have been distorted by underlying pathology. Considering the separate benefits of the MRI depiction of anatomy, neuronavigation, and neuroendoscopy, MRI-guided neuroendoscopic surgery will play an increasingly important role in the future.

Serial Imaging and Brain-Shift

In the closed-bore magnet, access to the patient is restricted. As a consequence, the main intervention takes place outside the magnet, and the surgical procedure must be interrupted by imaging to update changes related to intraoperative shifts and deformations.[44] Mechanical factors, physiologic motions, and pathophysiologic processes such as edema or hemorrhage typically cause these displacements.[44] For neurosurgery to be its most successful, surgeons must intraoperatively identify diseased tissue as well as critical brain tissue. The brain has few landmarks within the parenchyma to guide the surgeon, and diseased tissue is often difficult to differentiate from surrounding normal tissue. Critical brain tissue cannot be identified from visual inspection. The surgeon is often left guessing during the operation whether or not to remove more tissue. These problems become most difficult toward the end of the resection when brain shift has rendered reference images inaccurate, and the margin between diseased tissue and healthy tissue is being approached. Brain-shift is a continuous, dynamic process that evolves differently in distinct brain regions. Therefore, only serial imaging or continuous data acquisition can provide consistently accurate image guidance.

Intraoperative imaging updates the original preoperative (baseline) database to provide an effective solution; however, no scientific method thus far can optimize the frequency of serial imaging necessary to assess and take into account brain deformations.[33,45,51–53]

In practice, the neurosurgeon acquires new intraoperative images to study the configuration of the patient's brain and to monitor the progress of tumor resection. The first key limitation is that the neurosurgeon is required to make a subjective judgment as to when to obtain a new volumetric acquisition, a judgment that involves a subjective estimate of the quality of navigation information available from the existing data based on the surgeon's assessment of the amount of brain-shift and tumor resection that has occurred since the last acquired MRI. Furthermore, a second key limitation of existing state-of-the art systems is an inability to present key preoperatively acquired data fused with the patient's intraoperative position when the brain has undergone significant deformation. Rather, the surgeon must fuse the information from preoperative fMRI and DTI by mentally projecting it through the 3D spatial and temporal changes the patient's brain has undergone. A bridge to this clinical gap must focus on how to compensate for intraoperative brain-shift. Although MRI is effective in spatial localization, it lacks efficacy as a real-time monitor during surgery because real-time scanning cannot take place during surgical activities (e.g., dural opening, lesion resection, and biopsy). The typical protocol for MRI-guided surgery requires the cessation of surgical procedures and the clearing of metallic tools from the surgical field to minimize image artifacts. The time added to the overall duration of a procedure and to the time during which a patient is under general anesthesia increases significantly. Virtually all iMRI set-ups require moving the patient or the magnet, thereby adding to both procedure duration and risk.

Due to these inherent MRI deficiencies, surgeons are required to weigh the benefit of scanning time with diagnostic potential before ordering an intraoperative scan. The goal is to develop an adjunct continuous monitoring method that can quantify ongoing brain-shift, alert the clinical team when a predetermined threshold of movement of a monitored structure has been reached, and signal unexpected changes.

Various methods of intraoperative monitoring during neurosurgery can be used for detecting brain-shift including US and surface tracking. Tracking brain deformation as the case proceeds could allow the surgeon to know when structures are likely to have moved appreciably and can indicate the need to obtain updated information with intraoperative imaging. US imaging has potential advantages over other existing imaging modalities for intraoperative monitoring, yet US is not used for continuous monitoring during neurosurgery largely because it requires imaging through the craniotomy and interrupts the flow of surgery. Several groups have investigated the use of intraoperative US to provide data that could be used to update preoperative models to account for brain-shift.[54–58] Rather than the landmark-based methods, most have used full volume, intensity-based registration and 3D US.[54–57]

◆ Navigation

Intraoperative navigation is essential for image-guided neurosurgery. As intraoperative visualization matures, the need increases for an integrated system of navigation, visualization, and monitoring. Such a system can create an augmented reality visualization of the intraoperative configuration of the patient's brain merged with high-resolution preoperative imaging data, including DTI and fMRI to better localize the tumor and critical healthy tissues.[59,60] During the early phases of MRI-guided procedure development, a modular software tool, 3D-Slicer, with image segmentation, registration, surgical instrument tracking, and multi-layered display capabilities was developed and deployed in an MRI-equipped operating suite. The 3D-Slicer's capabilities reach far beyond real-time tracking of different surgical instruments by providing image segmentation, registration, and multilayered display capabilities. Its integration in the MR therapy delivery system has enabled the use of higher-quality, volumetric

intraoperative image updates for neuronavigation. The implementation of the 3D-Slicer in the MRT has paved the way for the next key development: the implementation of multi-modality image-based neuronavigation combined with intraoperative image updates. Since its integration in the MRT in 1999, the 3D-Slicer has been used for surgical guidance not only for over 1,000 neurosurgical procedures (craniotomies, biopsies), but also for other surgical procedures and imaging applications.[59,61]

Preoperative Surgical Planning versus Intraoperative Decision Making

Surgical decision making relies heavily on the availability of patient-specific morphologic, functional, and metabolic information that cannot be provided by any single iMRI parameter or any single modality. For instance, anatomic MRI does not detect cortical activity nor does it offer information on white matter structure. However, the availability of such information is essential when attempting to achieve maximal tumor removal while preserving neurologic function. Although anatomic MRI is highly sensitive for intracranial pathology, its specificity is limited. Different pathologies may have a very similar appearance on anatomic MRI. For instance, differentiating between radiation necrosis and active tumor or between reactive peritumoral edema and tumor infiltration based on anatomic MRI is difficult. Hence patient-specific atlases obtained by fusing anatomic MRI, functional MRI (cortical activity), diffusion tensor MRI (white matter structure), and metabolic imaging (MRS, PET) are needed to have the most complete information for intraoperative decision making.

The acquisition and processing of fMRI, diffusion tensor MRI (DTI), and metabolic imaging occurs before surgery. Although it is possible to acquire fMRI and (DTI) intraoperatively, the acquisition and processing times often stretch beyond the acceptable time constraints imposed by the surgical procedure. In the case of fMRI, a study requires an awake, cooperative patient. Electrocortical testing could be performed, preventing the need for functional imaging, except for research applications. Additional technical challenges arise from the need to preserve the accuracy of the multimodal imaging data throughout the procedure. Brain-shift inevitably occurs to some extent in response to surgical manipulation and anesthesia, rendering preoperative images inaccurate in the absence of mechanisms capable to compensate for these changes.

One strategy is to employ nonrigid registration algorithms for compensating for brain-shift and for preserving the accuracy of multimodal datasets. The surface deformation of the brain and cerebral ventricles is captured from intraoperative volumetric image updates. In the next step, this deformation field is applied to the multimodal image data using a finite element-based biomechanical simulation. Despite massive computational needs, this algorithm can be executed online on a multiprocessor platform during surgical procedures within a reasonable time (< 5 minutes), fast enough to be useful for surgical guidance.[62,63]

◆ Image-Based Navigation for Robotic Devices

MRI-compatible robotic systems and manipulators are being developed to enhance many types of neurosurgical procedures. MRI imposes severe restrictions on the mechanical devices to be used in or around the scanners. A solution to this challenging environment of the closed-bore scanner is to develop robotic systems to assist surgeons in performing complex neurosurgical procedures.[64-66] The manipulators already developed make use of different methods of actuation, and they belong to four main groups: actuation transmitted through hydraulics, pneumatic actuators, ultrasonic motors based on the piezoceramic principle, and remote manual actuation. Several compatibility issues concerning material selection have been resolved, and different tracking and actuation techniques have been tried.[64,65] Only a small number of developed systems have made it to the clinical level, revealing that the field has not yet reached maturity. Most systems lack the clinical validation needed to become commercial products.[67] An image-guided MRI-compatible surgical robot can execute not only for biopsies but also during complex surgical manipulations. MRI-compatible neurosurgical robots are under development and in the early stages of investigational clinical use.[68-70] A need exists to develop novel methods for tracking the motion of robotic devices during MRI-guided procedures and to integrate these methods into an advanced, generalized interface for image-guided planning, navigation, and targeting.[71] Robot-assisted interventions require fast and precise registration and tracking of devices in the image space, with a view toward achieving minimally invasive needle insertions for diagnosis and therapy, specifically in the brain. A uniform graphical interface in robot-assisted interventions displays the preacquired image volume for convenient target and entry-point selection. The computer then immediately calculates the inverse kinematics and displays the motion parameters (typically translation, rotation, insertion depth) for the robot.

◆ Thermal Ablations

MRI-Guided, Probe-Delivered Thermal Ablations

Thermal coagulation by heating or freezing of tumors is a minimally invasive alternative to surgical removal. These ablation methods have been developed using interstitial laser, radiofrequency, and microwave energy sources connected to heating and freezing probes for cryoablation. Their development significantly advanced the thermal ablation applications by allowing percutaneous treatment, especially with MRI guidance.[72] The probe-delivered thermal ablation methods, like interstitial laser therapy (ILT), deposit energy at a large tissue volume within which there is a wide temperature gradient with high temperature at the probe and lower temperature at the periphery.[7,31,72] Due to this large gradient, the biologic effects are also variable

within the treated volume and the boundary within which the tissue is irreversibly destroyed is, unfortunately, ill defined. In thermal ablations the spatial and temporal monitoring of the temperature distribution within the targeted tumor volume is important to reach the threshold of cell destruction to safely protect the outside area away from the volume. This temperature mapping and monitoring requires a temperature-sensitive imaging method, such as image-based quantitative thermometry that can be used for feedback or closed-loop control of energy deposition. If the localization of the tumor volume is accurate and the targeting of treatment volumes is correct, the thermal damage must be limited to the target. The size and shape of the thermal coagulation has to be conformed to the 3D extent and configuration of the tumor.

MRI-guided radiofrequency ablations and laser ablations of brain tumors have been tested and their feasibility established.[7,31,32,73-76] Laser-induced interstitial thermal therapy (LITT) of brain tumor can be monitored and controlled by MRI using MRI thermometry.[77,78] Real-time monitoring of temperature changes is particularly useful to maximize the coverage of tumor ablation and to minimize damage to critical structures around the tumor. In the near future, more MRI-guided probe-delivered thermal ablation will be used in neurosurgery for the minimally invasive treatment of various brain tumors. Although the indication today is restricted to malignancies, mostly recurrent gliomas and metastases, this well-controlled and safe method will eventually be used for benign tumors.

MRI-Guided Focused US Surgery (MRgFUS)

A promising MRI-guided thermal ablation treatment method developed over the last decade is MRI-guided thermal ablation using noninvasive focused US surgery, also called MRgFUS.[79-81]

Unlike the above-mentioned probe-delivered thermal energy deposition methods, MRgFUS uses extracorporeal acoustic energy for heating tissue only within the focal volume where most of the energy is absorbed. FUS does not require the insertion of a probe for energy delivery. In FUS, the treatment volume is small but the thermal gradient is very narrow, thus ensuring a more complete coagulation of the targeted tissue volume. Correct targeting is achieved by identifying the temperature elevations at the targeted tissue volume below the level of thermal coagulation (under 56°C), and, if the alignment is correct, repeating the sonication at a higher temperature to assure the desired tissue kill effect. MRI-based targeting and temperature-sensitive imaging provides closed-loop control of this thermal ablation method. The feasibility of MRgFUS was originally demonstrated in a series of animal experiments, followed by the treatment of benign tumors like the fibroadenoma of the breast and uterine fibroids using a commercial system (Exablate 200, Insightec, Haifa, Israel).[82-86] Based on the initial experience treating more than 4,000 patients worldwide, the system showed significant potential for replacing invasive tumor surgery and radiosurgery.

Several decades ago it was recognized that FUS fulfills the requirement for an "ideal surgery" for brain tumors because it has no invasive trajectory to the target, does not damage normal tissue adjacent to the tumor, and its tissue-killing effect was limited to the ablated tumor. Due to these advantages, FUS has had a long development history for the treatment of brain tumors.[87] Early attempts were made to treat using US through open craniotomy but the skull was impenetrable for the acoustic beams. Further, having the skull open negated the advantages of a minimally invasive technique.[88] Therefore, intensive research efforts have been made to resolve US penetration and to focus US through the intact skull to develop a FUS system for brain treatments.

If US beams can be focused so as to increase temperature over a threshold, a complete ablation can be accomplished. The beams, however, are distorted by the irregular thickness of the bone. Focusing can be realized through the use of large hemispheric phased arrays placed over the head and adjusting the phase of each phased array element according to the thickness of the underlying bone.[89,90]

Insightec (Haifa, Israel) and SuperSonic Imagine (Aix en Provence, France) are developing MRgFUS systems for brain treatment. A phase I clinical trial for the treatment of primary and metastatic malignancies of the brain has started with the Insightec system (Exablate 3000).[91]

MRgFUS treatment of intracranial lesions through the intact skull provides numerous advantages over currently available treatment, including shorter lengths of stay and less pain. Another example is that, compared with stereotactic radiosurgery, MRgFUS offers nonionizing radiation, repeatability, and real-time guidance and control of treatment. Real-time control of temperature achieved through MRI makes this technique safe, controllable, and accurate. In the future, due to this control, MRgFUS can be performed adjacent to critical structures like nerves and used for cases in which conventional surgery or radiosurgery have failed, including the removal of benign tumors in inaccessible locations (i.e., brainstem) or immediately adjacent to cranial nerves (skull base tumors).

FUS methods are also suited to functional neurosurgical applications, such as movement disorders, epilepsy, or pain. MRI-based targeting could replace or augment stereotactic methods of targeting ablation using invasive electrodes. FUS may also be applicable for functional localization because acoustic energy can block electrochemical nerve cell conduction, an effect called local acoustic anesthesia that can be used for pain control and reversible nerve block.[92] Also a possibility for US used at lower power levels is reversible stimulation.[93] Although these functional effects have been described in peripheral nerves, the central neural pathways in the brain can also be affected through FUS neuromodulation.[94] If developed in the future, this method can be applied to functional testing and, compared with the other available noninvasive method, transcranial magnetic stimulation (TMS) mapping, achieve better localization and targeting, and reach deeper subcortical regions in the brain.

In addition to heating, US has other bioeffects that can be used to alter brain structure and/or function. At high acoustic intensities, microbubbles interact with the US field, a process known as cavitation. Using short high-intensity pulses or a high-intensity pulse followed by a low-power sonication, one can use cavitation to increase the focal temperature rise while maintaining a relatively low power. Using this process to enhance heating could be especially helpful in areas where blood perfusion is high or the US absorption is relatively low. Although cavitation-enhanced heating offers some advantages over heating alone, it has an important drawback: bubbles can violently collapse producing jets and shock waves. This so-called inertial cavitation can cause hemorrhage and tissue damage. Cavitation-enhanced ablation, therefore, should be kept at a minimal level.

Using intravenously administered microbubbles and FUS, safe and noninvasive focal opening of the blood–brain barrier (BBB) can be accomplished.[95–97] The acoustic energy levels required for this technique are much less than those needed for thermal ablation. The disruption of the BBB is reversible within a few hours without neuronal damage. Drugs or other substances may be delivered into a desired anatomic location, effectively influencing local function or structure without affecting brain physiology beyond the targeted area. This method is suited to frequencies needed for transcranial application.

When used with tumor ablation, this approach can have significant clinical applications, including the delivery of large molecules that cannot pass the BBB in a normal brain to the targeted focal delivery of antibodies, chemotherapeutic agents, and neuroprotective substances.[98–100] This method requires MRI guidance. Because the temperature does not increase, it is necessary to image the small displacements caused by the acoustic pressure waves using MR acoustic radiation force imaging, or ARFI. ARFI has the potential to guide US therapies that use low-power pulsed US exposures, such as drug delivery.[101,102]

The targeted delivery of tissue-protective drugs, growth factors, and genes may have clinical use in stroke and spinal cord injury. The nonthermal effects of FUS can induce thrombolysis with or without thrombolytic drugs. Although the risk of associated cavitation-induced hemorrhage is great, transcranial FUS has the potential to treat ischemic stroke and to dissolve intracerebral hematomas into fluid is another possible use of transcranial MRgFUS.[103] Using FUS with and without microbubbles can be used to close arteries and veins noninvasively so as to treat hemostasis and some vascular malformations.[104,105]

◆ Molecular Imaging

Molecular Imaging-Guided Surgery Using Multimodality Imaging

Limiting ourselves to only one imaging method, namely MRI, does not address all the needs of IGT. Multimodality image-guided therapies provide comprehensive information derived from different physical and biologic properties of tissues. Combining multiple modalities offers anatomic, metabolic, and functional information that can be complemented with newly developed molecular imaging methods and techniques.

Advances in medical imaging are increasingly made possible through the development of multimodal imaging platforms and the use of multiple molecular probes and/or contrast agents. Therefore, we must expand our imaging platform for image-guided neurosurgery and include new modalities, especially those applicable for molecular imaging (PET, MRI, optical imaging).

Detection of Surgical Margins

Precisely determining tumor margins is critically important to the management of brain tumors. Surgical excision of any visible abnormality is often attempted, despite the consensus view that conventional MRI used to guide this excision tends to cause clinicians to underestimate the extent of the tumor, which in turn may lead to suboptimal treatment.[106,107] The majority of malignant gliomas recur within 2 cm of the enhancing edge of the original tumor.[108] The infiltration appears to follow the main fiber bundles, possibly along the vessel channels, without disrupting the BBB. Beyond direct visualization in open surgery, seeing tumor margins in vivo, especially for brain tumors, is nearly impossible. Further, MRI may not distinguish edema from tumor. On MRIs used for surgical guidance, nonenhancing lesions can be relatively poorly defined. MRI sensitivity in detecting tumor infiltrating normal brain is limited. MRI may, therefore, be inadequate as a standalone modality to predict the true extent of glioma and should be complemented by more sensitive molecular imaging methods and/or local measurements by various probes. More options are clearly needed. Several investigators are exploring paradigms on surgical margin detection using molecular imaging methods and multimodality platforms. However, no simple or effective methods available today address the surgical margin detection problem. DTI more than other MRI parameters may better delineate the tumor margin in gliomas.[109] But MRI can be complemented with even additional modalities to improve sensitivity, specificity, or both.

Nuclear Imaging

Various radioactive tracers may be useful to intraoperatively determine tumor boundaries and residual disease. Due to the high glucose metabolism in normal brain tissue, ^{18}F-fluorodeoxyglucose (18F-FDG) is not the ideal tracer to detect gliomas. Methyl-11C-l-methionine (11C-MET) is better suited for imaging the extent of gliomas because it aggregates specifically into tumors and far less significantly in normal brain tissue. The use of [11C]L-methionine PET (METPET) for surgical imaging guidance has provided, better than MRI guidance alone, independent and complementary information to assess brain tumor extent, select surgical targets, and plan tumor resection.[110] Given that its uptake in normal brain is low, 3′-deoxy-3′-18F-fluorothymidine (18F-FLT) has been introduced as a proliferation marker in a variety of neoplasias and has promising potential for the detection of brain tumors.[111] 11C-MET and fluorodopa (FDOPA) showed similar performance for the targeting of solid and infiltrative tumor foci in homogeneous and heterogeneous MRI nonenhancing and enhancing brain tumors.[112] 11C-MET and FDOPA have high detection sensitivity, especially for lower-grade astrocytomas.

Optical Imaging

Molecular imaging with a fluorescence-labeled compound, including the use of handheld optical probes for the sensitive detection of fluorescence, is a method that can be used in open surgery to detect the presence of tumor within the exposed surface layer. For molecular imaging, it is a relatively low-cost solution. If the probe is tracked, the measurements can be integrated into the image-guidance system.

5-Aminolevulinic (5-ALA) is a nonfluorescent prodrug that leads to intracellular accumulation of fluorescent protoporphyrins IX (PpIX) in a malignant glioma. The PpIX tends to accumulate in pathologic lesions and emit red fluorescence when excited by blue light. Several studies indicate the usefulness of 5-ALA-induced tumor fluorescence for guiding tumor resection. The completeness of resection, as determined intraoperatively from residual tissue fluorescence, is related to postoperative MRI findings and to survival in patients suffering from glioblastoma multiforme.[113]

5-ALA-induced fluorescence combined with the 3D MRI of a brain tumor has been incorporated into a robotic laser ablation neurosurgery system.[114] With laser excitation, the ALA fluorescence illuminates, enabling intraoperative identification of the position of a tumor and guidance for resection with laser photocoagulation. The information provided by the MRI is enhanced by the 5-ALA fluorescence data and integrated into a robotic laser ablation system in which the fluorescence assists in detecting malignant brain tumors intraoperatively and improving their removal.

Indocyanine green (ICG), an FDA-approved photosensitive tricarbocyanine dye with a molecular weight of 775 g/mol dye that is frequently used in angiography, has recently been successfully used to label brain tumor.[115] ICG rapidly binds to plasma proteins including albumin and globulins. In both animal models and human gliomas, ICG angiography improves tumor localization and enables assessment of postresection margins with high sensitivity and specificity.[115]

Advanced Multimodality Image-Guided Operating Room (AMIGO)

The National Center for IGT (NCIGT) at the Brigham and Women's Hospital and Harvard Medical School is in the process of integrating the components of a rich multimodal and translational clinical research environment to carry out open and minimally invasive surgeries and percutaneous interventions in a high-tech surgical environment called the Advanced Multimodality Image-Guided Operating Room (AMIGO) (**Fig. 21.1**). In this complex technologic infrastructure, multimodality imaging will be coupled with open and minimally invasive surgeries and interventional procedures. The AMIGO will be equipped with high-field 3.0 T MRI, CT, PET, x-ray fluoroscopy, 3D US, optical imaging, as well as

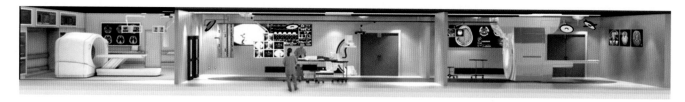

Fig. 21.1 Advanced Multimodality Image-Guided Operating Room (AMIGO) at Brigham and Women's Hospital, Harvard Medical School, Boston, MA.

image-guided robots, endoscopes, and advanced therapy devices for thermal energy delivery using radiofrequency, microwave, laser, cryoablation, and noninvasive MRgFUS.

The AMIGO will be the first site where molecular IGT will be performed in a multimodal surgical setting within which imaging tools and molecular imaging agents will be validated. During invasive surgeries, multiple tissue samples will be obtained for pathology to then compare these findings with imaging findings and local measurements from probes at the same location. Navigational and registration methods developed for multimodal registration can be used to compare multiple probes (optical, nuclear, mass spectroscopy) that are measuring the same tissue region.

The overall objective of multimodality IGT and the AMIGO project is to improve efficacy and reduce the morbidity of minimally invasive procedures and surgeries by providing the physician with image-based anatomic and physiologic information in real-time, intraoperatively or intraprocedurally. The aim is to develop highly innovative technology that optimizes and simplifies morphologic and correlated functional data derived from various imaging modalities. In the AMIGO it will be possible to refine and expand the resources of existing image-guided clinical procedures as well as to develop technology to enable new procedures that will benefit from a multimodality approach. The multimodality-based image guidance system will be complemented with a variety of high-performance computational methods including automatic segmentation and rigid and nonrigid registration. It will be possible to apply novel tracking methods and navigational technologies to catheter-based procedures and neuroendoscopy. We also foresee the optimized use of molecular imaging technology; direct measures of tissue characterization (i.e., PET or optical measurements and/or imaging); and the integration of the next generation of image-guided robotic systems. Endovascular procedures will be assisted by both fluoroscopy and MRI. The application of intraoperative image guidance for monitoring and controlling open surgeries, endoscopic procedures, thermal ablations, brachytherapy, and targeted drug delivery will consolidate minimally invasive therapies. In the new AMIGO environment, we anticipate fundamental change occurring for neurosurgical techniques; image data and surgical and interventional procedures will more closely integrate. The new knowledge and techniques emerging from within the AMIGO will enable clinicians to better understand areas of interest; to plan, monitor or change treatment; navigate through a procedure or operation; or know how, where, and when to best apply a novel therapy.

◆ Conclusion

The further development of intraoperative MRI in neurosurgery requires innovative approaches, the efficient use of MRI, computing technologies, and the integration of advanced diagnostic and therapy devices. This creation can only be accomplished with a multifocused, multidisciplinary effort aimed at developing and implementing these MRI-guided procedures. We anticipate that the further integration of iMRI guidance and computer-assisted surgery will greatly accelerate the clinical utility of IGT in general and iMRI in particular. Within the near future, given the rapid advancement of technology, high field strength 3.0 T magnets may become the standard in neurosurgery. In clinical practice, a wide range of surgical procedures should be tested to expand the number of applications (benign tumors, vascular lesions, spine surgery, neuroendoscopy, etc). The cost and technical support required for an iMRI system, however, presently limits its use to only a limited number of sites worldwide. As new technology is developed, both researchers and clinicians must explore and refine iMRI to make it cost-effective and widely accessible to users. Preoperative fMRI and DTI, for example, provide extremely valuable information for guiding neurosurgical resection and, therefore, should be intraoperatively integrated with MRI-guidance. When fused with the intraoperative configuration of the patient, such information can dramatically improve neurosurgical decision making by delineating regions of normal connectivity critical to normal function and margins suitable for resection.

These systems for capturing brain-shift are limited in their ability to account for resection by the data rate of iMRI and by their reliance on subjective neurosurgical judgment to control that data rate. To accurately capture brain-shift, whole-brain MRI to MRI nonrigid registration systems should be built to demonstrate the feasibility of utilizing sophisticated models. A successful new system without the limitations of current systems will significantly improve neurosurgical decision making and enable more complete removal of tumor while better preserving eloquent cortex and critical fiber tracts. To date, several investigators have demonstrated the great utility of iMRI to ensure a complete resection, particularly of low-grade tumors. Numerous techniques presently under development offer more opportunities to expand the role of iMRI in many directions. As MRI and other modalities improve visualization in pathology, physiology, structure, and function, neurosurgeons can deploy new techniques to improve therapy. These remarkable advances in neurosurgery will also serve as frontrunners as they form the basis for approaches that will impact other areas of medical intervention.

References

1. Jolesz FA, Shtern F. The operating room of the future: report of the National Cancer Institute workshop—imaging guided stereotactic tumor diagnosis and treatment. Invest Radiol 1992;27(4):326–328

2. Schenck JF, Jolesz FA, Roemer PB, et al. Superconducting open-configuration MR imaging system for image-guided therapy. Radiology 1995;195(3):805–814

3. Black PM, Alexander E III, Martin C, et al. Craniotomy for tumor treatment in an intraoperative magnetic resonance imaging unit. Neurosurgery 1999;45(3):423–431, discussion 431–433

4. Schwartz RB, Hsu L, Wong TZ, et al. Intraoperative MR imaging guidance for intracranial neurosurgery: experience with the first 200 cases. Radiology 1999;211(2):477–488

5. Jolesz FA, Talos IF, Schwartz RB, et al. Intraoperative magnetic resonance imaging and magnetic resonance imaging-guided therapy for brain tumors. Neuroimaging Clin N Am 2002;12(4):665–683

6. Dimaio SP, Archip N, Hata N, et al. Image-guided neurosurgery at Brigham and Women's Hospital. IEEE Eng Med Biol Mag 2006; 25(5):67–73

7. Kettenbach J, Silverman SG, Hata N, et al. Monitoring and visualization techniques for MR-guided laser ablations in an open MR system. J Magn Reson Imaging 1998;8(4):933–943

8. Silverman SG, Tuncali K, Adams DF, et al. MR imaging-guided percutaneous cryotherapy of liver tumors: initial experience. Radiology 2000;217(3):657–664

9. Fried MP, Topulos G, Hsu L, et al. Endoscopic sinus surgery with magnetic resonance imaging guidance: initial patient experience. Otolaryngol Head Neck Surg 1998;t;119(4):374–380

10. Hsu L, Fried MP, Jolesz FA. MR-guided endoscopic sinus surgery. AJNR Am J Neuroradiol 1998;19(7):1235–1240

11. D'Amico AV, Cormack R, Tempany CM, et al. Real-time magnetic resonance image-guided interstitial brachytherapy in the treatment of select patients with clinically localized prostate cancer. Int J Radiat Oncol Biol Phys 1998;42(3):507–515

12. Steinmeier R, Fahlbusch R, Ganslandt O, et al. Intraoperative magnetic resonance imaging with the Magnetom open scanner: concepts, neurosurgical indications, and procedures: a preliminary report. Neurosurgery 1998;43(4):739–747, discussion 747–748

13. Hall WA, Martin AJ, Liu H, et al. High-field strength interventional magnetic resonance imaging for pediatric neurosurgery. Pediatr Neurosurg 1998;29(5):253–259

14. Sutherland GR, Kaibara T, Louw D, Hoult DI, Tomanek B, Saunders J. A mobile high-field magnetic resonance system for neurosurgery. J Neurosurg 1999;91(5):804–813

15. Schulder M, Liang D, Carmel PW. Cranial surgery navigation aided by a compact intraoperative magnetic resonance imager. J Neurosurg 2001;94(6):936–945

16. Bradley WG. Achieving gross total resection of brain tumors: intraoperative MR imaging can make a big difference. AJNR Am J Neuroradiol 2002;23(3):348–349

17. Lewin JS, Metzger AK. Intraoperative MR systems. Low-field approaches. Neuroimaging Clin N Am 2001;11(4):611–628

18. Nimsky C, Ganslandt O, Kober H, et al. Integration of functional magnetic resonance imaging supported by magnetoencephalography in functional neuronavigation. Neurosurgery 1999;44(6):1249–1255, discussion 1255–1256

19. Talos IF, Zou KH, Ohno-Machado L, et al. Supratentorial low-grade glioma resectability: statistical predictive analysis based on anatomic MR features and tumor characteristics. Radiology 2006; 239(2):506–513

20. Nimsky C, Ganslandt O, Von Keller B, Romstöck J, Fahlbusch R. Intraoperative high-field-strength MR imaging: implementation and experience in 200 patients. Radiology 2004;233(1):67–78

21. Truwit CL, Hall WA. Intraoperative magnetic resonance imaging-guided neurosurgery at 3-T. Neurosurgery 2006; 58(4 Suppl 2)ONS-338–ONS-345

22. Hall WA, Martin AJ, Liu H, Nussbaum ES, Maxwell RE, Truwit CL. Brain biopsy using high-field strength interventional magnetic resonance imaging. Neurosurgery 1999;44(4):807–813, discussion 813–814

23. Moriarty TM, Quinones-Hinojosa A, Larson PS, et al. Frameless stereotactic neurosurgery using intraoperative magnetic resonance imaging: stereotactic brain biopsy. Neurosurgery 2000;47(5):1138–1145, discussion 1145–1146

24. Bernays RL, Kollias SS, Khan N, Brandner S, Meier S, Yonekawa Y. Histological yield, complications, and technological considerations in 114 consecutive frameless stereotactic biopsy procedures aided by open intraoperative magnetic resonance imaging. J Neurosurg 2002; 97(2):354–362

25. Martin AJ, Hall WA, Roark C, Starr PA, Larson PS, Truwit CL. Minimally invasive precision brain access using prospective stereotaxy and a trajectory guide. J Magn Reson Imaging 2008;27(4):737–743

26. Martin C, Alexander E III, Wong T, Schwartz R, Jolesz F, Black PM. Surgical treatment of low-grade gliomas in the intraoperative magnetic resonance imager. Neurosurg Focus 1998;4(4):e8

27. Hall WA, Liu H, Truwit CL. Functional magnetic resonance imaging-guided resection of low-grade gliomas. Surg Neurol 2005;64(1):20–27, discussion 27

28. Pergolizzi RS Jr, Nabavi A, Schwartz RB, et al. Intra-operative MR guidance during trans-sphenoidal pituitary resection: preliminary results. J Magn Reson Imaging 2001;13(1):136–141

29. Kelly JJ, Hader WJ, Myles ST, Sutherland GR. Epilepsy surgery with intraoperative MRI at 1.5 T. Neurosurg Clin N Am 2005;16(1):173–183

30. Schwartz RB, Hsu L, Black PM, et al. Evaluation of intracranial cysts by intraoperative MR. J Magn Reson Imaging 1998;8(4):807–813

31. Bettag M, Ulrich F, Schober R, et al. Stereotactic laser therapy in cerebral gliomas. Acta Neurochir Suppl (Wien) 1991;52:81–83

32. Leonardi MA, Lumenta CB, Gumprecht HK, von Einsiedel GH, Wilhelm T. Stereotactic guided laser-induced interstitial thermotherapy (SLITT) in gliomas with intraoperative morphologic monitoring in an open MR-unit. Minim Invasive Neurosurg 2001;44(1):37–42

33. Nabavi A, Black PM, Gering DT, et al. Serial intraoperative magnetic resonance imaging of brain shift. Neurosurgery 2001;48(4):787–797, discussion 797–798

34. Claus EB, Horlacher A, Hsu L, et al. Survival rates in patients with low-grade glioma after intraoperative magnetic resonance image guidance. Cancer 2005;103(6):1227–1233

35. Skirboll SS, Ojemann GA, Berger MS, Lettich E, Winn HR. Functional cortex and subcortical white matter located within gliomas. Neurosurgery 1996;38(4):678–684, discussion 684–685

36. Jolesz FA, Talos IF, Schwartz RB, et al. Intraoperative magnetic resonance imaging and magnetic resonance imaging-guided therapy for brain tumors. Neuroimaging Clin N Am 2002;12(4):665–683

37. Golby AJ, McConnell KA. Functional brain mapping options for minimally invasive surgery. In: Black PM, Proctor M, eds. Minimally Invasive Neurosurgery. *Totawa*, NJ: Humana Press; 2004: 87–106

38. Mittal S, Black PM. Intraoperative magnetic resonance imaging in neurosurgery: the Brigham concept. Acta Neurochir Suppl (Wien) 2006;98:77–86

39. Keles GE, Chang EF, Lamborn KR, et al. Volumetric extent of resection and residual contrast enhancement on initial surgery as predictors of outcome in adult patients with hemispheric anaplastic astrocytoma. J Neurosurg 2006;105(1):34–40

40. Nimsky C, Fujita A, Ganslandt O, Von Keller B, Fahlbusch R. Volumetric assessment of glioma removal by intraoperative high-field magnetic resonance imaging. Neurosurgery 2004;55(2):358–370, discussion 370–371

41. Fahlbusch R, Ganslandt O, Buchfelder M, Schott W, Nimsky C. Intraoperative magnetic resonance imaging during transsphenoidal surgery. J Neurosurg 2001;95(3):381–390

42. Ahn JY, Jung JY, Kim J, Lee KS, Kim SH. How to overcome the limitations to determine the resection margin of pituitary tumours with low-field intra-operative MRI during trans-sphenoidal surgery: usefulness of gadolinium-soaked cotton pledgets. Acta Neurochir (Wien) 2008;150(8):763–771, discussion 771

43. Schwartz TH, Stieg PE, Anand VK. Endoscopic transsphenoidal pituitary surgery with intraoperative magnetic resonance imaging. Neurosurgery 2006; 58(1, Suppl)ONS44–ONS51, discussion ONS44–ONS51

44. Dort JC, Sutherland GR. Intraoperative magnetic resonance imaging for skull base surgery. Laryngoscope 2001;111(9):1570–1575

45. Mamata Y, Mamata H, Nabavi A, et al. Intraoperative diffusion imaging on a 0.5 Tesla interventional scanner. J Magn Reson Imaging 2001;13(1):115–119

46. Gralla J, Ganslandt O, Kober H, Buchfelder M, Fahlbusch R, Nimsky C. Image-guided removal of supratentorial cavernomas in critical brain

areas: application of neuronavigation and intraoperative magnetic resonance imaging. Minim Invasive Neurosurg 2003;46(2):72–77

47. Muir KW, Buchan A, von Kummer R, Rother J, Baron JC. Imaging of acute stroke. Lancet Neurol 2006;5(9):755–768

48. Kaibara T, Hurlbert RJ, Sutherland GR. Transoral resection of axial lesions augmented by intraoperative magnetic resonance imaging. Report of three cases. J Neurosurg 2001; 95(2, Suppl)239–242

49. Schoenenberger AW, Steiner P, Debatin JF, et al. Real-time monitoring of laser diskectomies with a superconducting, open-configuration MR system. AJR Am J Roentgenol 1997;169(3):863–867

50. Hong J, Hata N, Konishi K, Hashizume M. Real-time magnetic resonance imaging driven by electromagnetic locator for interventional procedure and endoscopic therapy. Surg Endosc 2008;22(2):552–556

51. Ferrant M, Nabavi A, Macq B, et al. Serial registration of intraoperative MR images of the brain. Med Image Anal 2002;6(4):337–359

52. Nimsky C, Ganslandt O, Hastreiter P, Fahlbusch R. Intraoperative compensation for brain shift. Surg Neurol 2001;56(6):357–364, discussion 364–365

53. Nimsky C, Ganslandt O, Cerny S, Hastreiter P, Greiner G, Fahlbusch R. Quantification of, visualization of, and compensation for brain shift using intraoperative magnetic resonance imaging. Neurosurgery 2000;47(5):1070–1079, discussion 1079–1080

54. Comeau RM, Sadikot AF, Fenster A, Peters TM. Intraoperative ultrasound for guidance and tissue shift correction in image-guided neurosurgery. Med Phys 2000;27(4):787–800

55. Coenen VA, Krings T, Weidemann J, et al. Sequential visualization of brain and fiber tract deformation during intracranial surgery with three-dimensional ultrasound: an approach to evaluate the effect of brain shift. Neurosurgery 2005; **56**(1, Suppl)133–141, discussion 133–141

56. Lindner D, Trantakis C, Renner C, et al. Application of intraoperative 3D ultrasound during navigated tumor resection. Minim Invasive Neurosurg 2006;49(4):197–202

57. Letteboer MM, Willems PW, Viergever MA, Niessen WJ. Brain shift estimation in image-guided neurosurgery using 3-D ultrasound. IEEE Trans Biomed Eng 2005;52(2):268–276

58. White PJ, Whalen S, Tang SC, Clement GT, Jolesz F, Golby AJ. An intraoperative brain shift monitor using shear mode transcranial ultrasound: preliminary results. J Ultrasound Med 2009;28(2):191–203

59. Jolesz FA, Kikinis R, Talos IF. Neuronavigation in interventional MR imaging. Frameless stereotaxy. Neuroimaging Clin N Am 2001;11(4):685–693, ix

60. Gering DT, Nabavi A, Kikinis R, et al. An integrated visualization system for surgical planning and guidance using image fusion and an open MR. J Magn Reson Imaging 2001;13(6):967–975

61. Nabavi A, Gering DT, Kacher DF, et al. Surgical navigation in the open MRI. Acta Neurochir Suppl (Wien) 2003;85:121–125

62. Warfield SK, Haker SJ, Talos IF, et al. Capturing intraoperative deformations: research experience at Brigham and Women's Hospital. Med Image Anal 2005;9(2):145–162

63. Clatz O, Delingette H, Talos IF, et al. Hybrid formulation of the model-based non-rigid registration problem to improve accuracy and robustness. Med Image Comput Comput Assist Interv 2005;8(Pt 2):295–302

64. Elhawary H, Zivanovic A, Davies B, Lampérth M. A review of magnetic resonance imaging compatible manipulators in surgery. Proc Inst Mech Eng [H] 2006;220(3):413–424

65. Elhawary H, Tse ZT, Hamed A, Rea M, Davies BL, Lamperth MU. The case for MR-compatible robotics: a review of the state of the art. Int J Med Robot 2008;4(2):105–113

66. Chinzei K, Miller K. Towards MRI guided surgical manipulator. Med Sci Monit 2001;7(1):153–163

67. DiMaio SP, Pieper S, Chinzei K, et al. Robot-assisted needle placement in open MRI: system architecture, integration and validation. Comput Aided Surg 2007;12(1):15–24

68. Masamune K, Kobayashi E, Masutani Y, et al. Development of an MRI-compatible needle insertion manipulator for stereotactic neurosurgery. J Image Guid Surg 1995;1(4):242–248

69. Sutherland GR, Latour I, Greer AD. Integrating an image-guided robot with intraoperative MRI: a review of the design and construction of neuroArm. IEEE Eng Med Biol Mag 2008;27(3):59–65

70. Sutherland GR, Latour I, Greer AD, Fielding T, Feil G, Newhook P. An image-guided magnetic resonance-compatible surgical robot. Neurosurgery 2008;62(2):286–292, discussion 292–293

71. Chinzei K, Warfield S, Hata N, Tempany C, Jolesz F, Kikinis R. Planning, simulation and assistance with intraoperative MRI. Minim Invasive Ther Allied Technol 2003;12(1):59–64

72. McDannold NJ, Jolesz FA. Magnetic resonance image-guided thermal ablations. Top Magn Reson Imaging 2000;11(3):191–202

73. Anzai Y, Lufkin R, DeSalles A, Hamilton DR, Farahani K, Black KL. Preliminary experience with MR-guided thermal ablation of brain tumors. AJNR Am J Neuroradiol 1995;16(1):39–48, discussion 49–52

74. Ascher PW, Justich E, Schröttner O. Interstitial thermotherapy of central brain tumors with the Nd:YAG laser under real-time monitoring by MRI. J Clin Laser Med Surg 1991;9(1):79–83

75. Fan M, Ascher PW, Schröttner O, Ebner F, Germann RH, Kleinert R. Interstitial 1.06 Nd:YAG laser thermotherapy for brain tumors under real-time monitoring of MRI: experimental study and phase I clinical trial. J Clin Laser Med Surg 1992;10(5):355–361

76. Kahn T, Bettag M, Ulrich F, et al. MRI-guided laser-induced interstitial thermotherapy of cerebral neoplasms. J Comput Assist Tomogr 1994;18(4):519–532

77. Kuroda K, Oshio K, Chung AH, Hynynen K, Jolesz FA. Temperature mapping using the water proton chemical shift: a chemical shift selective phase mapping method. Magn Reson Med 1997;38(5):845–851

78. Stollberger R, Ascher PW, Huber D, Renhart W, Radner H, Ebner F. Temperature monitoring of interstitial thermal tissue coagulation using MR phase images. J Magn Reson Imaging 1998;8(1):188–196

79. Jolesz FA, Hynynen K. Magnetic resonance image-guided focused ultrasound surgery. Cancer J 2002;8(Suppl 1):S100–S112

80. Jolesz FA, Hynynen K, McDannold N, Tempany C. MR imaging-controlled focused ultrasound ablation: a noninvasive image-guided surgery. Magn Reson Imaging Clin N Am 2005;13(3):545–560

81. Jolesz FA, McDannold N. Current status and future potential of MRI-guided focused ultrasound surgery. J Magn Reson Imaging 2008;27(2):391–399

82. Cline HE, Hynynen K, Watkins RD, et al. Focused US system for MR imaging-guided tumor ablation. Radiology 1995;194(3):731–737

83. Hynynen K, Vykhodtseva NI, Chung AH, Sorrentino V, Colucci V, Jolesz FA. Thermal effects of focused ultrasound on the brain: determination with MR imaging. Radiology 1997;204(1):247–253

84. McDannold N, Hynynen K, Wolf D, Wolf G, Jolesz F. MRI evaluation of thermal ablation of tumors with focused ultrasound. J Magn Reson Imaging 1998;8(1):91–100

85. Hynynen K, Pomeroy O, Smith DN, et al. MR imaging-guided focused ultrasound surgery of fibroadenomas in the breast: a feasibility study. Radiology 2001;219(1):176–185

86. Tempany CM, Stewart EA, McDannold N, Quade BJ, Jolesz FA, Hynynen K. MR imaging-guided focused ultrasound surgery of uterine leiomyomas: a feasibility study. Radiology 2003;226(3):897–905

87. Jagannathan J, Sanghvi NT, Crum LA, et al. High-intensity focused ultrasound surgery of the brain: part 1—A historical perspective with modern applications. Neurosurgery 2009;64(2):201–210, discussion 210–211

88. Ram Z, Cohen ZR, Harnof S, et al. Magnetic resonance imaging-guided, high-intensity focused ultrasound for brain tumor therapy. Neurosurgery 2006;59(5):949–955, discussion 955–956

89. Clement GT, Hynynen K. A non-invasive method for focusing ultrasound through the human skull. Phys Med Biol 2002;47(8):1219–1236

90. Pernot M, Aubry JF, Tanter M, et al. In vivo transcranial brain surgery with an ultrasonic time reversal mirror. J Neurosurg 2007;106(6):1061–1066

91. McDannold N, Clement GT, Black P, Jolesz FA, Hynynen K. Transcranial MRI-guided focused ultrasound surgery of brain tumors: Initial findings in three patients. Neurosurgery, 2010;66(2):323–332

92. Colucci V, Strichartz G, Jolesz F, Vykhodtseva N, Hynynen K. Focused ultrasound effects on nerve action potential in vitro. Ultrasound Med Biol 2009;35(10):1737–1747

93. Currier DP, Greathouse D, Swift T. Sensory nerve conduction: effect of ultrasound. Arch Phys Med Rehabil 1978;59(4):181–185

94. Yoo SS, Lee JH, Zhang Y, et al. FUS-mediated reversible modulation of region-specific brain function. Paper presented at: MRGFUS 2008; October 6–7; Washington, DC

95. Hynynen K, McDannold N, Vykhodtseva N, Jolesz FA. Noninvasive MR imaging-guided focal opening of the blood-brain barrier in rabbits. Radiology 2001;220(3):640–646

96. Vykhodtseva N, McDannold N, Hynynen K. Induction of apoptosis in vivo in the rabbit brain with focused ultrasound and Optison. Ultrasound Med Biol 2006;32(12):1923–1929

97. McDannold NJ, Vykhodtseva NI, Hynynen K. Microbubble contrast agent with focused ultrasound to create brain lesions at low power levels: MR imaging and histologic study in rabbits. Radiology 2006;241(1):95–106

98. Kinoshita M, McDannold N, Jolesz FA, Hynynen K. Targeted delivery of antibodies through the blood-brain barrier by MRI-guided focused ultrasound. Biochem Biophys Res Commun 2006;340(4):1085–1090

99. Kinoshita M, McDannold N, Jolesz FA, Hynynen K. Noninvasive localized delivery of Herceptin to the mouse brain by MRI-guided focused ultrasound-induced blood-brain barrier disruption. Proc Natl Acad Sci U S A 2006;103(31):11719–11723

100. Treat LH, McDannold N, Vykhodtseva N, Zhang Y, Tam K, Hynynen K. Targeted delivery of doxorubicin to the rat brain at therapeutic levels using MRI-guided focused ultrasound. Int J Cancer 2007; 121(4): 901–907

101. Mitragotri S. Healing sound: the use of ultrasound in drug delivery and other therapeutic applications. Nat Rev Drug Discov 2005;4(3): 255–260

102. McDannold N, Maier SE. Magnetic resonance acoustic radiation force imaging. Med Phys 2008;35(8):3748–3758

103. Daffertshofer M, Gass A, Ringleb P, et al. Transcranial low-frequency ultrasound-mediated thrombolysis in brain ischemia: increased risk of hemorrhage with combined ultrasound and tissue plasminogen activator: results of a phase II clinical trial. Stroke 2005;36(7): 1441–1446

104. Hynynen K, Colucci V, Chung A, Jolesz F. Noninvasive arterial occlusion using MRI-guided focused ultrasound. Ultrasound Med Biol 1996;22(8):1071–1077

105. Hynynen K, Chung AH, Colucci V, Jolesz FA. Potential adverse effects of high-intensity focused ultrasound exposure on blood vessels in vivo. Ultrasound Med Biol 1996;22(2):193–201

106. Tovi M, Lilja A, Bergström M, Ericsson A, Bergström K, Hartman M. Delineation of gliomas with magnetic resonance imaging using Gd-DTPA in comparison with computed tomography and positron emission tomography. Acta Radiol 1990;31(5):417–429

107. Tovi M, Hartman M, Lilja A, Ericsson A. MR imaging in cerebral gliomas. Tissue component analysis in correlation with histopathology of whole-brain specimens. Acta Radiol 1994;35(5):495–505

108. Hochberg FH, Pruitt A. Assumptions in the radiotherapy of glioblastoma. Neurology 1980;30(9):907–911

109. Price SJ, Jena R, Burnet NG, et al. Improved delineation of glioma margins and regions of infiltration with the use of diffusion tensor imaging: an image-guided biopsy study. AJNR Am J Neuroradiol 2006;27(9):1969–1974

110. Ceyssens S, Van Laere K, de Groot T, Goffin J, Bormans G, Mortelmans L. [11C]methionine PET, histopathology, and survival in primary brain tumors and recurrence. AJNR Am J Neuroradiol 2006; 27(7): 1432–1437

111. Jacobs AH, Thomas A, Kracht LW, et al. 18F-fluoro-L-thymidine and 11C-methylmethionine as markers of increased transport and proliferation in brain tumors. J Nucl Med 2005;46(12):1948–1958

112. Becherer A, Karanikas G, Szabé M, et al. Brain tumour imaging with PET: a comparison between [18F]fluorodopa and [11C]methionine. Eur J Nucl Med Mol Imaging 2003;30(11):1561–1567

113. Stummer W, Reulen HJ, Meinel T, et al; ALA-Glioma Study Group. Extent of resection and survival in glioblastoma multiforme: identification of and adjustment for bias. Neurosurgery 2008;62(3):564–576, discussion 564–576

114. Liao H, Shimaya K, Wang K, et al. Combination of intraoperative 5-aminolevulinic acid-induced fluorescence and 3-D MR imaging for guidance of robotic laser ablation for precision neurosurgery. Med Image Comput Comput Assist Interv 2008;11(Pt 2):373–380

115. Haglund MM, Berger MS, Hochman DW. Enhanced optical imaging of human gliomas and tumor margins. Neurosurgery 1996; 38(2): 308–317

22

Equipment Integration: Neuronavigation

Christopher Nimsky and Oliver Ganslandt

Intraoperative imaging has attracted increasing interest in the last decade. The ability to objectively determine the extent of tumor removal during surgery is highly advantageous. If the resection is incomplete, one can attempt to remove the tumor residues that were initially missed during the same operation. In contrast to a subjective estimation by the neurosurgeon, intraoperative imaging allows an objective evaluation of the intraoperative situation, thus acting as quality control during surgery.[1-6] In addition to intraoperative imaging, an integral part of our concept of computer-aided surgery is the possibility to apply neuronavigation simultaneously.[5,7,8] Neuronavigation allows essentially visualizing the results of pre- and intraoperative imaging in the surgical field, so that the image data provide an immediate feedback. The most important aspect is to prevent increased neurologic deficits despite increased resections that might result from the attempt to remove initially overlooked tumor remnants that are detected by intraoperative imaging.

In standard neuronavigation, also known as frameless stereotaxy, the real space of the surgical field is registered to the three-dimensional (3D) image space, which is based on anatomic data only. We prefer the application of microscope-based navigation, where the extent and localization of a tumor is superimposed on the microscope field of view through contours using the heads-up display technology of the modern operating microscopes. Standard neuronavigation based on anatomic information only, which has become a routine tool in many neurosurgical departments, was developed further by the integration of further information from other modalities resulting in the so-called multimodal navigation.

A first step in the direction of multimodal navigation was the development of functional navigation, where preoperative data from magnetoencephalography (MEG)[9-11] and functional magnetic resonance imaging (fMRI)[5,12] defining localizations of cortical eloquent brain areas such as the motor and speech areas in individual patients, were integrated in the navigation set-up. This method of functional neuronavigation allowed for more thorough resection of tumors in risk zones with low morbidity. Integration of diffusion tensor imaging (DTI) data delineating the course of major white matter tracts extended this concept also to subcortical areas,[13-16] while the coregistration of positron emission tomography (PET) data and information from MR spectroscopy (MRS) added metabolic information leading to true multimodal navigation.[17-22]

◆ Implementation of Navigation in the Surgical Workflow

The neurosurgical operating room should be the integrative place where all patient data can be visualized in a surgeon-friendly fashion. Multimodal navigation – with the visualization of multimodal data on several screens close to the surgical site, as well as the parallel superimposition of the relevant structures visualized by contours in different colors in the microscope field of view – is the main tool to achieve this integration.

In contrast to pointer-based navigation, microscope-based navigation provides a more intuitive data visualization directly in the surgical field. Pointer-based systems only delineate the position of an instrument, for example, typically the tip of a pointer in the image space, so that during surgery when navigation information is needed the surgical workflow is interrupted by necessitating that the surgeon look away from the surgical field to a navigation screen. Microscope-based navigation has the advantage of heads-up displays superimposing additional information on the surgical field by color contours or semitransparent 3D objects. Furthermore, the position of an instrument, for example, the autofocus position of the microscope, may be additionally displayed on the navigation screen.

However, there is still much room for further enhancements of these display technologies. In most set-ups there is only a 2D visualization, lacking real depth information, which would be possible in a 3D image injection set-up. Also, the real-time rendering of the displayed objects in the current standard commercial systems does not represent what is now possible with near photo-realistic visualizations in other fields of computer graphics. One of the most important aspects in such systems is to avoid a confusion of the neurosurgeon by a potential information overload. Sophisticated systems have to be developed that present the most relevant information at a certain stage of surgery without impeding the surgical workflow and without distracting the neurosurgeon from his main task.

What are the navigation concepts in an intraoperative MRI (iMRI) environment? The MRI scanner may serve as a navigational device per se, as is the case with the 0.5 tesla (T) double-doughnut GE (General Electric Medical Systems, Waukesha, WI) scanner. The patient is operated directly in the scanner: the surgical space and imaging space were identical and an instrument in the surgical space could be tracked in image space without much additional effort.[1,23,24] Direct navigation in the MRI scanner is often based on real-time imaging, as in so-called prospective stereotaxy, a method for trajectory alignment for placements of catheters or sampling biopsies.[25–27]

Other systems that integrate iMRI and navigation result in a classical navigation set-up: image space and surgical space are not identical; hence some kind of patient registration has to be applied. Most set-ups implement navigation at the 5 gauss (G) line (**Fig. 22.1**), so that standard non-MRI-compatible instruments can be used. Ceiling-mounted solutions of the navigation camera and screens[5] are an optimal solution in the intraoperative scenario because placing a standard navigation system close to an MRI scanner increases the risk of potential magnetic accidents. To optimize the navigation workflow a close integration of imaging and navigation is necessary. For pre- and intraoperative registration an efficient data transfer between scanner and navigation computers is mandatory; an optimized order of the different imaging sequences allows navigation planning and preparation while scanning is still in process.

High navigation accuracy is a prerequisite if the navigation information is to be used at critical steps during the resection of a tumor. Among all errors contributing to the overall navigation accuracy, the initial patient registration process is mostly prone to errors. The most common strategy for patient registration relies on placement of skin-adhesive fiducials, which can be detected in the images, so that their position in virtual and real physical space can be correlated to define the registration coordinate system. Automatic registration set-ups, allowing a user-independent registration of patient space and image space, try to reduce the user-dependent errors.[28]

◆ Automatic Registration

Navigation accuracy is influenced by a variety of factors, among them are the so-called application accuracy, factors relating to a unwanted movement of the registration coordinate system

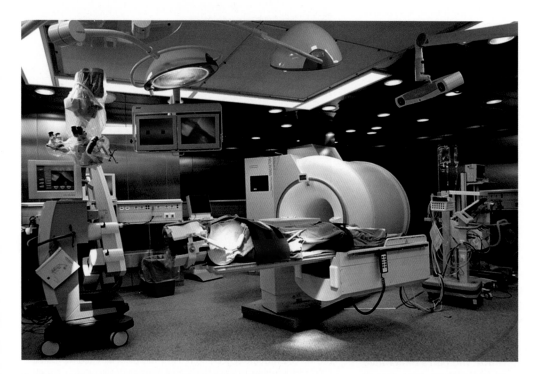

Fig. 22.1 Operating room set-up at the University Erlangen-Nuremberg with a 1.5 tesla magnetic resonance imaging (MRI) scanner and integrated microscope-based navigation. The navigation camera, as well as the navigation screens are ceiling mounted. The patient's head is placed at the 5 gauss (G) line, the head is fixed in an 8-channel MR coil/headholder combination with an attached registration matrix for automatic patient registration.

(positional shift), and intraoperative events like brain deformation, which is known as brain-shift. The application accuracy is influenced by the quality of imaging, by the technical accuracy of the system itself, and by the quality of patient registration, which defines the process of registering image space and real surgical space.[29] Although the spatial distortion of MR images, which is due to gradient field nonlinearities and resonance offsets (chemical shifts and magnetic field inhomogeneities),[30] and the technical accuracy of the navigation system are not easily influenced by the user, the patient registration process is very much user-dependent and is influenced by the individual registration strategy and user experience.

Standard patient registration can be achieved in different ways. There are "marker-fit" techniques using either extrinsic markers (so-called fiducials either self-adhesive or implanted in the skull bone) or anatomic landmarks for registration. There are also "surface-fit" techniques using the outer contour of the face and the skull for the referencing process. Several studies[31–34] have shown the reliability of these registration methods and rapid progress has been made toward automatic marker detection in image space and semiautomatic registration.[35] Nevertheless, the registration process itself still has to be performed manually; therefore it remains time-consuming and prone to error.

Automatic registration is based on paired-point registration but it spares the user all the error-prone steps associated with paired-point registration. The main task of automatic registration is to create an unambiguous relationship between the reference array and the acquired images used for navigation. The reference array is an important reflective marker structure rigidly attached to the patient head via the head clamp. It is used as a relative reference for the system to be able to track instruments, even when the stereoscopic camera is moved into a different position. Looking from the mathematical standpoint, the reference array and the volumetric images span two independent coordinate systems. One coordinate system is used to describe the position of tracked instruments in the surgical field or relative to the reference array, the other to render a 3D model of the tracked instrument in the volumetric images, which then is projected on a 2D view on a screen, or superimposed in the operating microscope, allowing the user to navigate on the images.

It is generally assumed that these two coordinate systems relate to each other via a rigid transformation matrix, describing the rotation and translation between these coordinate systems – or how to transform one position of the instrument, in the surgical space into a corresponding position in the virtual/image space. To be able to calculate the rotation and translational parameters, at least 3 points in the patient space and corresponding points in the virtual space have to be defined. A paired-point matching algorithm then optimizes the rotation and translational parameters to minimize the root mean square error between these point pairs or even to permute the pairs to achieve an optimal result. An additional indirection for fiducial registration is of importance to implement the automatic registration method. A so-called registration matrix is introduced, which already contains a fixed constellation of fiducials relative to a reflective marker structure, making it possible to use the registration matrix as a tracked instrument (**Fig. 22.2A**). The registration matrix is attached to the upper part of the head coil, so that the fiducials from the registration matrix are automatically imaged

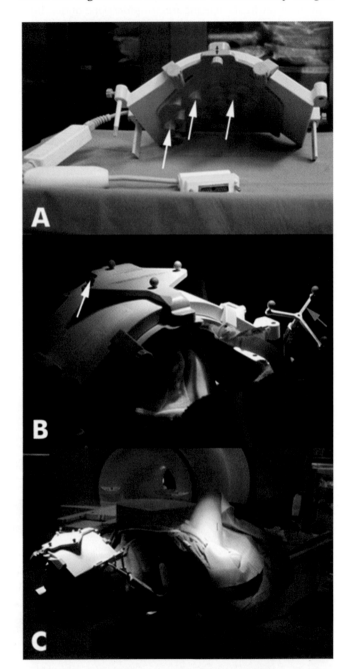

Fig. 22.2 Automatic patient registration. **(A)** The registration matrix is attached to the upper part of the head coil, the *white arrows* delineate the fixed integrated markers in the registration matrix, which can be detected automatically. **(B)** After the head is fixed in the magnetic resonance imaging- (MRI-) compatible headholder the upper part of the MR coil with the registration matrix is attached, reflective markers (*white arrow*) allow to track the spatial position of the reference matrix, the *gray arrow* points at the reference array (so-called reference star) that is rigidly attached to the headholder, so that the spatial relation between the head and the reference array is fixed. **(C)** Overview of patient placement with the head at the 5 G line just after preoperative scanning for initiation of automatic registration.

when placed close enough to the patient's head. Once the scan is completed and the acquired images are transferred to the navigation system, the user only has to adjust the navigation camera so that it can identify the reflective marker structure of the registration matrix and the reference array for a brief moment, so that the navigation system can determine the spatial relation between registration matrix and reference array (**Fig. 22.2B**). Once the acquisition of the reflective marker structures has been completed, an automatic marker detection algorithm detects the fiducials from the registration matrix in the image dataset. Because the system knows the exact arrangement and position of the fiducials integrated in the registration matrix this information can be used as input for the paired-point matching algorithm. Combining the information about where the registration matrix was in relation to the reference array and how the detected fiducials in the images relate to the fiducials of the registration matrix while also knowing how the fiducials from the registration matrix relate to the spatial position of the matrix itself by the defined construction, a transformation matrix can be calculated directly relating the reference array with the acquired images, so that the relation between image space and physical/surgical space is defined and navigation can be used (**Fig. 22.2C**). An additional skin fiducial that is not used for the registration

process is localized after patient registration to document a target registration error, which is typically in the range between 0.3 and 2.5 mm (**Fig. 22.3**). Phantom studies resulted in median localization errors between 0.88 and 2.13 mm for the automatic registration approach, which was at least not worse, in most test series even significantly better, than that of the standard registration no matter whether four or seven fiducial markers were used.[28]

◆ Multimodal Navigation

Low postoperative neurologic deficits are mandatory; especially in surgery of high-grade tumors it is of no benefit for the patient to maximize the extent of a resection to potentially increase the survival time by only some weeks, when risking permanent neurologic deficits right after surgery. It is absolutely mandatory to combine the goal of maximum resection with the goal of preservation of function. Intraoperative imaging helps not only to maximize the extent of resection but in combination with functional multimodal navigation also minimization of postoperative neurologic deficits is possible.[13,36] With the advances in surgical techniques and perioperative technology, it is now possible to maximally resect malignant intrinsic glial neoplasms, even

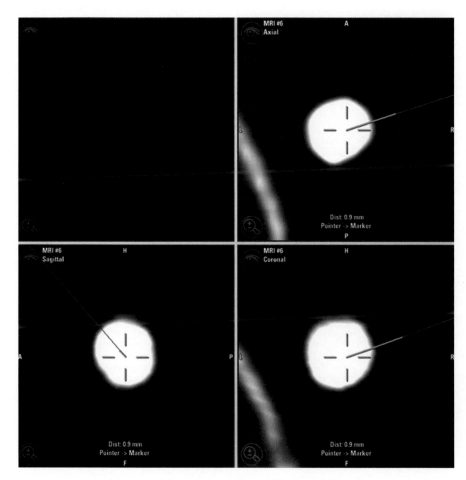

Fig. 22.3 A skin fiducial, which is not used for patient registration, allows to document the target registration error; after automatic registration the tip of a pointer is placed in the dip of the fiducial and its position is documented with the navigation system, which calculates the offset.

close to functionally critical areas, without increased morbidity. Studies have demonstrated a survival advantage of these lesions with a resection extent of 98% or greater, particularly in younger patients with good Karnofsky scores.[37]

To achieve this, functional neuronavigation (i.e., integrating functional data into anatomic navigational datasets) is an important add-on to iMRI because it prevents too extensive resections, which would otherwise result in new neurologic deficits. Meanwhile, data from MEG and fMRI are routinely integrated in functional navigation allowing identification of eloquent brain areas such as the motor area and speech-related areas.[11,12]

In a retrospective study, we focused on how the decision to resect a glioma was influenced by MEG.[9] In 5 consecutive years we have investigated every patient proposed for surgery, who harbored a lesion adjacent to an eloquent brain area. Altogether, 191 patients were examined, 119 of them harbored supratentorial gliomas. About every fourth patient (26.8%) yielded a severe possible danger of postoperative neurologic morbidity according to MEG and thus was not considered a good candidate for surgery. This is a corresponding result with published data where 12 out of 40 investigated patients (30%) with tumors and vascular malformations underwent nonsurgical therapy according to the MEG results.[38] When functional data were used in combination with frameless stereotactic devices the postoperative morbidity was as low as 2.3%. Overall

morbidity, however, was 6.8%. These data reflect the beneficial effects of functional navigation in comparison to data of other studies with morbidity rates varying from 6 to 31.7%.[39-43] These figures can also be interpreted as a result of a more careful patient selection through the help of preoperative brain mapping. Preoperative identification of eloquent brain areas has an impact in the risk evaluation in glioma surgery, as well as functional navigation reduces the risk for postoperative neurologic deficits. Besides identification of the motor strip, the localization of language areas is of great clinical impact.[44,45]

Functional data from MEG and fMRI only localize function at the brain surface. However, neurologic deficits can also occur during tumor resection due to damaging of deeper structures, such as major white matter tracts. DTI can be used not only to delineate tumor borders, but also to display the course of white matter tracts, such as the pyramidal tract. The knowledge of the course of major white matter tracts in relationship to a tumor helps to prevent new postoperative neurologic deficits.[46,47] Registration of diffusion data with the navigational dataset[16,48,49] facilitates the intraoperative preservation of these eloquent structures (**Fig. 22.4**). A prerequisite is that intraoperative changes of the brain anatomy, known as brain-shift, are taken into account. In contrast to the use of fMRI and MEG, brain-shift clinically effects much more of the DTI data

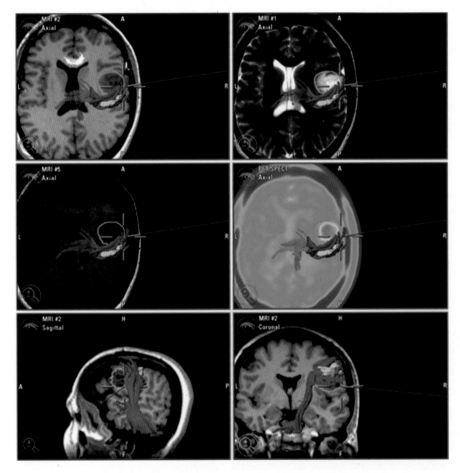

Fig. 22.4 Multimodal navigation set-up in a right precentral WHO grade III astrocytoma, functional magnetic resonance imaging (fMRI) activity delineating the motor cortex is displayed as a three-dimensional (3D) object (yellow). The reconstructed pyramidal tract is also visualized as a 3D object (blue). The tumor outline is segmented in orange as 2D contour, T1-, T2-weighted, and MR spectroscopy hybrid datasets are coregistered with positron emission tomography and functional data from fMRI and fiber tract data from diffusion tensor imaging.

because the intraoperative shifting of cortical areas during surgery can be well detected by the naked eye; however, changes in the depth of a resection cavity, close to major white matter tracts, is nearly undetectable for the neurosurgeon during tumor resection. Intraoperative DTI revealed a marked shifting of the pyramidal tract due to tumor resection.[15,50] As a consequence of this shifting, the preoperative functional data are no longer valid; hence navigation can no longer be relied on if this shifting is not compensated for. Therefore, it is necessary that not only intraoperative anatomic data are used to compensate for the effects of brain-shift, but also functional data have to be updated. Intraoperative acquisition of DTI data enables intraoperative fiber tracking to visualize how a tumor remnant is localized in relation to major white matter tracts.[15,50] Even intraoperative fMRI applying electrical stimulation of median and tibial nerves as a passive stimulation paradigm is possible and enables identification of the somatosensory cortex.[51]

Besides functional and structural data, further information is available for a multimodal navigation set-up. PET, MRS, and diffusion-weighted imaging may provide information on the diffuse tumor border. Integration of metabolic maps into the neuronavigation datasets enables a spatial correlation of metabolic data and histopathologic findings (**Fig. 22.5**).[52,53] Whether these techniques can also be used intraoperatively, so that these data can also be updated, is under investigation. Furthermore, upcoming techniques such as MR-based molecular imaging may find its role in the intraoperative imaging armamentarium.

◆ Navigation Updating

Tumor removal, brain swelling, the use of brain retractors, and cerebrospinal fluid (CSF) drainage all result in an intraoperative brain deformation – brain-shift.[24,54] Thus navigation systems relying on preoperative image data only have a decreasing accuracy during the surgical procedure. Intraoperative imaging offers the possibility to compensate for the effects of brain-shift because it provides a virtual reproduction of the actual intraoperative physical reality: on how the brain is deformed and on the achieved extent of tumor removal.[24,55–57] Compensation for brain-shift by intraoperative registration of the iMRI data to update the navigation set-up has been a cumbersome process.[56,57] In our low-field MRI setting, bone fiducial markers had to be placed around the craniotomy opening, which were then used for intraoperative patient reregistration. With the restricted image quality of the low-field MRI system, it was quite complicated to identify these markers in the intraoperative images. Furthermore, updating was a time-consuming process because these bone fiducials had to be placed around the

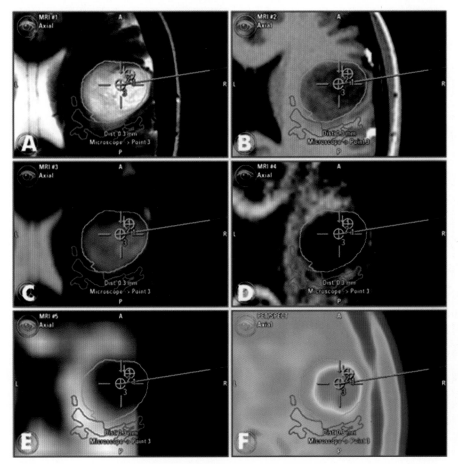

Fig. 22.5 Same patient as in Fig. 22.4. Prior to tumor resection, several biopsies were taken to correlate the histologic findings with the multimodal data; the position of the biopsy sites are recorded with the navigation system (numbers in circles). **(A)** T2-weighted, **(B)** T1-weighted with functional magnetic resonance imaging (fMRI) data superimposed, **(C)** diffusion data, **(D)** fractional anisotropy map, **(E)** magnetic resonance spectroscopy hybrid dataset, and **(F)** positron emission tomography (all axial images, the tumor is segmented in orange and the pyramidal tract in blue).

craniotomy opening; then they had to be identified and marked in the intraoperative images. After which they had to be individually identified in physical space using the tip of a pointer and correlated to the position in the intraoperative images to define the navigation coordinate system, i.e., intraoperative patient reregistration. This is the main reason why in only 16 out of 330 patients investigated with low-field MRI an actual navigation update was performed, despite the fact that intraoperative imaging had detected tumor remnants, e.g., gliomas underwent further resection in ~26% of the patients.[56,58]

The set-up integrating high-field MRI and microscope-based navigation offered to facilitate this intraoperative update procedure.[5] Besides the bone–fiducial placement for intraoperative reregistration two alternative patient registration methods and thus update strategies are available. A calibrated registration matrix can be attached to the upper part of the head coil and tracked by the navigation system.[28] This automatic registration matrix can be used for an initial patient registration. Before the patient registration, it is required that the anesthetized patient gets a preoperative 3D MRI scan after head fixation, which fully covers the registration matrix, so that all markers integrated in the registration matrix are visible and can be detected and used for registration. This approach also allows for registration of intraoperatively acquired images. A sterile registration matrix has to be connected to the sterile upper part of the head coil before it is attached to the head holder. This method serves as a backup approach if other registration strategies fail.

Navigation updating without an intraoperative patient reregistration is an even more straightforward approach. It is based on a rigid registration of the intraoperative image data with the preoperative image data, subsequent segmentation of the tumor remnant, and final restoring of the initial patient registration, so that the registration coordinate system of the preoperative image data are applied on the intraoperative images, allowing an immediate intraoperative image update. Updated image data allow a reliable identification of a tumor remnant or correction of a catheter. Microscope-based image injection with the direct visualization of the segmented tumor remnant in the surgical field plays a crucial role in the precise localization and orientation in the resection cavity (**Fig. 22.6**). Histologic analysis of the extended resections proved pathologic tissue in all cases; there were no false-positive findings. This is of course due to the fact that only areas of reliably identified tumor remnants were segmented and used for updating. The side-by-side analysis of pre- and intraoperative images greatly facilitates image interpretation and the ability to exclude misinterpretations due to surgically induced changes at the resection border.

The accuracy of intraoperative updating relying on the initial patient registration and subsequent rigid registration of pre- and intraoperative image data is dependent on whether there is positional shifting impairing the initial patient registration. In clinical practice this has not been a problem, as proven by landmark checks just after updating the navigation.

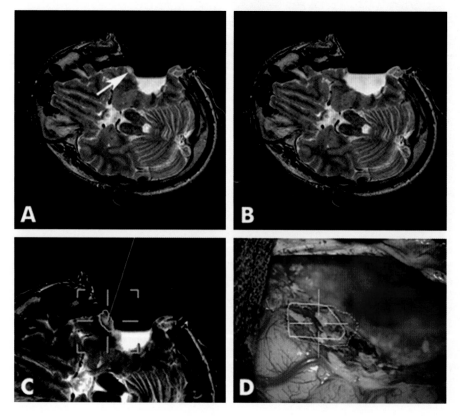

Fig. 22.6 In a right temporal lobe WHO III astrocytoma, intraoperative imaging revealed a small tumor remnant. **(A)** Intraoperative T2-weighted image; **(C)** after navigation update the remnant could be easily localized in the resection cavity, and **(D)** subsequently removed. **(B)** Proved by repeated intraoperative imaging, an identical scan to the first intraoperative scan, facilitating image comparison.

In the case of a positional shifting after initial patient registration, it is not their spatial position, but only the size of the segmented objects in the surgical field that is still displayed correctly and may serve as a guide for the extent of a tumor. To compensate for the errors in such a situation, either some intraoperative markers have to be placed around the craniotomy opening or the registration matrix for automatic registration has to be attached to the upper part of the head coil and the patient has to be rescanned, then a navigation based on the registration of the new intraoperative images is possible.

After updating a side-by-side display of pre-and intraoperative images visualizing the segmented tumor remnant in both of them is possible, facilitating orientation and image interpretation; therefore, the extent of brain-shift is also easily visible. Repeated landmark checks have proved that the rigid registration approach is a reliable approach to update the navigation system without a repeated patient registration. The rigid registration algorithm is robust enough to accomplish a registration that is not sensitive to the effects of brain-shift and the actual reduction of the tumor mass. This could be shown by analyzing the registration accuracy of structures that are not affected by brain-shift, such as the position of both orbits and the position of the skull fixation pins. An extensive analysis comparing the automatic registration, which is used to register pre- and intraoperative images, with an independent reference registration showed that the registration error is below 2 mm even in a worst case scenario.[59] Nevertheless, to prevent a misregistration a visual control after rigid registration of pre- and intraoperative images is mandatory.

Updating the navigation system with iMR image data seems to be the most reliable method to compensate for the effects of brain-shift. In contrast to previous set-ups this framework is also open to update multimodal information. Functional data, such as fMRI or DTI data can also be acquired intraoperatively and directly used for intraoperative updating, which in the clinical routine might be a time-consuming effort, especially when in the case of visualization of speech connecting fiber tracts, for example, some sophisticated time-consuming nonstandard tracking algorithms have to be applied.

Alternatively, either nonlinear registration techniques, as well as sophisticated techniques from pattern recognition analysis may allow a matching of preoperative MR datasets containing functional information with iMR image volumes.[60,61] This might also be a possibility in the case where iMRI is not available, but other imaging modalities provide intraoperative 3D information about the brain configuration, so that high-resolution multimodality data can be registered nonlinearly onto the "low-quality" intraoperative data. An alternative to iMRI might be intraoperative ultrasound, especially intraoperative 3D ultrasound.[62–64] Whether the image quality to evaluate the extent of a glioma resection is equivalent among the different imaging modalities is still controversial. However, without a doubt intraoperative ultrasound has the advantage of being a real-time modality. Ultrasound data may provide information on how to deform high-quality preoperative MR image data to represent the intraoperative "real" situation, thus compensating for the effects of brain-shift. This approach relies on the nonlinear registration of intraoperative ultrasound data with preoperative MR volume data. Consecutively, the MR data are deformed using a mathematical model describing the deformation of the brain during surgery.[65–69] Mathematical models trying to simulate brain-shift behavior will not be able to predict the actual intraoperative situation without further data. Intraoperative events such as the opening of the ventricular system and CSF drainage, patient positioning, and brain swelling all influence the extent and direction of brain-shift. However, mathematical models together with some sparse data describing the actual intraoperative 3D situation may be able to adjust high-quality preoperative data to represent the intraoperative reality.[67,69–71] Intraoperative high-field MRI with anatomic and functional imaging possibilities is the ideal tool to validate and refine these models.

◆ Conclusion

Microscope-based navigation serving as a common interface for the presentation of multimodal data in the surgical field in combination and close integration with intraoperative high-field MRI seems to be one of the most promising set-ups to avoid unwanted tumor remnants while preserving neurologic function. Multimodal navigation integrates standard anatomic, structural, functional, and metabolic data. Visualization of the initial extent of a lesion, identification of neighboring eloquent brain structures, as well as provision for the direct correlation of histology and multimodal data are the main tasks of navigation. After intraoperative imaging navigation data are updated, brain-shift may be compensated for and initially missed tumor remnants can be localized reliably.

References

1. Black PM, Moriarty T, Alexander E III, et al. Development and implementation of intraoperative magnetic resonance imaging and its neurosurgical applications. Neurosurgery 1997;41(4):831–842, discussion 842–845

2. Hall WA, Kowalik K, Liu H, Truwit CL, Kucharezyk J. Costs and benefits of intraoperative MR-guided brain tumor resection. Acta Neurochir Suppl 2003;85:137–142

3. Hall WA, Liu H, Martin AJ, Pozza CH, Maxwell RE, Truwit CL. Safety, efficacy, and functionality of high-field strength interventional magnetic resonance imaging for neurosurgery. Neurosurgery 2000; 46(3):632–641, discussion 641–642

4. Nimsky C, Ganslandt O, Fahlbusch R. Comparing 0.2 tesla with 1.5 tesla intraoperative magnetic resonance imaging analysis of setup, workflow, and efficiency. Acad Radiol 2005;12(9):1065–1079

5. Nimsky C, Ganslandt O, Von Keller B, Romstöck J, Fahlbusch R. Intraoperative high-field-strength MR imaging: implementation and experience in 200 patients. Radiology 2004;233(1):67–78

6. Sutherland GR, Kaibara T, Louw D, Hoult DI, Tomanek B, Saunders J. A mobile high-field magnetic resonance system for neurosurgery. J Neurosurg 1999;91(5):804–813

7. Nimsky C, Ganslandt O, Kober H, Buchfelder M, Fahlbusch R. Intraoperative magnetic resonance imaging combined with neuronavigation: a new concept. Neurosurgery 2001;48(5):1082–1089, discussion 1089–1091

8. Steinmeier R, Fahlbusch R, Ganslandt O, et al. Intraoperative magnetic resonance imaging with the Magnetom open scanner: concepts, neurosurgical indications, and procedures: a preliminary report. Neurosurgery 1998;43(4):739–747, discussion 747–748

9. Ganslandt O, Buchfelder M, Hastreiter P, Grummich P, Fahlbusch R, Nimsky C. Magnetic source imaging supports clinical decision making in glioma patients. Clin Neurol Neurosurg 2004;107(1):20–26

10. Ganslandt O, Steinmeier R, Kober H, et al. Magnetic source imaging combined with image-guided frameless stereotaxy: a new method in surgery around the motor strip. Neurosurgery 1997;41(3):621–627, discussion 627–628

11. Ganslandt O, Fahlbusch R, Nimsky C, et al. Functional neuronavigation with magnetoencephalography: outcome in 50 patients with lesions around the motor cortex. J Neurosurg 1999;91(1):73–79

12. Nimsky C, Ganslandt O, Kober H, et al. Integration of functional magnetic resonance imaging supported by magnetoencephalography in functional neuronavigation. Neurosurgery 1999;44(6):1249–1255, discussion 1255–1256

13. Nimsky C, Ganslandt O, Fahlbusch R. 1.5 T: intraoperative imaging beyond standard anatomic imaging. Neurosurg Clin N Am 2005;16(1):185–200, vii vii

14. Nimsky C, Ganslandt O, Fahlbusch R. Implementation of fiber tract navigation. Neurosurgery 2006; 58(4 Suppl 2):306–317

15. Nimsky C, Ganslandt O, Hastreiter P, et al. Preoperative and intraoperative diffusion tensor imaging-based fiber tracking in glioma surgery. Neurosurgery 2005;56(1):130–137, discussion 138

16. Nimsky C, Ganslandt O, Merhof D, Sorensen AG, Fahlbusch R. Intraoperative visualization of the pyramidal tract by diffusion-tensor-imaging-based fiber tracking. Neuroimage 2006;30(4):1219–1229

17. Ganslandt O, Stadlbauer A, Fahlbusch R, et al. Proton magnetic resonance spectroscopic imaging integrated into image-guided surgery: correlation to standard magnetic resonance imaging and tumor cell density. Neurosurgery 2005; 56(2, Suppl)291–298, discussion 291–298

18. Stadlbauer A, Ganslandt O, Buslei R, et al. Gliomas: histopathologic evaluation of changes in directionality and magnitude of water diffusion at diffusion-tensor MR imaging. Radiology 2006;240(3):803–810

19. Stadlbauer A, Moser E, Gruber S, Nimsky C, Fahlbusch R, Ganslandt O. Integration of biochemical images of a tumor into frameless stereotaxy achieved using a magnetic resonance imaging/magnetic resonance spectroscopy hybrid data set. J Neurosurg 2004;101(2):287–294

20. Stadlbauer A, Nimsky C, Buslei R, et al. Proton magnetic resonance spectroscopic imaging in the border zone of gliomas: correlation of metabolic and histological changes at low tumor infiltration—initial results. Invest Radiol 2007;42(4):218–223

21. Stadlbauer A, Nimsky C, Buslei R, et al. Diffusion tensor imaging and optimized fiber tracking in glioma patients: histopathologic evaluation of tumor-invaded white matter structures. Neuroimage 2007;34(3):949–956

22. Stadlbauer A, Prante O, Nimsky C, et al. Metabolic imaging of cerebral gliomas: spatial correlation of changes in O-(2-18F-fluoroethyl)-L-tyrosine PET and proton magnetic resonance spectroscopic imaging. J Nucl Med 2008;49(5):721–729

23. Black PM, Alexander E III, Martin C, et al. Craniotomy for tumor treatment in an intraoperative magnetic resonance imaging unit. Neurosurgery 1999;45(3):423–431, discussion 431–433

24. Nabavi A, Black PM, Gering DT, et al. Serial intraoperative magnetic resonance imaging of brain shift. Neurosurgery 2001;48(4):787–797, discussion 797–798

25. Truwit CL, Liu H. Prospective stereotaxy: a novel method of trajectory alignment using real-time image guidance. J Magn Reson Imaging 2001;13(3):452–457

26. Hall WA, Liu H, Truwit CL. Navigus trajectory guide. Neurosurgery 2000;46(2):502–504

27. Truwit CL, Hall WA. Intraoperative magnetic resonance imaging-guided neurosurgery at 3-T. Neurosurgery 2006; 58(4, Suppl 2) 338–345

28. Rachinger J, von Keller B, Ganslandt O, Fahlbusch R, Nimsky C. Application accuracy of automatic registration in frameless stereotaxy. Stereotact Funct Neurosurg 2006;84(2-3):109–117

29. Steinmeier R, Rachinger J, Kaus M, Ganslandt O, Huk W, Fahlbusch R. Factors influencing the application accuracy of neuronavigation systems. Stereotact Funct Neurosurg 2000;75(4):188–202

30. Sumanaweera TS, Adler JR Jr, Napel S, Glover GH. Characterization of spatial distortion in magnetic resonance imaging and its implications for stereotactic surgery. Neurosurgery 1994;35(4):696–703, discussion 703–704

31. Raabe A, Krishnan R, Wolff R, Hermann E, Zimmermann M, Seifert V. Laser surface scanning for patient registration in intracranial image-guided surgery. Neurosurgery 2002;50(4):797–801, discussion 802–803

32. Villalobos H, Germano IM. Clinical evaluation of multimodality registration in frameless stereotaxy. Comput Aided Surg 1999;4(1):45–49

33. Wolfsberger S, Rössler K, Regatschnig R, Ungersböck K. Anatomical landmarks for image registration in frameless stereotactic neuronavigation. Neurosurg Rev 2002;25(1-2):68–72

34. Barnett GH, Miller DW, Weisenberger J. Frameless stereotaxy with scalp-applied fiducial markers for brain biopsy procedures: experience in 218 cases. J Neurosurg 1999;91(4):569–576

35. Kozak J, Nesper M, Fischer M, et al. Semiautomated registration using new markers for assessing the accuracy of a navigation system. Comput Aided Surg 2002;7(1):11–24

36. Nimsky C, Ganslandt O, Fahlbusch R. Functional neuronavigation and intraoperative MRI. Adv Tech Stand Neurosurg 2004;29:229–263

37. Hentschel SJ, Sawaya R. Optimizing outcomes with maximal surgical resection of malignant gliomas. Cancer Control 2003;10(2):109–114

38. Hund M, Rezai AR, Kronberg E, et al. Magnetoencephalographic mapping: basis of a new functional risk profile in the selection of patients with cortical brain lesions. Neurosurgery 1997;40(5):936–942, discussion 942–943

39. Ammirati M, Galicich JH, Arbit E, Liao Y. Reoperation in the treatment of recurrent intracranial malignant gliomas. Neurosurgery 1987;21(5):607–614

40. Black PM. Surgery for cerebral gliomas: past, present and future. In: Howard III MA, Elliott JP, Haglund MM. McKhann II GM, eds. Clinical Neurosurgery. Boston: Lippincott Williams & Wilkins; 1999: 21–45

41. Cabantog AM, Bernstein M. Complications of first craniotomy for intra-axial brain tumour. Can J Neurol Sci 1994;21(3):213–218

42. Ciric I, Ammirati M, Vick N, Mikhael M. Supratentorial gliomas: surgical considerations and immediate postoperative results. Gross total resection versus partial resection. Neurosurgery 1987;21(1):21–26

43. Fadul C, Wood J, Thaler H, Galicich J, Patterson RH Jr, Posner JB. Morbidity and mortality of craniotomy for excision of supratentorial gliomas. Neurology 1988;38(9):1374–1379

44. Grummich P, Nimsky C, Pauli E, Buchfelder M, Ganslandt O. Combining fMRI and MEG increases the reliability of presurgical language localization: a clinical study on the difference between and congruence of both modalities. Neuroimage 2006;32(4):1793–1803

45. Kober H, Möller M, Nimsky C, Vieth J, Fahlbusch R, Ganslandt O. New approach to localize speech relevant brain areas and hemispheric dominance using spatially filtered magnetoencephalography. Hum Brain Mapp 2001;14(4):236–250

46. Hendler T, Pianka P, Sigal M, et al. Delineating gray and white matter involvement in brain lesions: three-dimensional alignment of functional magnetic resonance and diffusion-tensor imaging. J Neurosurg 2003;99(6):1018–1027

47. Clark CA, Barrick TR, Murphy MM, Bell BA. White matter fiber tracking in patients with space-occupying lesions of the brain: a new technique for neurosurgical planning? Neuroimage 2003;20(3):1601–1608

48. Coenen VA, Krings T, Mayfrank L, et al. Three-dimensional visualization of the pyramidal tract in a neuronavigation system during brain tumor surgery: first experiences and technical note. Neurosurgery 2001;49(1):86–92, discussion 92–93

49. Nimsky C, Grummich P, Sorensen AG, Fahlbusch R, Ganslandt O. Visualization of the pyramidal tract in glioma surgery by integrating diffusion tensor imaging in functional neuronavigation. Zentralbl Neurochir 2005;66(3):133–141

50. Nimsky C, Ganslandt O, Hastreiter P, et al. Intraoperative diffusion-tensor MR imaging: shifting of white matter tracts during neurosurgical procedures—initial experience. Radiology 2005;234(1):218–225

51. Gasser T, Ganslandt O, Sandalcioglu E, Stolke D, Fahlbusch R, Nimsky C. Intraoperative functional MRI: implementation and preliminary experience. Neuroimage 2005;26(3):685–693

52. Stadlbauer A, Moser E, Gruber S, Nimsky C, Fahlbusch R, Ganslandt O. Integration of biochemical images of a tumor into frameless stereotaxy achieved using a magnetic resonance imaging/magnetic resonance spectroscopy hybrid data set. J Neurosurg 2004;101(2):287–294

53. Stadlbauer A, Moser E, Gruber S, et al. Improved delineation of brain tumors: an automated method for segmentation based on pathologic changes of 1H-MRSI metabolites in gliomas. Neuroimage 2004;23(2):454–461

54. Hastreiter P, Rezk-Salama C, Nimsky C, et al. Registration techniques for the analysis of the brain shift in neurosurgery. Comput Graph 2000;24(3):385–389

55. Hastreiter P, Rezk-Salama C, Soza G, et al. Strategies for brain shift evaluation. Med Image Anal 2004;8(4):447–464

56. Nimsky C, Ganslandt O, Hastreiter P, Fahlbusch R. Intraoperative compensation for brain shift. Surg Neurol 2001;56(6):357–364, discussion 364–365

57. Wirtz CR, Bonsanto MM, Knauth M, et al. Intraoperative magnetic resonance imaging to update interactive navigation in neurosurgery: method and preliminary experience. Comput Aided Surg 1997;2(3-4):172–179

58. Nimsky C, Ganslandt O, Tomandl B, Buchfelder M, Fahlbusch R. Low-field magnetic resonance imaging for intraoperative use in neurosurgery: a 5-year experience. Eur Radiol 2002;12(11):2690–2703

59. Veyrat A. Automatic fusion of pre-and intraoperative patient data. A statistical evaluation of accuracy [doctoral dissertation]. Munich: Technical University; 2005

60. Archip N, Clatz O, Whalen S, et al. Non-rigid alignment of pre-operative MRI, fMRI, and DT-MRI with intra-operative MRI for enhanced visualization and navigation in image-guided neurosurgery. Neuroimage 2007;35(2):609–624

61. Wolf M, Vogel T, Weierich P, Niemann H, Nimsky C. Automatic transfer of preoperative fMRI markers into intraoperative MR-images for updating functional neuronavigation. IEICE T Inf Syst 2001;84(12):1698–1704

62. Comeau RM, Sadikot AF, Fenster A, Peters TM. Intraoperative ultrasound for guidance and tissue shift correction in image-guided neurosurgery. Med Phys 2000;27(4):787–800

63. Tirakotai W, Miller D, Heinze S, Benes L, Bertalanffy H, Sure U. A novel platform for image-guided ultrasound. Neurosurgery 2006;58(4):710–718, discussion 710–718

64. Letteboer MM, Willems PW, Viergever MA, Niessen WJ. Brain shift estimation in image-guided neurosurgery using 3-D ultrasound. IEEE Trans Biomed Eng 2005;52(2):268–276

65. Rasmussen IA Jr, Lindseth F, Rygh OM, et al. Functional neuronavigation combined with intra-operative 3D ultrasound: initial experiences during surgical resections close to eloquent brain areas and future directions in automatic brain shift compensation of preoperative data. Acta Neurochir (Wien) 2007;149(4):365–378

66. Arbel T, Morandi X, Comeau RM, Collins DL. Automatic non-linear MRI-ultrasound registration for the correction of intra-operative brain deformations. Comput Aided Surg 2004;9(4):123–136

67. Lunn KE, Paulsen KD, Lynch DR, Roberts DW, Kennedy FE, Hartov A. Assimilating intraoperative data with brain shift modeling using the adjoint equations. Med Image Anal 2005;9(3):281–293

68. Coenen VA, Krings T, Weidemann J, et al. Sequential visualization of brain and fiber tract deformation during intracranial surgery with three-dimensional ultrasound: an approach to evaluate the effect of brain shift. Neurosurgery 2005; 56(1, Suppl)133–141, discussion 133–141

69. Roberts DW, Miga MI, Hartov A, et al. Intraoperatively updated neuroimaging using brain modeling and sparse data. Neurosurgery 1999;45(5):1199–1206, discussion 1206–1207

70. Cao A, Thompson RC, Dumpuri P, et al. Laser range scanning for image-guided neurosurgery: investigation of image-to-physical space registrations. Med Phys 2008;35(4):1593–1605

71. Ding S, Miga MI, Thompson RC, et al. Estimation of intra-operative brain shift using a tracked laser range scanner. In: Conference Proceedings of the 29th Annual International Conference of the IEEE Engineering in Medicine and Biology Society. Piscataway, NJ: IEEE; 2007:848–851

23

Neurosurgical Robots: A Review

Shelly Lwu and Garnette R. Sutherland

The past two decades have witnessed an evolution in the robots developed for neurosurgery and spinal surgery. Although the earlier robots were machines capable of a limited number of specific and well-defined tasks, the newer generations of neurosurgical robots are designed to be able to perform more complex maneuvers and have more dexterity for enhanced tool manipulation. Up until the present time, manipulation of the robot has been under the direct control of the neurosurgeon. There is now, however, a trend toward automating some of the functions. We present here a review of the robots that have been developed for neurosurgery and spinal surgery, with an in-depth review of our project at the University of Calgary–neuroArm.

◆ Introduction

Neurosurgical robotics unifies the advantages of high-resolution imaging, neuronavigation, and robotic technology into a tool that can advance the diagnosis and treatment of brain and spinal pathologies. This was a logical evolution over the past several decades. The introduction of the operating microscope propelled the refinement in neurosurgical technique and instruments. The development of computed tomography (CT) and magnetic resonance imaging (MRI) provided enhanced lesion localization and anatomic detail. This allowed for the development of neuronavigation systems which link surgical procedure to the preoperative or intraoperatively acquired images, further increasing precision and accuracy. Together, these technologies provided the basis for progressively narrower surgical corridors, pushing surgeons toward the limits of their spatial orientation and technical ability. Image-guided robotics evolved as a means to overcome these limitations. Computers and robotics are able to process and utilize large amounts of quantitative information and are well-suited to tasks requiring high levels of accuracy, precision, and repetition.

We present here a review of the robots that have been developed for neurosurgery, with an in-depth review of neuroArm. Although this is by no means an exhaustive review, it includes systems that have contributed to the development of present day technology, which have clinical application (**Fig. 23.1**). The review also includes promising robotic systems that may be still in preclinical stages.

◆ Early Neurosurgical Robots

Programmable Universal Machine for Assembly

The programmable universal machine for assembly robot (PUMA; Advance Research and Robotics, Oxford, CT) was the first robot to be used in neurosurgical procedures. In 1985, Kwoh et al used the PUMA 200 robot in a stereotactic biopsy, where the robot was used to orient a cannula through which a needle was inserted.[1] In 1991, Drake et al used the PUMA 200 robot as a retractor holder in the resection of pediatric thalamic astrocytomas.[2]

The PUMA robot had a single arm with 6 degrees of freedom DOF.[1] The arm was capable of gripping and manipulating a biopsy cannula or a brain retractor. During surgery, a stereotactic frame base ring was placed on the patient and attached to the CT table. Following CT image acquisition, the stereotactic coordinates of the target lesion are computed, and based on three-dimensional (3D) reconstruction of the preoperative images, a desired trajectory was selected at the workstation.[2] The robot arm gripping the surgical instrument could then be programmed to move in line with and along the planned trajectory and the surgical instrument further manipulated with the computer interface. Calibration of the tool tip to the center of the stereotactic frame allowed for its position and orientation to be displayed in relation to the target lesion and the surrounding anatomic structures in 3D.

Despite early successes, the project was terminated because of safety concerns related to the operation of an industrial robot in an operating room.

Neurosurgical Robots:
First Published Clinical Use in Humans

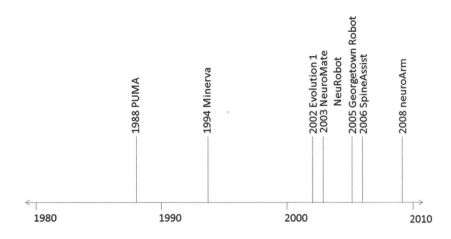

Fig. 23.1 Neurosurgical robots: first published clinical use in humans. This timeline denotes the neurosurgical robotic systems in the present review that have been used clinically. The year noted represents that of publication in a peer-reviewed journal of the first clinical use. The systems that are still in their preclinical stages have not been included in this timeline.

NeuroMate

NeuroMate (Integrated Surgical Systems, Davis, CA) was designed to assist with stereotactic procedures using image guidance.[3] It was based on earlier work by Benabid and colleagues at the Grenoble University Hospital in France in the mid 1980s.[4] In 1997, it received United States Food and Drug Administration (FDA) approval, for use in stereotactic neurosurgery.[5] NeuroMate has been successfully used in numerous stereotactic neurosurgical procedures, including tumor biopsy and placement of electrodes for deep brain stimulation.[6,7]

The robot has a single arm with 5 DOF and may be used in a frame-based or frameless mode for stereotaxy (**Fig. 23.2A**).[3] In the frameless mode, NeuroMate uses an ultrasound registration system. Preoperative imaging is obtained in the form of CT, MRI, digital subtraction angiography, or digitized radiographs. These are transferred to the planning computer workstation where the target trajectory is defined, using PC-based kinematic positioning software. The finalized plan is then transferred via Ethernet to the control workstation in the operating room. The surgeon uses the defined trajectory to command the robot arm holding the mechanical guide to move into target position, where it is

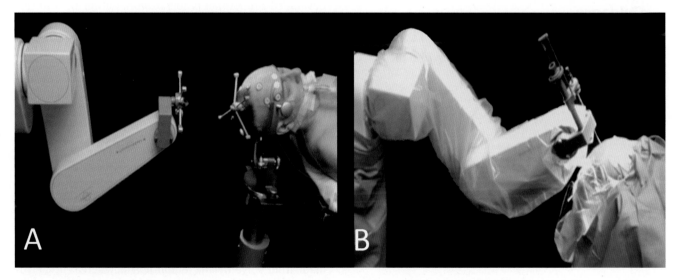

Fig. 23.2 NeuroMate (Integrated Surgical Systems, Davis, CA) was designed to assist with stereotactic neurosurgical procedures under image guidance. **(A)** For frameless stereotaxy, registration of the NeuroMate arm to the patient occurs using an ultrasound-based system. **(B)** After the planned trajectory is defined, NeuroMate moves into the surgical field in preparation for the biopsy. (Courtesy of Qing Hang Li, MD PhD, Wayne State University, Detroit, MI.)

fixed in place (**Fig. 23.2B**). The surgeon uses the mechanical guide to direct the trajectory of manual drilling or the insertion of a biopsy needle or an electrode. NeuroMate is not able to actuate a biopsy tool or other instruments. The main use of the NeuroMate system was to assist with lesion localization and targeting and provide tool stabilization and support.

Evolution 1

The Evolution 1 robot (Universal Robot Systems, Schwerin, Germany) was designed for precision in neurosurgical and endoscopic procedures. Evolution 1 has a single arm and utilizes hexapod platform with 6 DOF.[8] Positional accuracy is reported on the order of 10 μm.[9] Speed ranges from slow (0.5 mm/s) to fast (2 mm/s). The robot has a small working distance and therefore must be prepositioned by the surgeon ~5 cm above the entry point, in the general direction of use. User interface at the workstation is a touchscreen; intraoperative steering of the robot arm is performed with a joystick.

Use of Evolution 1 has been reported in neuroendoscopy as a tool for the positioning and maneuvering the ventriculoscope.[8,9] After navigation has been achieved using a combination of preoperative MRI and VectorVision system (BrainLab, Heimstetten, Germany), the skin incision and burr hole are performed manually by the neurosurgeon. The ventriculoscope is then maneuvered through the brain parenchyma into the ventricle, at which point the endoscope is inserted. It has also been adapted for endoscopic transsphenoidal resections of pituitary adenomas.[10] Robotic assistance with the endoscope in these cases allows the neurosurgeon to use two instruments simultaneously during surgery.

◆ Neurosurgical Robots with Image Guidance

The next logical step in the evolution of the neurosurgical robot was to couple intraoperative imaging with the robot to achieve more accuracy and precision during surgical dissection. The problem of brain-shift invalidates neuronavigation technology based on preoperative images. Intraoperative imaging, with up-to-date rendering of the brain, compensates for brain-shift that might occur during the procedure. In addition, real-time imaging allows the neurosurgeon to be able to make appropriate adjustments to the trajectory of the biopsy cannula or electrode during a stereotactic procedure. Initial efforts with an intraoperative CT system quickly stalled, soon to be followed by the more successful application of intraoperative MRI (iMRI).

Minerva

The Minerva robot (University of Lausanne, Lausanne, Switzerland) was the first real-time image-guidance system, designed solely for stereotactic neurosurgical procedures. The robot was designed to work within a CT scanner. This

meant that instrument position during a stereotactic procedure could be monitored by taking successive scans, producing real-time imaging.

Minerva is positioned behind the CT scanner with the arm operating inside the CT gantry.[11] The robot is linked to the CT table and moves freely along the longitudinal axis on rails. The stereotactic head frame is coupled to the scanner table to ensure precision with regard to the patient's head position. The robot arm has 5 DOF. Depth electrodes and biopsy instruments have been specially developed for use by the robot. Once the target lesion and trajectory have been selected, the authors claimed that skin incision, bone drilling, dural perforation, and probe manipulation could occur in an automated fashion.[12] Minerva offered the potential benefit of decreased total procedure time as the surgery could be performed within the scanner without having to transfer the patient from room to room and without the intermediate step of transferring and calculating coordinates.

The first clinical applications of Minerva were the successful aspiration and biopsy of malignant intracerebral cystic lesions in two patients.[11] The same group went on to report at least eight subsequent successful stereotactic biopsies.[12] Minerva has also been reported in use in phantom studies with 3D electrode probe placement at an accuracy of 1.3 mm.[13] Unfortunately, CT scanners can only obtain images in a single dimension, and repetitive scanning meant that the patient was exposed to large doses of radiation: this contributed to the termination of the project.

MRI-Compatible Robots

Harvard Medical School, the Surgical Planning Laboratory (SPL) at Brigham and Women's Hospital (Boston, MA), and the Surgical Assist Technology Group of the Agency of Industrial Science and Technology (AIST; Tsukuba, Japan) developed a robot that is able to work within an iMRI system (Signa SP/i, 0.5 tesla [T], General Electric Medical Systems, Waukesha, WI).[14] The open gantry parallel-facing donut-shaped magnets had an air gap of 56 cm, which provided enough room for a surgeon to work within the magnet. The main body of the robot and the actuators are mounted at the top of the magnet, above the head of the surgeon. The end-effector, which has 5 DOF, is attached to the main body of the robot by two rigid arms. The robot was built with titanium and plastics and includes piezoelectric actuators. Essentially, the robot functions as an aid for the precise positioning of probes and biopsy needles in stereotactic procedures. The main clinical use for the SPL/AIST robot has been in prostate biopsies and brachytherapy.[15,16]

Masamune et al at the Mechatronics Laboratory at the University of Tokyo developed an MRI-compatible needle manipulator for use in stereotactic neurosurgical procedures.[17] The manipulator arm and frame attachment are made from polyethylene terephthalate, whereas nonferromagnetic materials, such as brass, aluminum, polyoxymethylene (Delrin; DuPont, Wilmington, DE), ceramics, and polyetheretherketone were used for the bearings, screws, and gears. Piezoelectric ultrasonic motors are used for the actuators. The manipulator and frame, with 6 DOF, are mounted on an XYZ-base stage that is attached to the scanner bed for precision. The entire system fits within an MRI gantry of 60 cm in diameter. Using a personal computer at the workstation, the target lesion can be localized and a trajectory can be selected. Data transfer from workstation to the robot occurs by way of a direct cable connection.

◆ Neurosurgical Robots for Enhanced Tool Manipulation

Although the earlier neurosurgical robots functioned mainly as mechanical guides for stereotactic procedures, more recent systems saw the development of the robot as a tool for microsurgery. Newer robots incorporated various features to enhance the dexterity of the end-effector, such as haptic feedback, tremor filters, and motion scaling. They had specially designed instruments to be able to accomplish specific tasks. They were designed to enhance microsurgical techniques and procedures.

Robot-Assisted Microsurgery System

The robot-assisted microsurgery system (RAMS) was designed by the National Aeronautic and Space Administration's Jet Propulsion Laboratory (Pasadena, CA) in collaboration with MicroDexterity Systems, Inc. (Memphis, TN). RAMS is based on a master–slave control system and is neither MRI-compatible or image-guided. The single robot arm is designed to simulate the movements of a human upper extremity.[18] The slave robot has 10 joints and 6 DOF and is controlled by a master robot input handle, which has eight joints and 6 DOF. A laptop computer at the workstation uses a graphics user interface (GUI) for configuration of system parameters.

The robot arm is 34.6 cm long, from base to tip, and 2.5 cm in diameter, allowing for a large working field.[18] It is mounted on a cylindrical base and driven by tendons. Together, the arm and the base weigh 2.5 kg, and can sustain a load of over 3 pounds. Its working area is 30 cm diameter. While force scaling, motion scaling and tremor filtering have been incorporated into the system; there is no haptic feedback to the neurosurgeon.[19]

RAMS was designed to enhance the surgeon's performance. The neurosurgeon holds the master input handle the same way he would hold a conventional surgical instrument, in either his right or left hand, to command the slave robot in the manipulation of tissues or sutures.[20] Le Roux et al conducted feasibility studies regarding the use of RAMS for microvascular anastomosis in neurosurgery.[20] Rat carotid arteriotomies were performed and closed using either RAMS or conventional microsurgical techniques by surgeons, students, and engineers. Performance was measured in terms of vessel patency, surgical time, and surgical errors. Although RAMS could not be used to hold needles or to place sutures, it was used to manipulate the vessel or hold the vessel wall that was being sutured. The robot was also used to perform knot tying. All the procedures were successfully completed. RAMS was found to be as effective as the surgical group in all areas of performance except for the surgical time, which was twice as long.

Steady-Hand Robotics System

Taylor et al at Johns Hopkins University (Baltimore, MD) approached robotics systems as a tool to enhance the performance of the surgeon. With the Steady-Hand robotics system, the surgeon manipulates tools that are held by the robot, while the robot controls for the forces exerted and scales down motion amplitude (**Fig. 23.3**).[21] Low-threshold silicon strain gauges situated within the handles of the tools

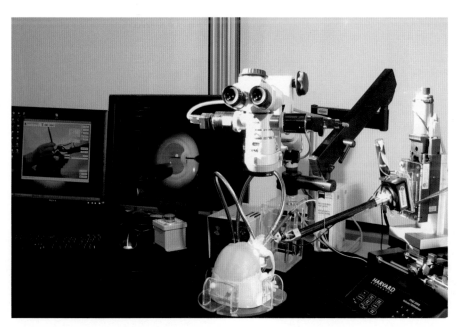

Fig. 23.3 The Steady-Hand robotic system (Johns Hopkins University, Baltimore, MD) was designed to "fine-tune" the surgeon's movements by scaling down force and motion. The third-generation robot, a video microscope, a two-dimensional display monitor, and a second monitor displaying system configuration comprise the current workstation. (Courtesy of Russell Taylor, PhD, Johns Hopkins University, Baltimore, MD.)

detect the force applied by the surgeon as well as the resistance from the tissue. The control system processes this information and then responds accordingly with force adjustments. In such a way, the robot can assist the surgeon to achieve smooth and tremor-free tissue manipulation with precision and the gentlest touch. At present, there is no available literature on clinical application.

NeuRobot

NeuRobot (Shinshu University School of Medicine, Matsuoto, Japan) was developed as a telecontrolled micromanipulator system for neurosurgery. NeuRobot has four main parts: a slave micromanipulator arm, a manipulator supporting device, a master operation-input device, and a 3D display monitor (**Fig. 23.4A**).[22] The micromanipulator arm is a long thin tube of 10 mm in external diameter, which houses three micromanipulators and a rigid 3D endoscope, of 1 and 4 mm in diameter, respectively (**Fig. 23.4B**). Each micromanipulator has 3 DOF and can be fitted with specially designed microinstruments, such as forceps, laser tips, scalpels, and dissectors as needed during surgery. The

microforceps attachment allows for a payload of 60 g. Several openings near the micromanipulators and endoscope can be adapted for suction and irrigation. The manipulator supporting device has six motor-driven joints, which provide 6 DOF. The joints are driven by ultrasonic motors.

NeuRobot is telecapable. Using the control panel, the neurosurgeon can move the manipulator arm into position by pressing direction-indicating arrows or inputting digits for each joint of the manipulator supporting device.[22] Using the master operation-input device that consists of three levers, each with 3 DOF, the neurosurgeon can operate the three micromanipulators from a remote location while viewing the 3D display monitor with polarizing lenses.

NeuRobot has been used in cadaveric studies as well as in surgery. NeuRobot was used to perform the opening of a sylvian fissure and a third ventriculostomy in cadaver heads.[22] It was also used to partially resect a recurrent meningioma in a 54-year-old patient.[23] The craniotomy and dural opening were performed manually. To demonstrate the feasibility of NeuRobot in telesurgery, surgery on rat brains was performed in a hospital 40 km away from the workstation.[24]

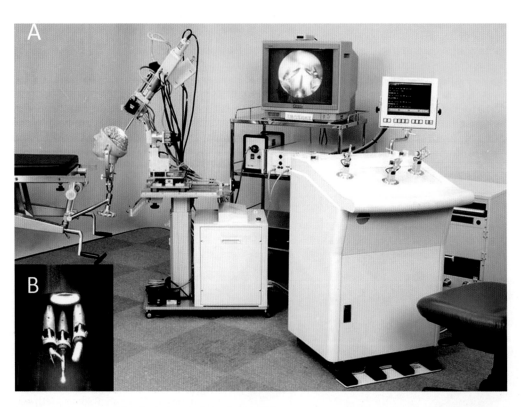

Fig. 23.4 NeuRobot (Shinshu University School of Medicine, Matsuoto, Japan) is a micromanipulator system designed for telesurgery. **(A)** The slave manipulator is positioned at the head of the operative table, while the workstation can be located remotely. The workstation comprises the three master hand controllers and the three-dimensional (3D) display monitor. **(B)** The slave manipulator arm houses three micromanipulators, which correspond to the three master hand controllers, and a rigid 3D endoscope. Microforceps, a laser tip, and a silicon tube attachment are shown. ([A] from Hongo K, Goto T, Miyahara T, et al. Telecontrolled micromanipulator system (NeuRobot) for minimally invasive neurosurgery. Acta Neurochir Suppl. 2006; 98: 64. [B] From Koyama J, Hongo K, Kakizawa Y, et al. Endoscopic telerobotics for neurosurgery: preliminary study for optimal distance between an object lens and a target. Neurol Res 2002; 24(4): 374. Reprinted with permission of Maney Publishing.)

◆ Spinal Surgery Robots

The trend toward minimally invasive spinal surgery is compatible with the development of robots dedicated to spinal surgery. Much like stereotactic neurosurgery, the goals in the placement of surgical hardware are accuracy and precision. The spinal surgical robots available at present function mainly as mechanical guides for the placement of needles and pedicle screws.

Georgetown Robot

Georgetown University Medical Center (Washington, DC), in collaboration with the Urology Robotics Laboratory of Johns Hopkins Medical Institutions at Johns Hopkins University (Baltimore, MD) developed a robotic needle driver for use in minimally invasive spine procedures.[25] The system is designed for use within an interventional suite, under biplane fluoroscopic guidance. The robot arm has 6 DOF and along with its joystick and touchscreen controls, is mounted on the scanner table. Once the robot arm is positioned manually near the skin entry point, the controls are switched over to joystick operation. Movement occurs in 1 DOF at a time. A personal computer chassis houses the main controls for the robot and is located in the back of the interventional suite. It is connected to the robot at the bedside by cables.

This robotic needle driver has been tested successfully in percutaneous facet blocks in both cadaveric and live patient studies.[26] In human studies, the positioning accuracy by the robot and the pain relief provided were comparable to that of the standard manual procedure.

SpineAssist

SpineAssist (MAZOR Surgical Technologies, Ltd., Caesarea, Israel) is a miniature robotic system developed as a guide for tool positioning and screw placement in spinal surgery. The robot measures 50 mm in diameter and 80 mm in height and weighs only 250 g (**Fig. 23.5**).[27] The robot has 6 DOF and is linked to the workstation by cables. The workstation uses specially designed GUI software in the registration of the preoperative CT images, the planning of optimal entry point and trajectory for the pedicle screw, and the control of the robot movements. Three different outrigger arm attachments are possible, each with a drill guide sleeve that can be attached to the upper moving platform.

In the preoperative planning stage, the surgeon chooses the screw to be used and plans the desired entry point and trajectory for each vertebra.[28] Virtual projections in three planes (axial, lateral, and anteroposterior) of each vertebra are reconstructed from the preoperative CT scans at the workstation. The surgeon then attaches the clamp system to the spinous process of a vertebra, in the proximity of the site of operation, through a 1.5-inch incision in the skin.[27] Alternatively, a minimally invasive Hover-T frame can be mounted to an iliac crest and one spinous process. An automatic CT-to-fluoroscopy registration process then follows, whereby the reconstructed CT images with the surgeon's

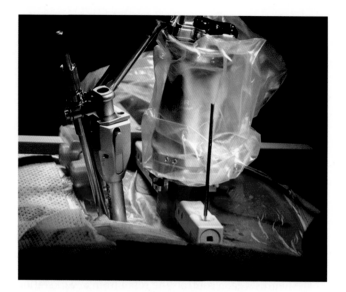

Fig. 23.5 SpineAssist (MAZOR Surgical Technologies, Ltd., Caesarea, Israel) is a miniature robotic system designed to aid in tool positioning and pedicle screw placement in spine surgery. The robot is mounted to a Hover-T frame, which is attached to the patient's iliac crest and spinous process. After automated computed tomography-to-fluoroscopy registration, the robot moves the cannulated guide into position, based on preoperatively defined entry points and trajectories. (Courtesy of Moshe Shoham, PhD, Israel Institute of Technology, Haifa, Israel.)

plans are matched to the intraoperative fluoroscopic images with the targeting device. Once the surgeon verifies and approves the plan, the targeting device used during registration is then replaced with a multilevel bridge onto which the robot is mounted. The robot then moves the cannulated guide into the desired entry point and trajectory based on the preoperative plan and locks in place. The surgeon can then proceed with the drilling or the introduction of a needle or guide-wire through the cannulated guide.

SpineAssist has been used successfully in clinical applications. In a series of 14 patients in which the SpineAssist system was used, 96% of the screws placed were within 1 mm of their planned trajectory.[29,30] Since receiving FDA approval for use in spinal surgery, it has become available commercially. The miniature robot from the SpineAssist system is also being developed for minimally invasive keyhole neurosurgery.[31] The robot attaches to a head clamp or directly to the patient's skull and acts as a mechanical guide for needle, probe, or catheter insertion. It uses an intraoperative 3D surface scan of the patient's facial features for registration. The robot then automatically positions itself based on targets defined on the preoperative CT or MRI images.

◆ NeuroArm

NeuroArm is the MR-compatible robot developed by the University of Calgary (Alberta, Canada).[32–35] NeuroArm unifies some of the best features of its predecessors and contemporaries. NeuroArm can operate within an intraoperative

MRI environment for stereotactic procedures as well as perform image-guided microsurgery outside of the magnet. For enhanced tool manipulation, neuroArm has incorporated features such as haptic feedback, tremor filter, and motion scaling. NeuroArm has two manipulators, or arms, that are able to mimic the performance of the primary neurosurgeon. The system is telecapable and includes a multisensory human–machine interface. Overall, neuroArm is a multifunctional and highly adaptable system.

NeuroArm's two manipulators are mounted on an adjustable mobile base along with a digitizing arm and a field camera (**Fig. 23.6**). Each manipulator has 7 DOF, including 1 DOF for tool actuation. During stereotactic procedures within the MRI gantry, either manipulator can be removed from the base unit and mounted onto a platform attached to the magnet. For MRI compatibility, the manipulators are made from titanium and polyetheretherketone, a plastic polymer.

The neurosurgeon controls the robot from a workstation located in a room adjacent to the operating room. The workstation is composed of a computer processor, two hand controllers for maneuvering the robot manipulators, a Spaceball 3D motion controller (3Dconnexion, Fremont, CA), four desk-mounted monitors, and a binocular visual display (**Fig. 23.7**). The robot operates under a master–slave control system, where the surgeon's movements of the hand controllers at the workstation are replicated by the robot arms. This, in turn, requires that the workstation

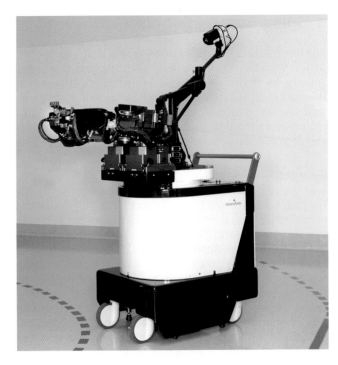

Fig. 23.6 NeuroArm has two manipulators, each with 7 DOF, to mimic the neurosurgeon. The manipulators are made from titanium, polyetheretherketone, and polyoxymethylene, all MRI-compatible materials. The manipulators, one digitizing arm, and a field camera are mounted on an adjustable mobile base.

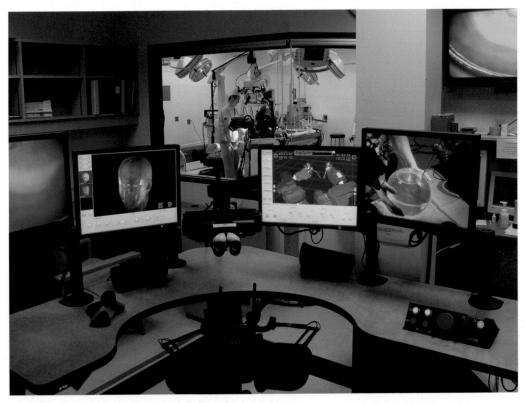

Fig. 23.7 Workstation. A computer processor, two force-feedback hand controllers, a Spaceball 3D motion controller (3Dconnexion, Fremont, CA), four desk-mounted monitors (two video monitors and two touchscreen displays), and a binocular stereoscopic display unit comprise the neuroArm workstation, which is located in an adjacent room.

provide the neurosurgeon with multisensory feedback in audio, visual, and tactile formats.

Two-way communication occurs between the members of the surgical team by way of a wireless intercom system (DX200 Digital Wireless Intercom system, HM Electronics, Inc., Poway, CA). Headsets are worn by the surgical team within the operating room, while the surgeon sitting at the workstation uses a desk-mounted microphone and speakers. In addition, a microphone mounted to the microscope transmits to the surgeon the sounds of surgical dissection. Digital encryption and a frequency-hopping spread spectrum ensure confidentiality of communication and at a frequency of 2.4 Hz, there is no interference with MRI.

Visual feedback is also reproduced with high fidelity at the workstation. Two high-definition cameras (Ikegami Tsushinki Co., Ltd., Tokyo, Japan) are mounted to the surgical microscope and transmit images to two miniature full-color monitors (Rockwell Collins Inc., Cedar Rapids, IA) fitted within the binocular display unit, at 1000 television lines (TVL) horizontal resolution. This provides a 3D stereoscopic view of the surgical site, reproducing the experience of looking directly into the microscope for the neurosurgeon. Two of the four video monitors display the field camera view and the single channel view from the left ocular piece of the stereoscopic display unit, both at XGA 1024 × 768 resolution. The other two monitors are interactive touchscreens. One of the touchscreen monitors displays 2D or 3D MR images that can be manipulated, using either touch or the Spaceball controller,

during surgical planning. The surgeon also has the option of adding a tool overlay to track tool position in relation to the target lesion. The other touchscreen is the control panel that displays information about system configuration.

Tactile feedback to the neurosurgeon is accomplished with force sensors at the neuroArm end-effectors and the two PHANTOM haptic hand controllers (SensAble Technologies Inc., Wobrun, MA) at the workstation. There are two titanium multiaxis force / torque sensors located directly between the tool and the end-effector. These, in turn, relay tool tip forces to the neurosurgeon's hand controllers. Each hand controller has 6 DOF and consists of a modified stylus. This design mimics the conventional way a neurosurgeon handles his tool (**Fig. 23.8A**). Each stylus has an index finger-activated lever for tool actuation (**Fig. 23.8B**). A foot-activated switch enables and disables the manipulators.

Force scaling, motion scaling, and tremor filters are additional features that can augment the surgeon's dexterity. Force and motion scaling can transform a much larger effort exerted at the hand controllers to a much diminished effect at the level of the end-effector so that tissues can be handled more gently and delicately. In addition, the option of tremor filtering can eliminate or at the very least diminish the human physiologic tremor that can get in the way especially when manipulating objects on a small scale. The end result of these features is more precision, accuracy, and the ability to work on a much smaller dimension than is humanly possible.

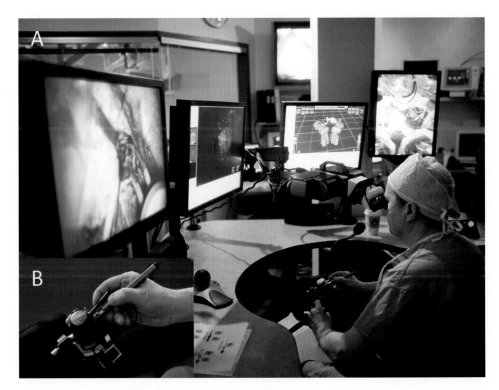

Fig. 23.8 Hand controllers. **(A)** The primary surgeon utilizes the two customized PHANTOM haptic hand controllers (SensAble Technologies Inc., Woburn, MA) at the workstation to operate the neuroArm manipulators. **(B)** Actuation of the tool occurs with an index finger-activated lever. Enabling and disabling the manipulators occurs with a foot-operated switch (not shown).

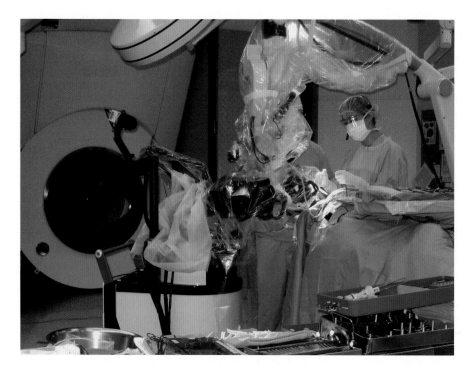

Fig. 23.9 Positioning of surgical team during microsurgery. NeuroArm is designed to take the place of the primary neurosurgeon at the head of the operating table. The microscope, the assistant, and the scrub nurse occupy the same positions as in a routine surgical set-up.

Safety has been designed into neuroArm, in terms of hardware and software. NeuroArm's ultrasonic piezoelectric motors have an average lifespan of 20,000 hours, a resolution of 1 nm. They brake if power is shut off to the system. The sine / cosine rotary encoders used for the manipulator joints are capable of error detection in case of failure. They also have the added benefit of retaining positional information when powered off for imaging. Antibacklash mechanics have also been incorporated for smooth motion in the forward and reverse directions. Collision detection software preempts potential collisions between the robot and operative site obstacles. Taking this one step further, virtual geometric regions can be outlined by the neurosurgeon within the 3D MR reconstructions to define safe surgical corridors and anatomic structures to be avoided. When these predefined boundaries of the "no-go" zone are reached, the surgeon feels a force feedback in the hand controller. In such a way, accidental movements can be prevented. Another safety feature is that safety-critical software actions, such as turning on power or enabling arm motion, always require additional hardware action as confirmation.

NeuroArm has four main software applications running concurrently on separate computers. The command status display provides the main graphic control interface with the 3D virtual scene of the robotic arms relative to the potential obstacles such as the radiofrequency (RF) coil and magnet bore. Another software application provides the 3D MRI reconstruction of the patient's anatomy with the virtual tool overly. The hand controller interface, the controller interfaces to the manipulator arms, and other required hardware are run with other software.

NeuroArm is designed to replace the main surgeon in the iMRI suite. Alternatively, neuroArm can also function as the assistant. The positions of all other operating room personnel and standard equipment are essentially the same (**Fig. 23.9**). This is based on the design concept of biomimicry, to replicate the way surgeons work during surgery. For microsurgery, after imaging and registration have been completed, neuroArm is positioned at the head of the operating table, occupying the same position that the primary surgeon would. Once in position, the mobile base is locked in place using a wheel brake. Even though microsurgery is performed outside the magnetic bore, intraoperative imaging can be performed at any time during the surgery after moving neuroArm outside of the 5 gauss (G) line.

Preoperative imaging is acquired using MRI-visible fiducials embedded in the RF coil headholder to facilitate registration. Once preoperative imaging has been acquired and the robot brought into position, registration is accomplished using a 6-DOF Microscribe MLX digitizing arm (Solution Technologies, Inc., Oella, MD) to identify the touchpoints on the manipulator arms and the RF coil. At the workstation, the MRI-visible fiducials are merged to those in a 3D model of the RF coil. This is followed by coordinate transformations to align the robotic coordinates with the MRI. Registration accuracy of less than 4 mm has been shown in initial clinical experiences. Reregistration is required each time the neuroArm base is repositioned.

NeuroArm's end-effector interacts with the surgical team in a similar fashion as the human arm of a neurosurgeon. Sterilized tool holders attach to the manipulator arms that are covered in sterile clear custom drapes. The tool holders accommodate a set of specially designed MRI-compatible tools, including bipolar forceps, needle drivers, suction, microscissors, and microdissectors. Tool exchange occurs at the request of the surgeon once the manipulator arm is moved out of the surgical field, and the scrub nurse manually exchanges the instruments. This part is designed to occur within a 20- to 30-second time frame to minimize disruption to the conventional routine of the procedure. Based on the maximum allowable time for tool exchange intraoperatively, the speed and payload requirements were determined to be 200 mm/s acceleration while carrying a payload of 500 g. Tool-free manual extraction of the surgical instrument ensures that safety is not compromised in the event of system failure.

NeuroArm is designed for use within the MRI gantry for stereotactic procedures. Either one of the manipulators can be transferred to a platform attached to the magnet for stereotaxy (**Figs. 23.10A,B**). Sequential MR images can be acquired intraoperatively displaying tool position in relation to the target lesion in real-time, effectively dealing with the problem of brain-shift. During stereotactic procedures, two MRI-compatible video cameras are also attached to the extension board of the operating table for patient monitoring.

NeuroArm's repertoire of skills, including biopsy needle insertion, microdissection, thermocoagulation, and fine suturing have been tested in cadaveric and animal studies. Recently, neuroArm has also been utilized in the surgical resections of tumors in five patients, successfully taking on more responsibility as the primary surgeon each time. Clinical studies remain an ongoing effort.

Clinical Trials

Phase I clinical trials have begun with NeuroArm. Clinical introduction occurred in a graded fashion, with the robot performing more tasks with each subsequent patient. For the first patient, the robot was draped and positioned for surgery to evaluate the effect on the assistant surgeon, the scrub nurse, and the anesthetist. The second patient had a left paracentral malignant astrocytoma. Following anesthesia

and patient positioning, intraoperative images were acquired. NeuroArm was brought into the surgical field and registered to the images. The robot was used for lesion localization and craniotomy placement. The robot was removed from the surgical field and draped for surgery. Following craniotomy, the robot was returned to the surgical field and reregistered to the patient. Holding bipolar forceps in the right manipulator and a suction in the left, the tools were manipulated by the surgeon located at the workstation. The third patient had a posterior left parafalcine meningioma. For this case, bipolar forceps were inserted into each manipulator. The surgeon working at the workstation was responsible for hemostasis and establishing a portion of the tumor–brain interface. The assistant surgeon operated the Cavitron ultrasonic aspirator (CUSA) and suction. The fourth patient had an olfactory groove meningioma arising from the left olfactory tract. For this case, neuroArm was used to remove the majority of the tumor. The fifth patient had a recurrent prepontine epidermoid tumor. Following a translabyrinthine exposure, neuroArm was used to remove the lesion.

iMRI Suite Upgrade

Subsequent to this initial clinical experience, the iMRI suite was shut down to upgrade the iMRI system from 1.5 to 3.0 T. In addition, neuroArm was integrated into this 3.0 T environment that included whole-room RF shielding. The new magnet has a 70-cm working aperture. This, together with RF shielding, provides considerably more room for the neuroArm manipulator during stereotaxy. Registration of the manipulator to the magnet isocenter greatly simplifies stereotactic biopsy. The clinical program has recently recommenced.

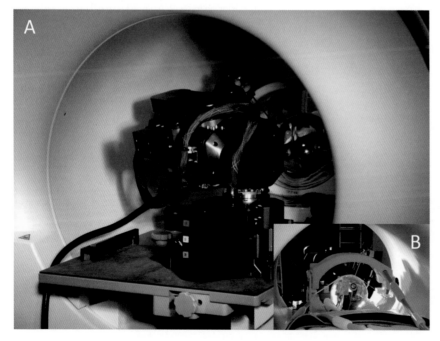

Fig. 23.10 Stereotaxy. Either of the manipulators can be transferred from the mobile base to the platform attached to the magnet for stereotactic procedures. **(A)** NeuroArm (MacDonald, Dettwiler & Assoc., Richmond, British Columbia) is shown here set up for a phantom experiment. **(B)** The view from inside the magnet bore demonstrates a large working aperture. Intraoperative magnetic resonance imaging can provide information of the tool tip in relation to the target lesion in real-time.

◆ Conclusion

Surgical robotics has the potential to advance neurosurgical diagnostic and therapeutic procedures. Certainly, the unifying goal among the systems presented in this review is the desire to refine surgery with superior preoperative planning and operative execution. Some systems were clearly built upon MR and CT imaging and neuronavigation systems to achieve accuracy and precision, whereas others have introduced new technologies, such as motion and force scaling and tremor filter, to enhance the performance of the human hand. Several robotics systems have also introduced the concept of telesurgery, that surgery can be performed remotely from the workstation where the surgeon is located.

At present time, few systems actually have FDA approval for use in patients and are available commercially. Most robotics systems are still undergoing clinical or preclinical studies. Clearly, there is still much work that remains to be done in the development of the surgical robot for neurosurgery and spinal surgery; however, the prospects are extraordinary.

References

1. Kwoh YS, Hou J, Jonckheere EA, Hayati S. A robot with improved absolute positioning accuracy for CT guided stereotactic brain surgery. IEEE Trans Biomed Eng 1988;35(2):153–160

2. Drake JM, Joy M, Goldenberg A, Kreindler D. Computer- and robot-assisted resection of thalamic astrocytomas in children. Neurosurgery 1991;29(1):27–33

3. Li QH, Zamorano L, Pandya A, Perez R, Gong J, Diaz F. The application accuracy of the NeuroMate robot—a quantitative comparison with frameless and frame-based surgical localization systems. Comput Aided Surg 2002;7(2):90–98

4. Benabid AL, Cinquin P, Lavalle S, Le Bas JF, Demongeot J, de Rougemont J. Computer-driven robot for stereotactic surgery connected to CT scan and magnetic resonance imaging. Technological design and preliminary results. Appl Neurophysiol 1987;50(1-6):153–154

5. The NeuroMate neurosurgical stereotactic robot. Available at: http://cedit.aphp.fr/servlet/siteCeditGB?Destination=reco&numArticle=00.06. Accessed March 2, 2009

6. Varma TRK, Eldridge PR, Forster A, et al. Use of the NeuroMate stereotactic robot in a frameless mode for movement disorder surgery. Stereotact Funct Neurosurg 2003;80(1-4):132–135

7. Varma TRK, Eldridge P. Use of the NeuroMate stereotactic robot in a frameless mode for functional neurosurgery. Int J Med Robot 2006;2(2):107–113

8. Zimmermann M, Krishnan R, Raabe A, Seifert V. Robot-assisted navigated neuroendoscopy. Neurosurgery 2002;51(6):1446–1451, discussion 1451–1452

9. Zimmermann M, Krishnan R, Raabe A, Seifert V. Robot-assisted navigated endoscopic ventriculostomy: implementation of a new technology and first clinical results. Acta Neurochir (Wien) 2004;146(7):697–704

10. Nimsky Ch, Rachinger J, Iro H, Fahlbusch R. Adaptation of a hexapod-based robotic system for extended endoscope-assisted transsphenoidal skull base surgery. Minim Invasive Neurosurg 2004;47(1):41–46

11. Fankhauser H, Glauser D, Flury P, et al. Robot for CT-guided stereotactic neurosurgery. Stereotact Funct Neurosurg 1994;63(1-4):93–98

12. Glauser D, Fankhauser H, Epitaux M, Hefti JL, Jaccottet A. Neurosurgical robot Minerva: first results and current developments. J Image Guid Surg 1995;1(5):266–272

13. Hefti JL, Epitaux M, Glauser D, Fankhauser H. Robotic three-dimensional positioning of a stimulation electrode in the brain. Comput Aided Surg 1998;3(1):1–10

14. Chinzei K, Miller K. Towards MRI guided surgical manipulator. Med Sci Monit 2001;7(1):153–163

15. Chinzei K, Warfield SK, Hata N, Tempany CMC, Jolesz FA, Kikinis R. Planning, simulation and assistance with intraoperative MRI. Minim Invasive Ther Allied Technol 2003;12(1):59–64

16. DiMaio SP, Pieper S, Chinzei K, et al. Robot-assisted needle placement in open MRI: system architecture, integration and validation. Comput Aided Surg 2007;12(1):15–24

17. Masamune K, Kobayashi E, Masutani Y, et al. Development of an MRI-compatible needle insertion manipulator for stereotactic neurosurgery. J Image Guid Surg 1995;1(4):242–248

18. Siemionow M, Ozer K, Siemionow W, Lister G. Robotic assistance in microsurgery. J Reconstr Microsurg 2000;16(8):643–649

19. Das H, Zak H, Johnson J, Crouch J, Frambach D. Evaluation of a telerobotic system to assist surgeons in microsurgery. Comput Aided Surg 1999;4(1):15–25

20. Le Roux PD, Das H, Esquenazi S, Kelly PJ. Robot-assisted microsurgery: a feasibility study in the rat. Neurosurgery 2001;48(3):584–589

21. Taylor RH, Jensen P, Whitcomb L, et al. A Steady-Hand robotic system for microsurgical augmentation. Int J Robot Res 1999;18(12):1201–1210

22. Hongo K, Kobayashi S, Kakizawa Y, et al. NeuRobot: telecontrolled micromanipulator system for minimally invasive microneurosurgery—preliminary results. Neurosurgery 2002;51(4):985–988, discussion 988

23. Goto T, Hongo K, Kakizawa Y, et al. Clinical application of robotic telemanipulation system in neurosurgery. Case report. J Neurosurg 2003;99(6):1082–1084

24. Hongo K, Goto T, Miyahara T, Kakizawa Y, Koyama J, Tanaka Y. Telecontrolled micromanipulator system (NeuRobot) for minimally invasive neurosurgery. Acta Neurochir Suppl (Wien) 2006;98:63–66

25. Cleary K, Stoianovici D, Patriciu A, Mazilu D, Lindisch D, Watson V. Robotically assisted nerve and facet blocks: a cadaveric study. Acad Radiol 2002;9(7):821–825

26. Cleary K, Watson V, Lindisch D, et al. Precision placement of instruments for minimally invasive procedures using a "needle driver" robot. Int J Med Robot 2005;1(2):40–47

27. Lieberman IH, Togawa D, Kayanja MM, et al. Bone-mounted miniature robotic guidance for pedicle screw and translaminar facet screw placement: Part I—Technical development and a test case result. Neurosurgery 2006;59(3):641–650, discussion 641–650

28. Shoham M, Lieberman IH, Benzel EC, et al. Robotic assisted spinal surgery—from concept to clinical practice. Comput Aided Surg 2007;12(2):105–115

29. Sukovich W, Brink-Danan S, Hardenbrook M. Miniature robotic guidance for pedicle screw placement in posterior spinal fusion: early clinical experience with the SpineAssist. Int J Med Robot 2006;2(2):114–122

30. Barzilay Y, Liebergall M, Fridlander A, Knoller N. Miniature robotic guidance for spine surgery—introduction of a novel system and analysis of challenges encountered during the clinical development phase at two spine centres. Int J Med Robot 2006;2(2):146–153

31. Joskowicz L, Shamir R, Freiman M, et al. Image-guided system with miniature robot for precise positioning and targeting in keyhole neurosurgery. Comput Aided Surg 2006;11(4):181–193

32. Greer AD, Newhook P, Sutherland GR. Human-machine interface for robotic surgery and stereotaxy. IEEE/ ASME Transactions on Mechatronics 2008; 13(3): 355–361.

33. Louw DF, Fielding T, McBeth PB, Gregoris D, Newhook P, Sutherland GR. Surgical robotics: a review and neurosurgical prototype development. Neurosurgery 2004;54(3):525–536, discussion 536–537

34. Sutherland GR, Latour I, Greer AD. Integrating an image-guided robot with intraoperative MRI: a review of the design and construction of neuroArm. IEEE Eng Med Biol Mag 2008;27(3):59–65

35. Sutherland GR, Latour I, Greer AD, Fielding T, Feil G, Newhook P. An image-guided magnetic resonance-compatible surgical robot. Neurosurgery 2008;62(2):286–292, discussion 292–293

24

MRI-Guided Focused Ultrasound Surgery in the Brain

Rivka R. Colen and Ferenc A. Jolesz

◆ MRgFUS: Introduction and History

Magnetic resonance imaging-guided focused ultrasound (MRgFUS) is expected to revolutionize disease treatment including, but not limited to, the ablation of benign and malignant tumors and vascular malformations as well as the nonablative targeted delivery of therapeutic drugs, genes, and antibodies. Coupling magnetic resonance imaging (MRI) guidance with advanced phased-array ultrasound (US) technology, coined MRgFUS, has allowed FUS therapy to emerge as a viable noninvasive alternative to invasive and minimally invasive treatment.

In 1880 Pierre and Jacques Curie described the basic tenet on which modern US is founded, the piezoelectric effect (the production of acoustic energy when electric current is applied to a piezoelectric crystal).[1] However, it was not until 40 years later, in 1918, with the development of technologic advances in electronics, that US, as we know it today, was created. This era of modern US began when Paul Langevin, a physicist, designed the sonar for submarine detection by interposing a mosaic of thin quartz crystals glued between two steel plates.[2,3] In 1938, Raimar Pohlman noted the first "therapeutic effect" of US on human tissue using low-intensity US to treat patients with inflammatory conditions.[4] Langevin subsequently went on to make the first observations of high-intensity focused ultrasound (HIFU) by demonstrating alterations in the swimming patterns of fishes during the emission of sound waves.[2] The first demonstrated use of HIFU on biologic tissue occurred when Lynn and Putman treated 37 animals by delivering targeted FUS to specific areas of the brain.[5–7] Fry then accentuated the potential of FUS as an alternative to open neurosurgery[8–10] following the demonstration of successful pinpoint ablations through a craniotomy window in primates. Even though their clinical results were mixed, Fry and Heimburger subsequently went on to establish the safety of HIFU to destroy brain tumors after craniectomy.[11,12] Additionally, in 1955 Barnard et al led

the first study of US-induced disruption of the blood–brain barrier (BBB).[13] Similar research was subsequently performed by the Ballantine and Lele team,[14] which described the biologic effects of FUS on sonicated brain tissue.[15,16]

Inspired by the results of previous research and clinical trials, Petter Lindstrom, considered by many as one of the pioneers of "bloodless surgery," used HIFU lesioning to treat patients with psychiatric disorders, epilepsy, and intractable pain from carcinomatosis.[17] Introduced to this functional neurosurgical method by Lindstrom, Leksell, the acknowledged pioneer of radiosurgery, was the first to develop a special adapted frame for an US transducer for the purpose of HIFU lesioning. For Leksell, the major limitation precluding the use of HIFU as a therapeutic device included the (1) need for a craniotomy, (2) lack of reliable imaging tool to plan treatment, and (3) lack of real-time intraoperative feedback and assessment of the targeted lesions. He subsequently abandoned HIFU as a lesioning device and focused on ionizing radiation, an effort that resulted in the development of the gamma knife in 1967.[18] The above-mentioned limitations have been successfully addressed with the development of magnetic resonance imaging (MRI) by Lauterbach and colleagues in the 1980s. This was a significant contribution to the advancement of FUS as an image-guided therapeutic instrument. MRI is a proven reliable and sensitive imaging modality used to define the target (i.e., tumors) and to plan treatment preoperatively. Coupled with the development of MRI thermometry[19–23] in the early 1990s, MRI can provide real-time intraprocedural feedback, permitting a controlled treatment environment. MRI thermometry detects temperature changes with marked accuracy and sensitivity based on shifts of proton resonance frequency.[24] Subsequent research found that temperature elevations correlated well with the degree of tissue damage,[25,26] making MRI thermal imaging the modality of choice for intraprocedural evaluation of treatment performance. At the same time, the development of phased-array transducers[27–29] led to the potential of transcranial delivery of therapeutic US through an intact skull, precluding the need for craniotomy. Alongside MRI, FUS makes a strong case as a safe, noninvasive, and practical alternative to conventional invasive treatment options.

◆ MRgFUS: General Concepts, Advantages, and Limitations

MRgFUS combines and integrates two modalities into a single image-guided therapy delivery system. FUS is the therapeutic instrument causing direct US-induced changes in the targeted tissue that include nonthermal (nonablative) and thermal (ablative) tissue changes. As an ablative tool, FUS ablates deep tissue volumes without disturbing the overlying tissue (near-field tissue).[30,31] Coupled with the latter, MRI provides both guidance and immediate postprocedural evaluation of the treatment. It is used preoperatively to accurately identify the target tissue, intraoperatively to monitor treatment in real-time via MR thermometry and postoperatively to validate treatment success. As nonablative therapy, FUS can reversibly disrupt the BBB, resulting in an increase in cerebrovascular capillary permeability and, therefore, an increase of the flux of relatively larger, non-lipophilic, and high-molecular-weight molecules that would otherwise not cross the BBB.[32,33]

MRgFUS offers clear, unambiguous advantages over other current treatment modalities. It is noninvasive and does not deliver ionizing radiation to either patient or physician. In contrast to the gamma knife, which lends itself to only a single treatment session (irrelevant of the treatment success) due to its toxic cumulative effects, FUS allows for unlimited treatments in a single session as well as unlimited repeated sessions over time. Unlike in both surgery and radiotherapy, real-time noninvasive intraprocedural monitoring can be performed with remarkable accuracy using MR thermometry, which gives outstanding anatomic definition of the target site. MRI thermal imaging is the sole modality available to evaluate thermal tissue effects; it is used to determine the therapeutic endpoint in FUS ablation, and the success of treatment.[34,35] Secondary neoplasms, caused by radiosurgery and radiotherapy, are not seen with FUS therapy. Furthermore, the thermal gradients of FUS are much narrower than the dose-curves in radiosurgery; therefore, they are more precise and less thermally damaging to the adjacent tissues.

However, both technical and inherent limitations remain, including lengthy treatment sessions largely due to small focal volumes of ablation per sonication and to relatively long cooling times that prevent the accumulation of heat beyond the focal volumes.

Ongoing research is striving to annihilate or at least decrease to a certain extent these limitations. Long treatment times reflect the small volume of ablation per sonication, and the cooling time and MRI thermometry acquisition needed between each sonication. However, increased volumes can be obtained by creating multiple focal points as well as overlapping sonications. Due to the absence of an adequate acoustic window for the transmission of sound waves, as opposed to the creation of an acoustic window through a craniotomy site, the intact osseous skull creates two major challenges when performing transcranial FUS: (1) heating caused by the absorptive properties of bone, and (2) the inability to establish a focal point of convergence due to scatter, resulting in inaccurate targeting and uncontrolled energy deposition. Current phased-array transducers address these challenges by allowing for transcranial focusing[28,36] without overheating the skull by using models derived from preprocedural computed tomography (CT) scans used to compute and correct for skull thickness and density.[27] Organ motion during treatment is important as small motion can cause large shifts in focal points, resulting in an imprecise and incorrect zone of ablation. For the latter, intraprocedural MRI and adaptation of the phased-array transducer elements are enjoined to retarget and refocus, yielding for a controlled, precise deposition of heat to the intended target lesion. Organ motion also prevents correct temperature measurements with phase difference-based thermometry. For the treatment of moving organs like liver and kidney, more research is necessary to achieve the same precise treatment that is possible in the brain. By addressing the above-mentioned limitations, the procedure will decrease in complexity, require less manpower, and translate into an increased acceptance of clinical applications by clinicians.

◆ MRgFUS: Mechanism of Action

Thermal (Ablation) Effects

The thermal effects of FUS on tissue depend on the acoustic intensity and the absorption coefficient of the tissue. The ablative effects on tissue are caused by thermal heating that is predominantly a product of the absorption coefficient of the tissues. Given the dependency on the acoustic intensity of the US beam, generation of thermal energy is mostly on the focal point of convergence where the intensity is highest. Using temperatures higher than 56 to 60°C, focused sonication with only a few seconds duration causes thermal coagulation.[29] This nonselective tissue coagulation necrosis results in the killing of both neoplastic and nonneoplastic cells; it is an unambiguous heat-induced cell death occurring secondary to protein denaturation that beckons the need for a reliable and sensitive imaging method for monitoring tissue changes. Given that it can accurately detect fluctuations of less than 2 to 3°C, MR temperature-sensitive imaging (MR thermometry) fits these criteria.[34,35]

The all-or-none ablative effect of FUS irrespective of tissue type resembles surgical treatment. However, unlike surgery, the nonablated region is preserved. In contrast, hyperthermia, which also has tissue ablative effects, delivers relatively lower temperatures (43°C) over a longer period of time (30–60 minutes),[37,38] thereby causing more selective cell damage. Percutaneous heat-conducting probes cause a shallow temperature gradient due to the steep heat sink effects from perfusion and blood flow that dissipate heat farther from the single source probe. These probes, therefore, need long exposures to increase the ablative volume.

Additionally, unlike FUS, the probe ablation zone cannot be tailored to fit the geometry of the target volume. Regardless of the ablative source, therefore, to monitor therapy and avoid under- and overtreatment, spatial and temporal monitoring of thermal heating is of utmost importance.

Nonthermal (Nonablation) Effects

The nonthermal, nonablative effects of FUS on soft tissue are due to multiple complex mechanisms, the most important mechanism being cavitation that results in the following: (1) acoustic streaming, (2) mechanical (acoustic radiation) forces, and (3) inertial (transient) cavitation.[39-42] Inertial cavitation is likely responsible for most of the nonthermal biologic effects. These mechanisms result from the interaction of microbubbles with US.[43,44] Microbubbles can be induced by the high-intensity US itself and generated within the native sonicated tissue, or preformed microbubbles (clinically used US imaging contrast agents) can be intravenously administered, the latter termed microbubble-enhanced therapeutic ultrasound.[45-48]

At low acoustic power, oscillating microbubbles contribute to disruption of the BBB by producing shear stresses on the cells by microstreaming fluid around the bubble.[43,44] Mechanical radiation forces cause the bubble to move in the direction of the wave propagation, exerting force on the endothelium perpendicular to the direction of the blood flow and length of the vessel.[49] This action causes localized stretching of the cell membrane and stimulation of the endothelial cells, inducing its biologic effects on the BBB. At high acoustic pressures, FUS causes oscillation and the rapid growth of bubbles, that on implosion (violent collapse; also known as inertial cavitation), unpredictably release stored energy in the form of shock waves.[33,43,44] It also produces high velocity jets[50] and free radicals.[51] These biologic effects disrupt the cell membrane and endothelial tight junctions, allowing uncontrolled deposition of thermal heat. Due to its unpredictable, nonlinear effects on heating that can lead to hemorrhage and unwanted tissue destruction,[52] cavitation is an undesirable effect of thermal ablation where precise, controlled targeted lesion ablation is needed. In nonthermal ablations, however, the effects of cavitation can be exploited. For example, disrupting the BBB, at lower energy levels can increase cell and vascular permeability. With the development of contrast microbubble agents,[42,45,53] disruption of the BBB can be performed at even lower acoustic pressure levels, decreasing the above-mentioned side effects of uncontrolled heating including hemorrhage and unwanted tissue destruction.[40]

◆ MRgFUS: Approach

Preprocedure Stage: Planning and Localization

Preprocedural planning is critical to evaluate and precisely define the anatomy of the desired target lesion and adjacent structures, determine the procedural approach, and plan a viable trajectory for the delivery of focused sonications. Given the ability to visualize lesions, MRI and CT scanning are pivotal in planning, optimizing, and controlling treatment.

With its superior signal-to-noise ratio (SNR) and ability to provide a three-dimensional spatial map of the targeted tissue volume, MRI remains the imaging method of choice for surgical and procedural planning including the defining of correct anatomic (and functional) localization and mapping, spatial volume, size and extent of the targeted lesion, the margins of the lesion itself and surrounding critical anatomic structures, as well as providing exquisite tissue characterization. MRI's accuracy and reliability far outperform other imaging modalities. Furthermore, by increasing SNR that results in superior resolution, higher field strengths provided by 3.0 T confer added sensitivity over 1.5 T MRI systems with consequent improvement in tumor margin delineation. However, because of the inherent infiltrative nature of most malignant tumors and the limited sensitivity of MRI to detect microscopic infiltration of tumor cells into normal-appearing tissue, precise definition of the margins of malignant tumors remains a challenge and incomplete treatment can result.

Similar in importance to MRI for preprocedural planning, the CT scan of the head is pivotal for planning transcranial MRgFUS therapy. Given its high acoustic attenuation coefficient, bone represents a relative barrier that is not impenetrable to the transmission of US sound waves and acoustic energy deposition,[54] unlike air- and gas-containing cavities that represent absolute barriers to acoustic energy deposition. The high acoustic impedance of the osseous skull is proportional to skull thickness and density. It is evaluated and computed from the information obtained by the CT scan.[27] The acoustic impedance is a result of and due to multiple factors including but not limited to scatter and absorption of most of the energy.[55]

Absorption of energy by bone also contributes to the heating of the skull, an important limitation in transcranial FUS. Heating of the skull due to energy absorption and severe aberration and phase distortion due to scatter is corrected by current phased-array transducers via acoustic modeling.[27,29,36,56] The elements of the phased-array US may correct and compensate for phase distortions, a consequence of bone density and thickness inhomogeneities. Overheating is addressed by means of two methods used by the first MRgFUS brain system developed by Insightec (Haifa, Israel). A helmet-type, hemispherically configured phased-array transducer and a cold water cap containing circulating degassed water chilled to ~15°C are placed over the patient's head. The hemispherical transducer provides an active cooling system for the skull.[30,31] The spreading of phased-array elements onto a semicircular hemispherical helmet that operates at a low frequency (<1 MHz) distributes the thermal energy across a larger surface area, decreasing superficial heating and resulting in sufficient thermal heat at the focal point of convergence (the target lesion). The phased-array configuration also permits adjustments of the elements to correct for skull-induced aberration.

Intraprocedure Stage: Targeting and Monitoring

After placement of the cranial apparatus consisting of the hemispherical phased-array transducer and underlying chilled, degassed water cap over the patient's head, MRI is performed once more. This time the scans are done along with the stereotactic apparatus with the objective of retargeting the desired lesion and evaluating surrounding critical anatomic structures. Subsequently, noncoagulative low-power-focused sonications are delivered to define the target tissue. MRI guidance, specifically MR thermometry, detects noncoagulative tissue changes to confirm the focal point on the target lesion.

After retargeting, high-power-focused sonications (500–20,000 W/cm^2) of short duration (1–60 seconds) are administered. Short ablation times are preferred to circumvent cooling effects from perfusion, diffusion, blood flow, and steep thermal gradients that would otherwise result in longer sessions to obtain adequate treatment and to reduce the buildup of heat in pathway nontargeted tissues traversing through the trajectory site. Although negligible, these cooling effects should be recognized to avoid risk of undertreatment. Using MRI guidance for beam path visualization and to ensure a controlled treatment, overlapping sonications are delivered to the target tissues, generating heat at the focal point that induces thermal necrosis of ~2 mm in diameter (perpendicular to the beam) and 10 mm in length (parallel to the beam).[29]

Given the small focal point of ablation per sonication, multiple overlapping sonications in a single session are performed. Strategies to increase the focal volume per sonication include dynamic steering of the focal point or creating multiple focal points, both of which can be done with phased-array transducers. Each sonication is followed by MR thermometry that provides accurate temperature information from the treated area.[57] Using temperature as a surrogate for tissue viability[25,26] this modality, unlike other imaging modalities, allows for controlled energy deposition by providing immediate observation and evaluation of treatment performance with unprecedented sensitivity. This immediate feedback is a true closed-loop treatment imaging system that allows immediate retreatment of areas in which suboptimal temperature elevation has occurred. Multiple sonications are performed until adequate treatment is deemed complete. Unlike radiosurgery, which is a single-session, one-shot deal, FUS therapy has the added advantage of being delivered over multiple sessions.

Postprocedure Stage: Validation

Once satisfactory treatment is achieved, postcontrast MRI is obtained for accurate treatment validation and assessment. Expected posttreatment changes in thermal ablations include a focal region of nonenhancement corresponding to the region of necrosis.[57] In nonthermal ablations, such as in the disruption of the BBB, expected adequate posttreatment changes include enhancement of the sonicated area, reflecting increased permeability.[58]

◆ MRgFUS: Clinical Applications

Thermal (Ablative) Applications

Brain Tumor Ablation

The concept of "ideal surgery" refers to a procedural technique in which the entire tissue volume of the targeted lesion is removed with anatomic and functional preservation of the surrounding tissue. Unlike primary malignant central nervous system (CNS) neoplasms, particularly glioblastomas multiforme that have microscopic infiltration of the normal appearing parenchyma, benign tumors and metastatic disease present well-defined boundaries, making these ideal target lesions. The first clinical application of MRgFUS was done in benign breast fibroadenomas.[59] In some instances, a decrease in tumor volume and tumor debulking rather than complete removal can be considered a satisfactory outcome in some patients. Such outcomes are satisfactory when treating uterine fibroids[60] for which the U.S. Food and Drug Administration has already approved MRgFUS as a treatment.[60-63] If regrowth occurs, retreatment can be performed.

Given the critical function of the brain, preservation of adjacent structures is imperative to any technique that claims to qualify as an "ideal modality" for treatment of brain tumors. In turn, given its critical biologic function, the brain makes a compelling case as the ideal organ for MRgFUS therapy. Efforts to treat malignant brain tumors through an open craniotomy without[15,64] and with MRI guidance[65] have shown some success. However, as a completely noninvasive technique, trancranial MRgFUS through an intact skull, pioneered by Jolesz et al,[27] is considered the revolutionary change needed to treat brain disease.

Other Applications

FUS can also be used for accurate targeting of functional neurologic disorders such as movement disorders, epilepsy, or pain (**Figs. 24.1, 24.2,** and **24.3**).[4] Localized thermal energy can inhibit nerve conduction, making it useful for pain control and the treatment of spastic diseases.[66] Several studies have shown these effects to be reversible,[67-69] raising the possibility that FUS may have a future as a tool for noninvasive functional testing and mapping similar to the following currently investigated modality, transcranial magnetic stimulation (TMS).

Nonthermal (Nonablative) Applications

Blood–Brain Barrier Disruption

The ability of MRgFUS to reversibly disrupt the BBB, thereby increasing permeability, can potentially transform and replace the current nonselective drug delivery methods that cause systemic toxicity. Such toxicity is an important limiting factor in chemotherapy. US's cause of an increase in BBB permeability can enable the delivery of targeted chemotherapy drugs into the region of interest that would otherwise not enter the desired site due to almost complete impermeable

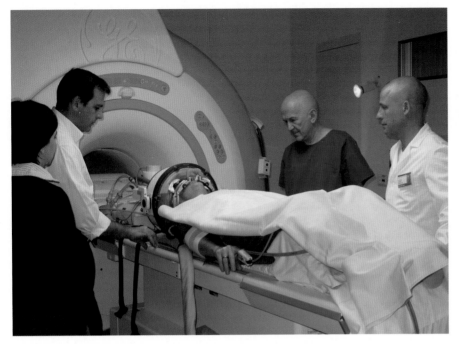

Fig. 24.1 Patient ready for the high-intensity focused ultrasound (HIFU) intervention. The patient is positioned on the table of a 3.0 tesla magnetic resonance imaging (MRI) scanner. In the background is the bore of the scanner. The head is fixated in a stereotactic frame (metal frame with black poles and white pins). Monitoring is attached. The head is placed inside the helmet-like ultrasound-transducer (white cylinder behind head). The transducer is filled with degassed water for transmitting the ultrasound waves from the transducer to the skull surface and for cooling the skin. A gray flexible membrane seals the water between transducer and patient's head. (Courtesy of Insightec, Haifa, Israel.)

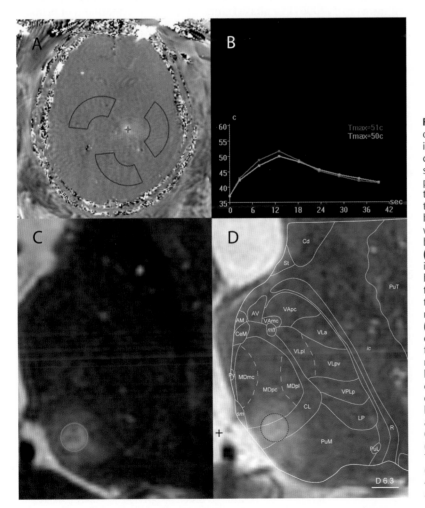

Fig. 24.2 **(A)** Thermal map on axial plane at the level of the third ventricle. Thermal maps are refreshed at intervals of 3 to 5 seconds to monitor localization and dynamics of temperature rise during sonication and subsequent temperature relaxation during cooling period. The blue circle delineates the planned sonication target in the posterior part of the central lateral thalamic nucleus. The red cross marks the pixel with the highest temperature at the end of sonication. The three wedge shaped forms are placed by the operator to balance background noise in thermal calculations. **(B)** Red: temperature evolution during a therapeutic sonication of 12-second duration using 850 W in the voxel of highest temperature; time resolution 4 seconds, monitored cooling period after sonication 30 seconds. Green: temperature evolution of average temperature within neighboring voxels around the temperature maximum. **(C)** Red circle: contour line of a standardized thermal dose corresponding to 17 equivalent minutes at 43°C at the target location superimposed on the T2-weighted magnetic resonance image (T2WI MRI) obtained at 48 hours after treatment. **(D)** Stereotactic reconstruction of MRI-guided high-intensity focused ultrasound-guided central lateral thalamotomy (CLT). The dotted circle outlines the coagulation zone (3- to 5-millimeter diameter) according to the temperature map. The location of the CLT is determined by projecting the corresponding atlas (6.3 mm dorsal to intercommissural plane) onto the T2WI MRI using the position of the posterior commissure (black cross) for anteroposterior alignment. Scale bars = 4 mm. (Courtesy of E. Martin, D. Jeanmonod, E. Zadicario, and B. Werner, University of Zurich.)

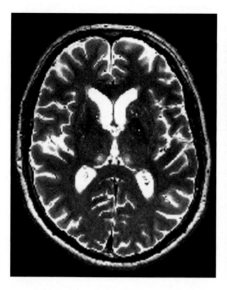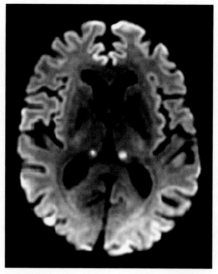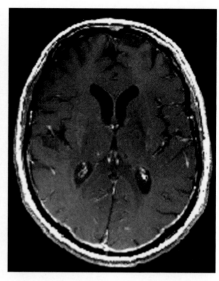

A

Fig. 24.3 A 71-year-old patient with chronic lumbar pain syndrome following a disk hernia operation L4/L5, 10 years ago. **(A)** Axial T2-weighted magnetic resonance (MR) image, **(B)** isotropic diffusion tensor image, and **(C)** postcontrast T1-weighted MR image, respectively, obtained 48 hours after bilateral central lateral thalamotomy with transcranial MRI-guided high-intensity focused ultrasound. The sonications were placed bilaterally in the posterior parts of the central lateral thalamic nuclei. (Courtesy of E. Martin, D. Jeanmonod, E. Zadicario, and B. Werner, University of Zurich.)

tight junctions at the BBB.[53,70] Furthermore, although the chemotherapeutic drug continues to be administered intravenously, the drug can be encapsulated in bubbles or liposomes and attached to nanoparticles before administration.[71–74] At the moment of bubble rupture, the drug is released locally in the sonicated region. This, compounded with the opening of the BBB, makes for an unparalleled combination. Studies are investigating the ability of large molecular drugs, such as Herceptin (Genentech, South San Francisco, CA) and doxorubicin, to pass through the BBB after sonication, with the hope that this method can be successfully used in the future to treat primary and secondary CNS malignancies.[70,75] Due to the noninvasiveness of the procedure and the potential to enhance therapeutic delivery of drugs, this technique may translate into clinical practice with relative ease.

MRgFUS also carries a potential role for targeted gene,[76–80] antibody,[81] and Parkinson's and Alzheimer's disease therapy.[81,82] Furthermore, in patients with acute stroke, the coupling of thermal effects of FUS on thrombolytic drugs increases thrombolysis, thereby increasing the effectiveness of therapy.[83–86] However, the risk of cavitation-induced hemorrhage is great in ischemic stroke,[87] and multiple studies are under way in an attempt to decrease this risk by using FUS-induced closure of the hemorrhaging vessels to induce hemostasis.[88–90]

In terms of the use of the "negative" side effects of cavitation in ablative therapy, a research protocol using "cavitation-enhanced ablation" of large uterine fibroids is ongoing to enhance the volume of thermal ablations at a lower temperature.

◆ MRgFUS: Going Forward

Insightec (Haifa, Israel) and SuperSonic Imagine (Aix en Provence, France) are developing an MRgFUS system for the treatment of brain tumors. At the Brigham and Women's Hospital (Boston, MA), use of the Insightec system (Exablate 4000) in a phase I clinical trial for the treatment of primary and secondary (metastatic) brain malignancies is under way.[91,92] So far, four patients have been treated. Thalamotomy using MRgFUS was also performed in 10 patients in Zurich for the treatment of intractable pain.[93] Preclinical research is under way for the targeted delivery of chemotherapeutic drugs that normally do not cross the BBB.

Although many challenges remain, MRgFUS has emerged as a noninvasive alternative therapy that provides unparalleled control in a closed-loop treatment program. Inspired by recent advances in the transcranial delivery of FUS therapy that has few proven side effects, researchers around the country and worldwide have shown a marked interest in both thermal and nonthermal effects of this therapy. By causing targeted delivery of molecules secondary to BBB disruption, MRgFUS may be instrumental in changing the way chemotherapy and other CNS drugs are delivered or enhanced. Furthermore, the ability of MRgFUS to ablate tissue and spare surrounding tissues is thought to be revolutionary to the treatment of brain tumors.

References

1. Curie P, Curie J. Crystal physics: development by pressure of polar electrics in hemihedral crystals with inclined faces. C R Acad Sci 1880:91
2. Briquard P, Paul Langevin. Ultrasonics 1972;10(5):213–214
3. Van Tiggelen R, Pouders E. Ultrasound and computed tomography: spin-offs of the world wars. JBR-BTR 2003;86(4):235–241
4. Meyers R, Fry WJ, Fry FJ, Dreyer LL, Schultz DF, Noyes RF. Early experiences with ultrasonic irradiation of the pallidofugal and nigral complexes in hyperkinetic and hypertonic disorders. J Neurosurg 1959; 16(1):32–54
5. Lynn JG, Zwemer RL, Chick AJ. The biological application of focused ultrasonic waves. Science 1942;96(2483):119–120
6. Lynn JGPT, Putnam TJ. Histology of cerebral lesions produced by focused ultrasound. Am J Pathol 1944;20(3):637–649

7. Lynn JGZR, Zwemer RL, Chick AJ, Miller AE. A new method for the generation and use of focused ultrasound in experimental biology. J Gen Physiol 1942;26(2):179–193

8. Fry WJ, Mosberg WH Jr, Barnard JW, Fry FJ. Production of focal destructive lesions in the central nervous system with ultrasound. J Neurosurg 1954;11(5):471–478

9. Fry WJ, Barnard JW, Fry FJ, Brennan JF. Ultrasonically produced localized selective lesions in the central nervous system. Am J Phys Med 1955;34(3):413–423

10. Fry FJ. Precision high intensity focusing ultrasonic machines for surgery. Am J Phys Med 1958;37(3):152–156

11. Heimburger RF. Ultrasound augmentation of central nervous system tumor therapy. Indiana Med 1985;78(6):469–476

12. Heimburger RF. An encounter with stereotactic brain surgery. Neurosurgery 2005;56(6):1367–1373, discussion 1373–1374

13. Barnard JW, Fry WJ, Fry FJ, Krumins RF. Effects of high intensity ultrasound on the central nervous system of the cat. J Comp Neurol 1955; 103(3):459–484

14. Bakay L, Ballantine HT Jr, Hueter TF, Sosa D. Ultrasonically produced changes in the blood–brain barrier. AMA Arch Neurol Psychiatry 1956;76(5):457–467

15. Lele PP. A simple method for production of trackless focal lesions with focused ultrasound: physical factors. J Physiol 1962;160:494–512

16. Lele PP. Production of deep focal lesions by focused ultrasound—current status. Ultrasonics 1967;5:105–112

17. Lindstrom PA. Prefrontal ultrasonic irradiation–a substitute for lobotomy. AMA Arch Neurol Psychiatry 1954;72(4):399–425

18. Leksell L. Cerebral radiosurgery. I. Gammathalanotomy in two cases of intractable pain. Acta Chir Scand 1968;134(8):585–595

19. Cline HE, Schenck JF, Watkins RD, Hynynen K, Jolesz FA. Magnetic resonance-guided thermal surgery. Magn Reson Med 1993;30(1): 98–106

20. Cline HE, Hynynen K, Hardy CJ, Watkins RD, Schenck JF, Jolesz FA. MR temperature mapping of focused ultrasound surgery. Magn Reson Med 1994;31(6):628–636

21. Hynynen K, Vykhodtseva NI, Chung AH, Sorrentino V, Colucci V, Jolesz FA. Thermal effects of focused ultrasound on the brain: determination with MR imaging. Radiology 1997;204(1):247–253

22. Jolesz FA, Hynynen K. Magnetic resonance image-guided focused ultrasound surgery. Cancer J 2002;8(Suppl 1):S100–S112

23. Jolesz FA, Hynynen K, McDannold N, Tempany C. MR imaging-controlled focused ultrasound ablation: a noninvasive image-guided surgery. Magn Reson Imaging Clin N Am 2005;13(3):545–560

24. Cline HE, Hynynen K, Schneider E, et al. Simultaneous magnetic resonance phase and magnitude temperature maps in muscle. Magn Reson Med 1996;35(3):309–315

25. Chen L, Bouley D, Yuh E, D'Arceuil H, Butts K. Study of focused ultrasound tissue damage using MRI and histology. J Magn Reson Imaging 1999;10(2):146–153

26. Chen L, Bouley DM, Harris BT, Butts K. MRI study of immediate cell viability in focused ultrasound lesions in the rabbit brain. J Magn Reson Imaging 2001;13(1):23–30

27. Hynynen K, Jolesz FA. Demonstration of potential noninvasive ultrasound brain therapy through an intact skull. Ultrasound Med Biol 1998;24(2):275–283

28. Hynynen K, Clement GT, McDannold N, et al. 500-Element ultrasound phased array system for noninvasive focal surgery of the brain: a preliminary rabbit study with ex vivo human skulls. Magn Reson Med 2004;52(1):100–107

29. Hynynen K, McDannold N, Clement GT, et al. Pre-clinical testing of a phased array ultrasound system for MRI-guided noninvasive surgery of the brain—a primate study. Eur J Radiol 2006;59(2):149–156

30. Hynynen K, McDannold N, Clement G, et al. Pre-clinical testing of a phased array ultrasound system for MRI-guided noninvasive surgery of the brain—a primate study. Eur J Radiol 2006;59(2):149–156

31. McDannold N, Moss M, Killiany R, et al. MRI-guided focused ultrasound surgery in the brain: tests in a primate model. Magn Reson Med 2003;49(6):1188–1191

32. Hynynen K, McDannold N, Vykhodtseva N, et al. Focal disruption of the blood–brain barrier due to 260-kHz ultrasound bursts: a method for molecular imaging and targeted drug delivery. J Neurosurg 2006;105(3):445–454

33. Vykhodtseva N, McDannold N, Hynynen K. Progress and problems in the application of focused ultrasound for blood–brain barrier disruption. Ultrasonics 2008;48(4):279–296

34. Hynynen K, Vykhodtseva NI, Chung AH, Sorrentino V, Colucci V, Jolesz FA. Thermal effects of focused ultrasound on the brain: determination with MR imaging. Radiology 1997;204(1):247–253

35. Vykhodtseva N, Sorrentino V, Jolesz FA, Bronson RT, Hynynen K. MRI detection of the thermal effects of focused ultrasound on the brain. Ultrasound Med Biol 2000;26(5):871–880

36. Clement GT, Sun J, Giesecke T, Hynynen K. A hemisphere array for non-invasive ultrasound brain therapy and surgery. Phys Med Biol 2000; 45(12):3707–3719

37. Diederich CJ, Hynynen K. Ultrasound technology for hyperthermia. Ultrasound Med Biol 1999;25(6):871–887

38. Hynynen K. Biophysics and technology of ultrasound hyperthermia. In: Gautherie M, ed., Methods of External Hyperthermic Heating. New York: Springer-Verlag; 1990;61–116

39. Deng CX, Sieling F, Pan H, Cui J. Ultrasound-induced cell membrane porosity. Ultrasound Med Biol 2004;30(4):519–526

40. Hynynen K, McDannold N, Vykhodtseva N, Jolesz FA. Noninvasive MR imaging-guided focal opening of the blood-brain barrier in rabbits. Radiology 2001;220(3):640–646

41. Mitragotri S. Healing sound: the use of ultrasound in drug delivery and other therapeutic applications. Nat Rev Drug Discov 2005;4(3):255–260

42. Sheikov N, McDannold N, Vykhodtseva N, Jolesz F, Hynynen K. Cellular mechanisms of the blood–brain barrier opening induced by ultrasound in presence of microbubbles. Ultrasound Med Biol 2004;30(7):979–989

43. Nyborg WL. Mechanisms for nonthermal effects of sound. J Acoust Soc Am 1968;44(5):1302–1309

44. Nyborg WL. Biological effects of ultrasound: development of safety guidelines. Part II: general review. Ultrasound Med Biol 2001;27(3): 301–333

45. Hynynen K, McDannold N, Martin H, Jolesz FA, Vykhodtseva N. The threshold for brain damage in rabbits induced by bursts of ultrasound in the presence of an ultrasound contrast agent (Optison). Ultrasound Med Biol 2003;29(3):473–481

46. McDannold N, Vykhodtseva N, Hynynen K. Targeted disruption of the blood-brain barrier with focused ultrasound: association with cavitation activity. Phys Med Biol 2006;51(4):793–807

47. McDannold N, Vykhodtseva N, Raymond S, Jolesz FA, Hynynen K. MRI-guided targeted blood-brain barrier disruption with focused ultrasound: histological findings in rabbits. Ultrasound Med Biol 2005; 31(11):1527–1537

48. McDannold NJ, Vykhodtseva NI, Hynynen K. Microbubble contrast agent with focused ultrasound to create brain lesions at low power levels: MR imaging and histologic study in rabbits. Radiology 2006; 241(1):95–106

49. Leighton TG. The Acoustic Bubble. San Diego: Academic Press; 1994

50. Brujan EA, Ikeda T, Matsumoto Y. Jet formation and shock wave emission during collapse of ultrasound-induced cavitation bubbles and their role in the therapeutic applications of high-intensity focused ultrasound. Phys Med Biol 2005;50(20):4797–4809

51. Riesz P, Kondo T. Free radical formation induced by ultrasound and its biological implications. Free Radic Biol Med 1992;13(3):247–270

52. Vykhodtseva NI, Hynynen K, Damianou C. Histologic effects of high intensity pulsed ultrasound exposure with subharmonic emission in rabbit brain in vivo. Ultrasound Med Biol 1995;21(7):969–979

53. Sheikov N, McDannold N, Sharma S, Hynynen K. Effect of focused ultrasound applied with an ultrasound contrast agent on the tight junctional integrity of the brain microvascular endothelium. Ultrasound Med Biol 2008;34(7):1093–1104

54. Connor CW, Hynynen K. Patterns of thermal deposition in the skull during transcranial focused ultrasound surgery. IEEE Trans Biomed Eng 2004;51(10):1693–1706

55. Fry FJ, Barger JE. Acoustical properties of the human skull. J Acoust Soc Am 1978;63(5):1576–1590

56. Clement GT, White PJ, King RL, McDannold N, Hynynen K. A magnetic resonance imaging-compatible, large-scale array for trans-skull ultrasound surgery and therapy. J Ultrasound Med 2005;24(8):1117–1125

57. McDannold NJ, King RL, Jolesz FA, Hynynen KH. Usefulness of MR imaging-derived thermometry and dosimetry in determining the threshold for tissue damage induced by thermal surgery in rabbits. Radiology 2000;216(2):517–523

58. McDannold N, Vykhodtseva N, Hynynen K. Effects of acoustic parameters and ultrasound contrast agent dose on focused-ultrasound induced blood–brain barrier disruption. Ultrasound Med Biol 2008; 34(6):930–937

59. Hynynen K, Pomeroy O, Smith DN, et al. MR imaging-guided focused ultrasound surgery of fibroadenomas in the breast: a feasibility study. Radiology 2001;219(1):176–185

V Design, Equipment, and Logistics

60. Tempany CM, Stewart EA, McDannold N, Quade BJ, Jolesz FA, Hynynen K. MR imaging-guided focused ultrasound surgery of uterine leiomyomas: a feasibility study. Radiology 2003;226(3):897–905

61. Fennessy FM, Tempany CM, McDannold NJ, et al. Uterine leiomyomas: MR imaging-guided focused ultrasound surgery–results of different treatment protocols. Radiology 2007;243(3):885–893

62. Hindley J, Gedroyc WM, Regan L, et al. MRI guidance of focused ultrasound therapy of uterine fibroids: early results. AJR Am J Roentgenol 2004;183(6):1713–1719

63. Stewart EA, Gedroyc WM, Tempany CM, et al. Focused ultrasound treatment of uterine fibroid tumors: safety and feasibility of a noninvasive thermoablative technique. Am J Obstet Gynecol 2003;189(1):48–54

64. Fry WJ, Fry FJ. Fundamental neurological research and human neurosurgery using intense ultrasound. IRE Trans Med Electron 1960;ME-7: 166–181

65. Ram Z, Cohen ZR, Harnof S, et al. Magnetic resonance imaging-guided, high-intensity focused ultrasound for brain tumor therapy. Neurosurgery 2006;59(5):949–955, discussion 955–956

66. Foley JL, Little JW, Starr FL III, Frantz C, Vaezy S. Image-guided HIFU neurolysis of peripheral nerves to treat spasticity and pain. Ultrasound Med Biol 2004;30(9):1199–1207

67. Young RR, Henneman E. Functional effects of focused ultrasound on mammalian nerves. Science 1961;134:1521–1522

68. Fry FJ, Ades HW, Fry WJ. Production of reversible changes in the central nervous system by ultrasound. Science 1958;127(3289):83–84

69. Currier DP, Greathouse D, Swift T. Sensory nerve conduction: effect of ultrasound. Arch Phys Med Rehabil 1978;59(4):181–185

70. Kinoshita M, McDannold N, Jolesz FA, Hynynen K. Noninvasive localized delivery of Herceptin to the mouse brain by MRI-guided focused ultrasound-induced blood–brain barrier disruption. Proc Natl Acad Sci U S A 2006;103(31):11719–11723

71. Bednarski MD, Lee JW, Callstrom MR, Li KC. In vivo target-specific delivery of macromolecular agents with MR-guided focused ultrasound. Radiology 1997;204(1):263–268

72. Unger EC, McCreery TP, Sweitzer RH. Ultrasound enhances gene expression of liposomal transfection. Invest Radiol 1997;32(12):723–727

73. Unger EC, Porter T, Culp W, Labell R, Matsunaga T, Zutshi R. Therapeutic applications of lipid-coated microbubbles. Adv Drug Deliv Rev 2004;56(9):1291–1314

74. Li YS, Reid CN, McHale AP. Enhancing ultrasound-mediated cell membrane permeabilisation (sonoporation) using a high frequency pulse regime and implications for ultrasound-aided cancer chemotherapy. Cancer Lett 2008;266(2):156–162

75. Treat LH, McDannold N, Vykhodtseva N, Zhang Y, Tam K, Hynynen K. Targeted delivery of doxorubicin to the rat brain at therapeutic levels using MRI-guided focused ultrasound. Int J Cancer 2007;121(4): 901–907

76. Deckers R, Rome C, Moonen CT. The role of ultrasound and magnetic resonance in local drug delivery. J Magn Reson Imaging 2008;27(2): 400–409

77. Ferrara K, Pollard R, Borden M. Ultrasound microbubble contrast agents: fundamentals and application to gene and drug delivery. Annu Rev Biomed Eng 2007;9:415–447

78. Moonen CT. Spatio-temporal control of gene expression and cancer treatment using magnetic resonance imaging-guided focused ultrasound. Clin Cancer Res 2007;13(12):3482–3489

79. Frenkel V, Li KC. Potential role of pulsed-high intensity focused ultrasound in gene therapy. Future Oncol 2006;2(1):111–119

80. Frenkel V. Ultrasound mediated delivery of drugs and genes to solid tumors. Adv Drug Deliv Rev 2008;60(10):1193–1208

81. Kinoshita M, McDannold N, Jolesz FA, Hynynen K. Targeted delivery of antibodies through the blood–brain barrier by MRI-guided focused ultrasound. Biochem Biophys Res Commun 2006;340(4): 1085–1090

82. Raymond SB, Treat LH, Dewey JD, McDannold NJ, Hynynen K, Bacskai BJ. Ultrasound enhanced delivery of molecular imaging and therapeutic agents in Alzheimer's disease mouse models. PLoS One 2008; 3(5):e2175

83. Alexandrov AV, Molina CA, Grotta JC, et al; CLOTBUST Investigators. Ultrasound-enhanced systemic thrombolysis for acute ischemic stroke. N Engl J Med 2004;351(21):2170–2178

84. Alexandrov AV, Wojner AW, Grotta JC ; CLOTBUST Investigators. CLOTBUST: design of a randomized trial of ultrasound-enhanced thrombolysis for acute ischemic stroke. J Neuroimaging 2004;14(2):108–112

85. Daffertshofer M, Fatar M. Therapeutic ultrasound in ischemic stroke treatment: experimental evidence. Eur J Ultrasound 2002;16(1-2): 121–130

86. Molina CA, Ribo M, Rubiera M, et al. Microbubble administration accelerates clot lysis during continuous 2-MHz ultrasound monitoring in stroke patients treated with intravenous tissue plasminogen activator. Stroke 2006;37(2):425–429

87. Daffertshofer M, Gass A, Ringleb P, et al. Transcranial low-frequency ultrasound-mediated thrombolysis in brain ischemia: increased risk of hemorrhage with combined ultrasound and tissue plasminogen activator: results of a phase II clinical trial. Stroke 2005;36(7):1441–1446

88. Hynynen K, Chung AH, Colucci V, Jolesz FA. Potential adverse effects of high-intensity focused ultrasound exposure on blood vessels in vivo. Ultrasound Med Biol 1996;22(2):193–201

89. Hynynen K, Colucci V, Chung AH, Jolesz F. Noninvasive arterial occlusion using MRI-guided focused ultrasound. Ultrasound Med Biol 1996;22(8):1071–1077

90. Zderic V, Brayman AA, Sharar SR, Crum LA, Vaezy S. Microbubble-enhanced hemorrhage control using high intensity focused ultrasound. Ultrasonics 2006;45(1-4):113–120

91. McDannold NCG, Zadicario E, Black PM, Jolesz F, Hynynen K. Transcranial MRI guided focused ultrasound surgery in brain tumors: initial findings in patients. Paper presented at the 17th Scientific Meeting of the International Society for Magnetic Resonance in Medicine; April 18–24, 2009; Honolulu, HI

92. McDannold NCG, Zadicario E, Black PM, Jolesz F, Hynynen K. Transcranial MRI guided focused ultrasound surgery of brain tumors: Initial findings in three patients. Neurosurgery 2009; In press

93. Martin E, Jeanmonod D, Morel A, Zadicario E, Werner B. High intensity focused ultrasound for non-invasive functional neurosurgery. Ann Neurol 2009;66(6):858–861

25

Cost and Benefit Analysis of Intraoperative MRI-Guided Neurosurgery

William C. Broaddus, Zhijian Chen, G. T. Gillies, John Kucharczyk, and Wayne L. Monsky

Over the past two decades, there have been significant advances in intraoperative MRI-guided (iMRI) neurosurgical applications. The first dedicated open interventional MRI system was developed at Brigham and Women's Hospital during the mid-1980s. In 1996, the first intraoperative MRI-guided craniotomy was reported by the University Hospital in Heidelberg.[1] The first neurosurgical operation in a dedicated 3.0 tesla (T) MRI suite was performed at the University of Minnesota,[2] which also performed magnetic resonance spectroscopy (MRS) and functional MRI (fMRI) immediately prior to craniotomy.[3]

MRI-guided neurosurgical procedures now include stereotactic biopsy and resection of brain tumors, placement of deep brain stimulating electrodes, targeted drug and cell delivery, and various other procedures where localization of a probe, implant, or target structure is critical to the outcome.[4–6] MRI is generally well suited for such neurosurgical interventions because the submillimeter spatial resolution available in multiple projections allows the clinician to determine the optimal surgical trajectory, to avoid critical neural structures, and to evaluate the status and efficacy of the procedure intraoperatively.[7–9] MRI has an additional advantage over computed tomography (CT) because there is no radiation exposure to the patient or health care personnel. At the same time, the use of iMRI guidance has added several challenges to the already complex neurosurgery operating room (OR). The use of iMRI alters the surgical working environment and affects various diagnostic and surgical protocols and procedures in many ways. For example, sterile draping of the patient has to be modified, communications between OR personnel can be difficult because of noise from the scanner, and specialized MRI-compatible surgical instruments are often required because of the large magnetic fields and gradients produced by the scanner.[10,11]

As iMRI-guided procedures gain increasing acceptance in the neurosurgical community, medical centers around the world have launched evaluations of their investments in interventional MRI suites. Multiple interested parties, including insurance companies, hospital administrators, physicians, patient advocacy groups, and government representatives have become active participants in the ongoing debate about the cost effectiveness of MRI-guided interventions. However, to date, only a few studies have provided comparisons of the financial costs and clinical benefits of iMRI guidance relative to procedures performed in a conventional OR in terms of patient length of stay, hospital charges and costs, net health outcome, and other technology assessment criteria now generally demanded by managed care organizations, third-party coverage agencies, hospital administrations, and the relevant regulatory entities. In this chapter we summarize the available data on the cost efficacy of iMRI-guided neurosurgery and discuss the potential future role of iMRI guidance in the diagnosis and management of various neurologic diseases and disorders.

◆ Analyzing Cost Effectiveness

In the modern managed care environment, medical and surgical treatments are increasingly being subjected to evaluations of economic efficiency. A conventional cost-effectiveness analysis essentially measures the cost of a medical technology per unit of a defined health output. Such an analysis is useful for directly comparing competing medical treatments and enabling them to be ranked based on economic efficiency.[12] Components of a cost-effectiveness analysis typically include the costs of the procedure, the use of discounting for both costs and benefits, an appropriate viewpoint of the analysis, and a sensitivity analysis of the assumptions and probabilities that drive the analysis and underlie the results. The cost of adding an iMRI system to a hospital must also take into account its benefits to physician users, its ability to improve patient clinical outcome, and its capacity to favorably impact other hospital costs, including those associated with risk management. Cost–benefit analysis can be further complicated if an interventional MRI unit is purchased for multipurpose use, including diagnostic MRI, MRI-guided interventions, as well as iMRI-guided neurosurgery. At many hospitals and medical centers, multipurpose use of interventional MRI is in fact mandated as a practical economic requirement because MRI-guided neurosurgery is still performed relatively infrequently. Consideration of such detailed information is necessary to objectively evaluate whether iMRI-guidance is cost effective (particularly in terms of capital equipment expenses, suite constructions and renovations, and the associated personnel and maintenance costs).

◆ MRI-Guided Brain Biopsy and Tumor Resection

iMRI-guided systems were developed initially to facilitate safer and more effective neurosurgical procedures for brain biopsy and tumor resection. MRI guidance generally enables the neurosurgeon to take into account brain-shift after opening the skull, to more accurately localize the lesion to be resected, to determine the full extent of the lesion, and to establish a safe surgical approach to the lesion with reduced operative morbidity. However, with both frame-based and frameless neuronavigational systems, the radiologic images obtained before surgery do not necessarily provide the surgeon with information during the actual surgery that reflects the dynamic changes in the operative lesion and surrounding structures, especially brain-shift. During stereotactic brain biopsies, shift of the target by 5 mm or more has been reported,[13] which can result in significant loss of navigational accuracy. Many neurosurgical procedures have a very small margin for anatomic error, which has led to the development of several Food and Drug Administration-approved stereotactic computer-assisted guidance systems for various procedures.

Successful biopsy rates of 80 to 99% have been reported in recent studies of stereotactic biopsy procedures aided by iMRI guidance.[6] Bernays et al[14] obtained a histologic yield of 100% and a diagnostic yield of 97.4% in 114 consecutive frameless stereotactic biopsy procedures with iMRI guidance. Brain-shift was detected in 45% of the patients. Six complications, including one death and one case of a new neurologic deficit, were reported.

An early cost-effectiveness analysis of stereotactic radiosurgery versus resection for patients with solitary metastatic brain tumors revealed a lower uncomplicated procedure cost ($20,209 versus $27,587), a lower average complication cost per case ($2,534 versus $2,874), a lower total cost per procedure ($22,743 versus $30,461), a better overall cost effectiveness ($24,811 versus $32,149 per life year), and a better incremental cost effectiveness ($40,648 versus $52,384 per life year) for radiosurgery than for surgical resection.[15] However, controversy remains regarding the relative efficacy of radiosurgery in comparison to open surgery for metastatic disease, adding further complexity to attempts at comparing the two management alternatives.

Another early study that analyzed the cost effectiveness of anterior temporal lobectomy for intractable temporal lobe epilepsy found that surgery provided an average of 1.1 additional quality-adjusted life years (QALYs) compared with continued medical management at an additional cost of $29,800.[16] Anterior temporal lobectomy yielded a cost-effectiveness ratio of $27,200 per QALY, which was comparable to various high-volume therapeutic procedures such as total knee arthroplasty ($16,700/QALY) or coronary artery balloon arthroplasty ($40,800/QALY).[16]

An evaluative study performed at the University of Minnesota[17] compared the financial costs and clinical benefits of brain tumor resection performed in an interventional MRI suite compared with a conventional operating room (OR). To evaluate the comparative cost efficacy, financial data for 51 tumors resected under iMRI were compared with conventional OR data. Eighteen patients had a first brain tumor resection and another 29 patients underwent 33 tumor resections for recurrent disease. The iMRI data were analyzed together with 35 pediatric and 118 adult tumor resections performed in the OR. Comparisons were made for adults and children for length of stay, hospital charges and payments, hospital total direct and indirect costs, readmission rates, repeat resection interval, and net health outcome.

For adults, the length of stay associated with iMRI-guided surgery (3.7 days) was significantly shorter than for conventional OR surgery (8.2 days) for first resections. iMRI hospital charges were 12.2% lower ($4,063) for first resections and 4.1% lower ($922) for repeat resections than for OR surgery. Total MRI suite hospital costs associated with iMRI-guided procedures were 14.4% lower ($3,415) than for OR surgery for first resections and 3.3% lower ($723) than costs for repeat resections. Cost-to-charge ratio for first resections was 69.6% for iMRI procedures and 71.4% for OR procedures, but was not different for repeat resections. For children, the length of stay associated with iMRI-guided surgery (4.5 days) was significantly shorter than for OR surgery (14.1 days) for first resections, as well as for repeat resections (8.0 days vs 13.3 days, respectively). Hospital charges associated with iMRI-guided surgery were significantly lower than for OR surgery for both first resections and repeat resections. The iMRI-guided surgery costs were also significantly lower for first resections and repeat resections compared with OR surgery. Operative morbidity and mortality were not different with use of the iMRI procedures. Notably, no repeat resections followed iMRI surgery, whereas the OR repeat resection rate was 20% (adults) and 30% (children). The mean time from iMRI-guided surgery was 11.3 months (adults) and 18.0 months (children). For OR surgery, the mean time to repeat resection rate was 9.3 months (adults) and 13.3 months (children).

The results of the University of Minnesota study[17] provided some early evidence that iMRI-guided surgery can improve net health outcomes in terms of reduced hospital length of stay, reduced resection rate, and reduced hospital charges and costs. The length of stay for iMRI-patients was 31 to 68% lower compared with that of brain tumor patients undergoing resection in the OR. Hospital charges were 3 to

44% lower for iMRI-patients than for OR patients. Costs for iMRI-resection admissions were 3 to 46% lower for iMRI patients compared with OR patients. Patients that had iMRI-guided surgery were also found to have a lower repeat tumor resection rate after the initial resection or subsequent resections. Interpretation of the Minnesota study results is limited by the fact that the data was not obtained from a randomized, controlled trial. Nonetheless, the results do suggest that compared with conventional OR surgery, iMRI-guided surgery can reduce hospitalization length of stay, associated hospital charges, and repeat resection rate. Moreover, although neurosurgery for brain tumor resection performed in a conventional OR generally has a 20 to 50% repeat resection rate within one year, the Minnesota results found that iMRI-guided neurosurgery can have a much lower repeat resection rate during a comparable period.

Several studies have demonstrated that iMRI-guidance improves the extent of tumor resection for both low-grade and high-grade gliomas.[18-25] Most of these studies found no differences in outcome between the use of high-field versus low-field MRI guidance, although there are two reports that high-field iMRI-guidance led to a significant improvement in the extent of tumor resection compared with low-field MRI.[20,26] Survival studies suggest that iMRI can usefully guide total surgical resection of gliomas. The risk of low-grade glioma recurrence during a median follow-up of 3 years was found to be 1.4 times higher for patients who underwent subtotal resection, and the risk of death was 4.9-fold higher compared with patients who underwent gross total resection.[27] Wirtz et al[25] found that the mean survival time for patients with glioblastoma multiforme was 15.7 months for patients without residual tumor, which was an 83% improvement over the 8.6-month survival time for patients with residual tumor.

However, not all studies have found benefits associated with iMRI-guidance for surgical treatment of gliomas. Hirschberg et al,[28] for example, reported that although iMRI guidance can improve imaging of residual grade IV gliomas, it did not increase the efficacy of surgery or reduce the complication rate in patients compared with more conventional neurosurgery.

The benefits of iMRI guidance for resection of nonglioma intracranial tumors have been mixed. Gralla et al[29] reported that in 26 patients with supratentorial cavernomas, there was no difference in extent of tumor resection between patients undergoing iMRI-guided surgery versus conventional neurosurgery.

In another study of 21 patients undergoing resection of craniopharyngiomas, iMRI-guidance (0.2 T) facilitated monitoring of cyst puncture and aspiration and complete resection, but did not exclude recurrence of the tumor.[30]

Yrjana et al[31] recently reported their 7-year experience with 160 craniotomies in an operating theater equipped with a 0.23 T MRI scanner, which could be turned on and off during surgery. The tumors undergoing iMRI-guided resection included 87 low-grade and high-grade gliomas, 16 meningiomas, 13 benign tumors, along with various histologically miscellaneous subgroups. The authors of this study concluded that for many patients conventional neurosurgery, possibly aided by neuronavigation, offers benefits comparable to iMRI-guided surgery. However, Yrjana et al also found that for some patients with deep-seated tumors, or with tumors in critical locations, prognosis may be significantly enhanced by iMRI-guidance.

The impact of iMRI on surgical outcomes has also been evaluated in studies in which imaging updates were used during the procedure to see if further surgery was necessary. Measurements of usage rate or frequency (the percentage of procedures in which the surgeon decided to use intraoperative imaging) ranged from 17.5 to 73.6% in three studies reporting on 309 procedures.[32-34] Among 419 tumor resection procedures where iMRI was available, further resection based on updated imaging was beneficially performed in 14.8 to 63.4% of cases.

In a recent analysis of the impact of iMRI on health care costs, outcomes were compared in 102 patients who had undergone intracranial tumor resection with the use of preoperative and postoperative MRI alone versus 160 patients that underwent tumor resection with iMRI guidance.[35] Mean total costs, OR costs, and intensive care unit (ICU) costs were not significantly different between the two groups, although, importantly, length of hospital stay was reduced in glioma patients that had tumor resection with iMRI-guidance.

Lycette et al[36] compared hospital charges for iMRI-guided surgery with standard neurosurgery for 18 patients with glial neoplasms who underwent craniotomies. The iMRI group had an average operation time of 9.9 hours with an associated hospital charge of $8,840 and average material costs of $17,180. The standard OR group had an average operation time of 6.3 hours, hospital charge of $4,390, and material costs of $16,900. The majority of the cost difference between the two groups was attributable to the longer operation time for the iMRI group for which the hospital charged an hourly rate.

The impact of neuronavigation without iMRI update on surgical resection of brain tumors has also been evaluated in several studies.[37-41] These studies reported rates of 81.2 to 100% total removal of lesions. Extent of resection was confirmed with operative MRI or computed tomography (CT) within 48 hours of the surgical procedure. Three additional studies involved biopsies of cranial tumors with a combined sample size of 258 patients. Diagnostic accuracy, defined as the percentage of intraoperative smear diagnoses later corroborated by definitive histologic study, ranged from 87 to 96%.[42,43] Medical and surgical complication rates ranged from 8.8 to 14%.

In a prospective nonrandomized study, Dorward et al[42] compared 76 frameless procedures with 79 frame-based procedures, all without intraoperative imaging updates. Histopathologic results and the accuracy of smear diagnosis were comparable in the two groups. The frame-based group had a complication rate of 22%, significantly higher than the 14% complication rate in the frameless group. Germano et al[40] reported a mean of 7.5 days hospital length of stay when neuronavigation without imaging update was used for surgical resection of tumors, versus 10.8 days in patients undergoing conventional surgery, a more than 30% difference.

The standard treatment for glioblastoma remains biopsy and resection followed by radiotherapy and, in some cases, systemic chemotherapy. However, newer therapies, including local chemotherapy using implantable biodegradable polymers, immunotherapy, gene therapy, and anti-angiogenic agents, are under active, ongoing development.[44,45] Analyses of the costs of these newer approaches and interventions need to be performed in relation to the costs of standard neurosurgical treatment to get a more complete picture of the cost effectiveness of various approaches.

◆ MRI-Guided Functional Neurosurgery

Functional neurosurgery currently encompasses procedures that seek to improve patient status relative to movement disorders, psychiatric illness, pain, and epilepsy. These procedures have traditionally incorporated frame-based stereotactic localization, but are moving generally toward frameless techniques. The goals of iMRI-guidance are to localize the target accurately and quickly and to allow efficient surgical implantation of a lead, sensor, or other probe.

Advances in imaging, improvements in target localization, and increasingly sophisticated neuronavigational systems have stimulated interest in iMRI neurosurgical management for movement disorders in particular. Because iMRI guidance provides real-time visualization of target brain structures contemporaneous with intraoperative microelectrode recording, the opportunity exists to optimize deep brain stimulation (DBS) by correlating functional anatomy with the clinical and physiologic manifestations of movement disorders.

Until recently, stereotactic thalamotomy and posteroventral pallidotomy were the most commonly used neurosurgical procedures for movement disorders. Although ablative surgery remains an option, increasing attention is now focused on high-frequency DBS of the thalamus, globus pallidus interna, and subthalamic nucleus. Electrical stimulation of the subthalamic nucleus has become generally accepted as an effective treatment for advanced stage or otherwise medically refractory Parkinson's disease.[46–48]

In one early study, unilateral or bilateral iMRI-guided DBS was performed in 31 patients.[49] Preliminary data were obtained in the first 17 patients in whom 6-month follow-up had been completed. Ten underwent thalamic ventral intermediate nucleus DBS for essential or parkinsonian tremor. Based on tremor rating scales, nine of 10 patients had marked improvement (absent or minimal tremor) at 6-month follow up. All three parkinsonian patients who underwent globus pallidus DBS experienced significant improvement in their motor scores and a reduction in medication-induced dyskinesias. Three of four patients with subthalamic nucleus stimulation demonstrated marked improvement in motor scores and at least a 40% reduction in medication dosages. Complications occurred in two patients (11%), including a lead fracture and wound infection requiring lead replacement in each case. In two other studies involving 50 patients with movement disorders, iMRI provided reliable guidance for catheter or electrode placement and detected electrode placement errors.[50] These data suggest that the use of iMRI-guidance has the potential to improve the use of DBS to provide safe and effective treatment for medically refractory Parkinson's disease.

Further work may reveal the utility of DBS for diseases and syndromes other than movement disorders. One group has reported a patient with Parkinson's disease and associated profound depression who responded to modified placement of subthalamic DBS.[51,52] Another group has reported improvement in three out of four patients with obsessive compulsive disorder receiving DBS of the anterior limb of the internal capsule.[53] Such reports hold promise that a reversible and adjustable procedure such as DBS will become a treatment option for selected psychiatric disorders as it currently has for movement disorders.

iMRI guidance has been used in a small number of studies of medically intractable epilepsy.[54,55] In one study of 71 patients,[54] registration and surgical planning took place with the patient anesthetized using the same 1.5 T MRI unit that provided intraoperative imaging. iMRI revealed residual tissue that had been targeted for resection in 26% of all patients in the study and in 50% of patients undergoing selective resections of medial temporal structures. Seventy percent of patients remained seizure-free at 6-month follow-up.

Depth electrode placement, intraoperative verification of electrode location, and image-guided electrode repositioning can be performed in the iMRI suite without the use of a head frame. Depth electrodes have been implanted successfully in two patients under MRI guidance.[56] One patient was a 45-year-old right-handed woman with intractable seizures localized to the left posterior temporal/insular region. A depth electrode was successfully placed at the lesion site in the iMRI suite along with a grid for recording seizure focus and mapping of language and motor areas. Additional studies at several centers will be required to determine whether iMRI can provide a cost-effective alternative to traditional stereotactic implantation of depth electrodes in patients with epilepsy, especially those subject to grand mal seizures.

Future improvements in MRI-guided functional neurosurgery will likely focus on more efficient systems in which imaging time is reduced without loss of anatomic resolution. High-field systems that are mobile and allow better patient access are increasingly attainable with refinements in existing designs. With improved resolution and three-dimensional imaging, it seems possible that language, memory, and motor mapping can be performed to the detail required for epilepsy resections.

◆ MRI-Guided Drug and Cell Therapy

Targeted delivery of therapeutic agents directly to tissues can potentially improve therapeutic efficacy while minimizing systemic side effects. Delivery of therapeutic agents into the brain is complicated by the presence of the blood–brain barrier (BBB) and the inability to directly visualize the distribution of the active agent in vivo.[57] Historically, intraparenchymal infusion or the slow bolus injection of therapeutic agent has been accomplished by stereotactic guidance of a cannula, catheter, or other delivery device through a burr hole to the target intracranial site. MRI/CT imaging studies were often used preoperatively to estimate the optimal insertion trajectory. Infusion methodologies for both framed and frameless stereotaxis have now been developed, with forms of the latter optimized for use in the iMRI setting.

Convection-enhanced delivery (CED) was developed as a method to treat brain tumors by circumventing the selective behavior of the BBB on drug penetration into the brain's extracellular compartment.[58] The use of CED with various therapeutic agents, including immunotoxins, gene therapy vectors, and radioisotope-labeled antibodies, has been evaluated during the past decade in several phase I and phase II clinical trials. Phase III clinical trials are now under way at several hospitals and academic medical centers to define the best clinical practice for CED.[59]

iMRI guidance has been used for intraparenchymal delivery of agents for the treatment of intracranial tumors.[58–61] Numerous additional applications currently under investigation include MRI-guided delivery of antisense oligonucleotides for treatment of brain tumors,[62–64] remyelination therapy for multiple sclerosis,[65] regional infusion therapy for glioblastoma multiforme,[66–68] and MRI-guided stereotactic injections of cells or chemotherapeutic agents for recurrent primary or secondary brain tumors.[69–72]

MRI-guided delivery of cell transplants for the treatment of Parkinson's disease is undergoing human clinical testing and evaluation.[73–75] Selective excitotoxic ablation within the globus pallidus[76] and the infusion of viral vectors into striatal neurons to restore dopamine production[77] are also undergoing investigation.

Other restorative neurosurgical procedures that involve image-guided stereotactic cell delivery include neurotransplantation for Huntington disease[78] and stroke.[79] Preclinical animal studies also suggest the possibility of treating chemical dependency syndromes and appetite disorders via intraparenchymal infusion of dopaminergic agents.[80]

The cost efficacy of MRI-guided intraparenchymal drug and cell infusion will likely be best demonstrated by empirical proof that MRI guidance permits the attainment of an adequate dose of the therapeutic agent throughout a desired volume of distribution, such that all the target tissues are fully treated. Such detailed studies have yet to be performed. Measurements of the concentration and range of spread of the infusate will be needed, preferably both during and after treatment (i.e., in both the convective and diffusive stages of flow of the drug through the interstitial space). Image-based approaches offer the only noninvasive means of accomplishing this task. The choice of imaging modality will generally depend on the drug or cells to be delivered, the device or mechanism used for delivery, the rate at which updated images must be obtained, and the patient's clinical status.

If the therapeutic agent is tagged with an MRI-visible contrast agent, standard time course MR images will map the volume of distribution, with the resolution of the measurements ultimately limited by the voxel noise level of the imager and its sensitivity to the agent being resolved. However, this approach also presents difficulties in developing the labeling process, establishing the stability of the labeled therapeutic agent, understanding its rate of metabolism and clearance, and establishing its behavioral similarity to the unlabeled agent. Presumably for these reasons, infusion protocols that have been utilized in patients to date, including those that have attempted to incorporate an accurate MRI-based method for monitoring the distribution of the therapeutic agent during or after the infusion, are still regarded as being developmental in nature. One promising strategy along these lines incorporates the use of functionalized metallofullerenes (modified "buckyballs") as a nanoplatform serving as an enhanced contrast agent and as a platform for delivery of radiotherapeutics into malignant brain tumors.[81]

Other MRI approaches do not require contrast labeling of the therapeutic agent. For example, convection-enhanced drug delivery enables the drug agent to access the extracellular compartment of the brain, thus altering the behavior of resident tissue water protons.[58] Diffusion tensor imaging (DTI) can map changes in spatial and temporal distribution of interstitial water, from which the apparent diffusion coefficient of the infusate can be established quantitatively. DTI is already finding clinical application in several neuroradiologic applications, including assessment of multiple sclerosis lesions,[82] investigation of neuroanatomic abnormalities in Alzheimer patients,[83] and evaluation of neurophysiologic parameters of stroke patients.[84] Software packages for installation in clinical MRI scanners are available from several commercial vendors (e.g., MR Vision Co., Winchester, MA).

The infusion catheter itself can play a significant role in imaging the volume of distribution of the infusate. Image-guided placement of the tip of a drug delivery catheter directly into specific regions of the brain can initially produce maximal drug concentration close to the target tissue receptors. At the same time, the limited distribution of drug injected from a single catheter tip presents other problems. For example, delivery of a drug from a single point source limits the distribution of the drug by decreasing the effective radius of penetration of the drug agent into the surrounding tissue receptor population.[85] Catheter designs that are MRI-visible and have radiofrequency receiver microcoils incorporated into their tips have been developed to facilitate iMRI-guided drug and cell delivery into target tissues.[86–89]

Image-guided transparenchymal delivery of drugs and cells is an emerging approach that holds great promise for delivering a wide variety of agents directly across the BBB.[81,90] Large-scale, prospective, randomized, multicenter trials have not been conducted to establish the cost efficacy of iMRI-guidance in the delivery of therapeutic agents into the brain, but as approval of individual agents occurs, such trials will inevitably be needed.

◆ The Politics of Health Care Reform in the United States: Implications for Intraoperative MRI-Guided Neurosurgery

The rapid diffusion of new medical technologies into the health care systems of Western industrialized countries since the mid-1970s has generated ongoing controversy about their cost effectiveness. The response of legislators and politicians to this debate has been varied. Regulatory approaches have attempted to restrict technology diffusion in several countries, for example, Canada and Great Britain. In the United States, on the other hand, the planning, purchase, and siting of new medical technologies have been largely unrestricted by state or federal governments.

In the current political debate about health care reform in the United States, there is reasonably broad agreement about the principal issues that must be addressed. These include cost containment, improved access, and improved quality. There is little agreement, however, on the exact strategy to achieve these objectives. High-technology medicine generally and diagnostic imaging in particular have been labeled as major culprits in the failure to achieve better cost containment in health care spending. Numerous key politicians have pointed to high-tech medicine as a significant inflationary factor in rapidly escalating health care costs. Critics of the current "laissez-faire" system are actively discussing regionalization and rationing of expensive medical technologies, such as MRI. A major effort to counter the perception that iMRI is too expensive and unproven will be required. As a result, neurosurgeons and neuroradiologists, as well as equipment and pharmaceutical manufacturers, will need to provide evidence of the benefits of iMRI-guided interventions in relation to costs, health outcomes, and efficacy.

The rules governing the assessment and utilization of high-tech medicine are changing. Private sector and government insurers increasingly want to see data that permits objective conclusions to be drawn on health outcomes, proof that the new technology is superior to established technologies, and evidence that benefits are attainable outside of major medical centers. There is some evidence that managed care organizations are actually considering implementation of the concept of cost effectiveness as a coverage criterion for recipients of health insurance.

The eventual outcome of the current health care reform debate now under way in the United States could have an enormous impact on availability and reimbursement for interventional MRI. If an indiscriminate cost-containment effort is initiated at political levels, iMRI-guided surgery could be a highly visible target. Rationing of the use of MRI and regionalization of high-tech health care services may result. Technology assessment initiatives are therefore needed to compare the cost effectiveness of iMRI in relation to alternative approaches. In particular, double-blind, prospective randomized clinical trials should be performed to assess the costs, benefits, and utilization of iMRI-guided neurosurgery.

Acknowledgments The work at the University of Virginia was supported in part by a grant from the Kopf Family Foundation, Inc.

References

1. Wirtz CR, Bonsanto MM, Knauth M, et al. Intraoperative magnetic resonance imaging to update interactive navigation in neurosurgery: method and preliminary experience. Comput Aided Surg 1997;2(3-4): 172–179

2. Martin AJ, Hall WA, Liu H, et al. Brain tumor resection: intraoperative monitoring with high-field-strength MR imaging-initial results. Radiology 2000;215(1):221–228

3. Martin AJ, Liu H, Hall WA, Truwit CL. Preliminary assessment of turbo spectroscopic imaging for targeting in brain biopsy. AJNR Am J Neuroradiol 2001;22(5):959–968

4. Black PM, Moriarty T, Alexander E III, et al. Development and implementation of intraoperative magnetic resonance imaging and its neurosurgical applications. Neurosurgery 1997;41(4):831–842, discussion 842–845

5. Hall WA, Martin AJ, Liu H, Nussbaum ES, Maxwell RE, Truwit CL. Brain biopsy using high-field strength interventional magnetic resonance imaging. Neurosurgery 1999;44(4):807–813, discussion 813–814

6. Hall WA, Liu H, Martin AJ, Pozza CH, Maxwell RE, Truwit CL. Safety, efficacy, and functionality of high-field strength interventional magnetic resonance imaging for neurosurgery. Neurosurgery 2000;46(3):632–641, discussion 641–642

7. Hall WA, Galicich W, Bergman T, Truwit CL. 3-Tesla intraoperative MR imaging for neurosurgery. J Neurooncol 2005;29:1–7

8. Maurer CR Jr, Hill DLG, Martin AJ, et al. Investigation of intraoperative brain deformation using a 1.5-T interventional MR system: preliminary results. IEEE Trans Med Imaging 1998;17(5):817–825

9. Yrjänä SK, Tuominen J, Koivukangas J. Intraoperative magnetic resonance imaging in neurosurgery. Acta Radiol 2007;48(5):540–549

10. Archer DP, McTaggart Cowan RA, Falkenstein RJ, Sutherland GR. Intraoperative mobile magnetic resonance imaging for craniotomy lengthens the procedure but does not increase morbidity. Can J Anaesth 2002;49(4):420–426

11. Silverman SG, Jolesz FA, Newman RW, et al. Design and implementation of an interventional MR imaging suite. AJR Am J Roentgenol 1997; 168(6):1465–1471

12. Rutigliano MJ. Cost effectiveness analysis: a review. Neurosurgery 1995;37(3):436–443, discussion 443–444

13. Rubino GJ, Farahani K, McGill D, Van De Wiele B, Villablanca JP, Wang-Mathieson A. Magnetic resonance imaging-guided neurosurgery in the magnetic fringe fields: the next step in neuronavigation. Neurosurgery 2000;46(3):643–653, discussion 653–654

14. Bernays RL, Kollias SS, Khan N, Brandner S, Meier S, Yonekawa Y. Histological yield, complications, and technological considerations in 114 consecutive frameless stereotactic biopsy procedures aided by open intraoperative magnetic resonance imaging. J Neurosurg 2002;97(2): 354–362

15. Rutigliano MJ, Lunsford LD, Kondziolka D, Strauss MJ, Khanna V, Green M. The cost effectiveness of stereotactic radiosurgery versus surgical resection in the treatment of solitary metastatic brain tumors. Neurosurgery 1995;37(3):445–453, discussion 453–455

16. King JT Jr, Sperling MR, Justice AC, O'Connor MJ. A cost-effectiveness analysis of anterior temporal lobectomy for intractable temporal lobe epilepsy. J Neurosurg 1997;87(1):20–28

17. Hall WA, Kowalik K, Liu H, Truwit CL, Kucharczyk J. Costs and benefits of intraoperative MR-guided brain tumor resection. Acta Neurochir (Wien) 2002;85:137–142

18. Black PM, Alexander E III, Martin C, et al. Craniotomy for tumor treatment in an intraoperative magnetic resonance imaging unit. Neurosurgery 1999;45(3):423–431, discussion 431–433

19. McPherson CM, Bohinski RJ, Dagnew E, Warnick RE, Tew JM. Tumor resection in a shared-resource magnetic resonance operating room; experience at the University of Cincinnati. Acta Neurochir Suppl 2002;85:39–44

20. Nimsky C, Fujita A, Ganslandt O, Von Keller B, Fahlbusch R. Volumetric assessment of glioma removal by intraoperative high-field magnetic resonance imaging. Neurosurgery 2004;55(2):358–370, discussion 370–371

21. Nimsky C, Ganslandt O, Buchfelder M, Fahlbusch R. Glioma surgery evaluated by intraoperative low-filed magnetic resonance imaging. Acta Neurochir Suppl 2002;85:55–63

22. Nimsky C, Ganslandt O, von Keller B, Fahlbusch R. Preliminary experience in glioma surgery with intraoperative high-field MRI. Acta Neurochir Suppl (Wien) 2003;88:21–29

23. Schulder M, Carmel PW. Intraoperative magnetic resonance imaging: impact on brain tumor surgery. Cancer Control 2003;10(2):115–124

24. Sutherland GR, Kaibara T, Louw D. Intraoperative MR at 1.5 Tesla – experience and future directions. Acta Neurochir Suppl 2002;85:21–28

25. Wirtz CR, Knauth M, Staubert A, et al. Clinical evaluation and follow-up results for intraoperative magnetic resonance imaging in neurosurgery. Neurosurgery 2000;46(5):1112–1120, discussion 1120–1122

26. Bergsneider M, Sehati N, Villablanca P, McArthur D, Liau L. Extent of brain tumor resection using high-field (1.5-t) versus low-field (0.2-t) intraoperative magnetic resonance imaging. Neurosurgery 2004;55: 483–484

27. Claus EB, Horlacher A, Hsu L, et al. Survival rates in patients with low-grade glioma after intraoperative magnetic resonance image guidance. Cancer 2005;103(6):1227–1233

28. Hirschberg H, Samset E, Hol PK, Tillung T, Lote K. Impact of intraoperative MRI on the surgical results for high-grade gliomas. Minim Invasive Neurosurg 2005;48(2):77–84

29. Gralla J, Ganslandt O, Kober H, Buchfelder M, Fahlbusch R, Nimsky C. Image-guided removal of supratentorial cavernomas in critical brain areas: application of neuronavigation and intraoperative magnetic resonance imaging. Minim Invasive Neurosurg 2003;46(2):72–77

30. Nimsky C, Ganslandt O, Hofmann B, Fahlbusch R. Limited benefit of intraoperative low-field magnetic resonance imaging in craniopharyngioma surgery. Neurosurgery 2003;53(1):72–80, discussion 80–81

31. Yrjänä SK, Tuominen J, Koivukangas J. Intraoperative magnetic resonance imaging in neurosurgery. Acta Radiol 2007;48(5):540–549

32. Haberland N, Ebmeier K, Hliscs R, et al. Neuronavigation in surgery of intracranial and spinal tumors. J Cancer Res Clin Oncol 2000;126(9):529–541

33. Tuominen J, Yrjänä SK, Katisko JP, Heikkilä J, Koivukangas J. Intraoperative imaging in a comprehensive neuronavigation environment for minimally invasive brain tumour surgery. Acta Neurochir Suppl (Wien) 2003;85:115–120

34. Wirtz CR, Knauth M, Stamov M, et al. Clinical impact of intraoperative magnetic resonance imaging on central nervous system neoplasia. Tech Neurosurg 2002;7:326–331

35. Patel A. Intraoperative MRI: impact on health care cost. Newark, NJ: New Jersey Medical School; 2008:49

36. Lycette C, Rubino GJ, Van de Weile B, Villablanca JP, Farahani K. Comparison of hospital charges for interventional MRI guided surgery vs standard surgery. Proc Intl Soc Mag Res Med. 2000;8:65

37. Gumprecht H, Lumenta CB. Intraoperative imaging using a mobile computed tomography scanner. Minim Invasive Neurosurg 2003;46(6):317–322

38. Wagner W, Gaab MR, Schroeder HWS, Tschiltschke W. Cranial neuronavigation in neurosurgery: assessment of usefulness in relation to type and site of pathology in 284 patients. Minim Invasive Neurosurg 2000;43(3):124–131

39. Zhao JZ, Wang S, Wang DJ, et al. Application of frameless stereotaxy in craniotomy procedures. Clinical evaluation. Neurosurg Q 2003;13:51–55

40. Germano IM, Villalobos H, Silvers A, Post KD. Clinical use of the optical digitizer for intracranial neuronavigation. Neurosurgery 1999;45(2):261–269, discussion 269–270

41. Broaddus WC, Prabhu SS, Dreusicke MH, Wolber SB, Gillies GT. Use of intraoperative stereotactic navigation correlates with improved tumor resection. Abstract presented at: Poster Program of the 2000 Annual Meeting of the American Association of Neurological Surgeons; April 8–13, 2000; San Francisco, CA

42. Dorward NL, Paleologos TS, Alberti O, Thomas DG. The advantages of frameless stereotactic biopsy over frame-based biopsy. Br J Neurosurg 2002;16(2):110–118

43. Paleologos TS, Dorward NL, Wadley JP, Thomas DG. Clinical validation of true frameless stereotactic biopsy: analysis of the first 125 consecutive cases. Neurosurgery 2001;49(4):830–835, discussion 835–837

44. Brem H, Piantadosi S, Burger PC, et al; The Polymer-Brain Tumor Treatment Group. Placebo-controlled trial of safety and efficacy of intraoperative controlled delivery by biodegradable polymers of chemotherapy for recurrent gliomas. Lancet 1995;345(8956):1008–1012

45. Valtonen S, Timonen U, Toivanen P, et al. Interstitial chemotherapy with carmustine-loaded polymers for high-grade gliomas: a randomized double-blind study. Neurosurgery 1997;41(1):44–48, discussion 48–49

46. Bejjani BP, Dormont D, Pidoux B, et al. Bilateral subthalamic stimulation for Parkinson's disease by using three-dimensional stereotactic magnetic resonance imaging and electrophysiological guidance. J Neurosurg 2000;92(4):615–625

47. Benabid AL, Benazzouz A, Gao D, et al. Chronic electrical stimulation of the ventralis intermedius nucleus of the thalamus and of other nuclei as a treatment for Parkinson's disease. Tech Neurosurg 1999; 5:5–30

48. Benabid AL, Koudsié A, Benazzouz A, et al. Subthalamic stimulation for Parkinson's disease. Arch Med Res 2000;31(3):282–289

49. Chu RM, Tummala RP, Kucharczyk J, Truwit CL, Maxwell RE. Minimally invasive procedures. Interventional MR image-guided functional neurosurgery. Neuroimaging Clin N Am 2001;11(4):715–725

50. Nimsky C, Ganslandt O, Fahlbusch R. From intraoperative patient transport to surgery in the fringe field. Intraoperative application of magnetic resonance imaging using a 0.2 Tesla scanner: The Erlangen experience. Tech Neurosurg 2002;7:265–273

51. Bejjani BP, Damier P, Arnulf I, et al. Transient acute depression induced by high-frequency deep-brain stimulation. N Engl J Med 1999;340(19):1476–1480

52. Bejjani BP, Damier P, Agid Y. Transient acute depression induced by high-frequency deep-brain stimulation–Reply. N Engl J Med 1999;341(1):104

53. Nuttin B, Cosyns P, Demeulemeester H, Gybels J, Meyerson B. Electrical stimulation in anterior limbs of internal capsules in patients with obsessive-compulsive disorder. Lancet 1999;354(9189):1526

54. Kelly JJ, Hader WJ, Myles ST, Sutherland GR. Epilepsy surgery with intraoperative MRI at 1.5 T. Neurosurg Clin N Am 2005;16(1):173–183

55. Nimsky C, Ganslandt O, Von Keller B, Romstöck J, Fahlbusch R. Intraoperative high-field-strength MR imaging: implementation and experience in 200 patients. Radiology 2004;233(1):67–78

56. Chu RM, Tummala RP, Truwit CL, et al. Functional neurosurgery under magnetic resonance imaging guidance. Neuroimaging Clin N Am 2001;11:717–727

57. Arieff AI, Guisado R. Effects on the central nervous system of hypernatremic and hyponatremic states. Kidney Int 1976;10(1):104–116

58. Oldfield EH, Youle RJ. Immunotoxins for brain tumor therapy. Curr Top Microbiol Immunol 1998;234:97–114

59. Hall WA, Rustamzadeh E, Asher AL. Convection-enhanced delivery in clinical trials. Neurosurg Focus 2003;14(2):e2

60. Kopyov OV, Jacques S, Eagle KS. Fetal transplantation for the treatment of neurodegenerative diseases. Current status and future potential. CNS Drugs 1998;9:77–83

61. Thompson TP, Lunsford LD, Kondziolka D. Restorative neurosurgery: opportunities for restoration of function in acquired, degenerative, and idiopathic neurological diseases. Neurosurgery 1999;45(4):741–752

62. Broaddus WC, Prabhu SS, Gillies GT, et al. Distribution and stability of antisense phosphorothioate oligonucleotides in rodent brain following direct intraparenchymal controlled-rate infusion. J Neurosurg 1998;88(4):734–742

63. Broaddus WC, Prabhu SS, Wu-Pong S, Gillies GT, Fillmore H. Strategies for the design and delivery of antisense oligonucleotides in central nervous system. Methods Enzymol 2000;314:121–135

64. Kopyov OV, Jacques S, Lieberman A, Duma CM, Eagle KS. Safety of intrastriatal neurotransplantation for Huntington's disease patients. Exp Neurol 1998;149(1):97–108

65. Blakemore WF, Franklin RJ. Transplantation options for therapeutic central nervous system remyelination. Cell Transplant 2000;9(2):289–294

66. Laske DW, Youle RJ, Oldfield EH. Tumor regression with regional distribution of the targeted toxin TF-CRM107 in patients with malignant brain tumors. Nat Med 1997;3(12):1362–1368

67. Oldfield EH, Broaddus WC, Bruce J, et al. Phase II trial of convention-enhanced distribution of recombinant immunotoxin in patients with recurrent malignant gliomas. Abstract presented at: the 2000 Annual Meeting of the American Association of Neurological Surgeons; April 8–13, 2000; San Francisco, CA

68. Rand RW, Kreitman RJ, Patronas N, Varricchio F, Pastan I, Puri RK. Intratumoral administration of recombinant circularly permuted interleukin-4-*Pseudomonas* exotoxin in patients with high-grade glioma. Clin Cancer Res 2000;6(6):2157–2165

69. Oldfield EH, Ram Z, Culver KW, Blaese RM, DeVroom HL, Anderson WF. Gene therapy for the treatment of brain tumors using intra-tumoral transduction with the thymidine kinase gene and intravenous ganciclovir. Hum Gene Ther 1993;4(1):39–69

70. Ram Z, Culver KW, Oshiro EM, et al. Therapy of malignant brain tumors by intratumoral implantation of retroviral vector-producing cells. Nat Med 1997;3(12):1354–1361

71. Bouvier G, Penn RD, Kroin JS, Beique R, Guerard MJ. Direct delivery of medication into a brain tumor through multiple chronically implanted catheters. Neurosurgery 1987;20(2):286–291

72. Walter KA, Tamargo RJ, Olivi A, Burger PC, Brem H. Intratumoral chemotherapy. Neurosurgery 1995;37(6):1128–1145

73. Freed CR, Breeze RE, Rosenberg NL, et al. Survival of implanted fetal dopamine cells and neurologic improvement 12 to 46 months after transplantation for Parkinson's disease. N Engl J Med 1992;327(22):1549–1555

74. Palfi S, Nguyen JP, Brugieres P, et al. MRI-stereotactical approach for neural grafting in basal ganglia disorders. Exp Neurol 1998;150(2):272–281

75. Clarkson ED, Freed CR. Development of fetal neural transplantation as a treatment for Parkinson's disease. Life Sci 1999;65(23):2427–2437

76. Lonser RR, Corthésy ME, Morrison PF, Gogate N, Oldfield EH. Convection-enhanced selective excitotoxic ablation of the neurons of the globus pallidus internus for treatment of parkinsonism in nonhuman primates. J Neurosurg 1999;91(2):294–302

77. Bankiewicz KS, Eberling JL, Kohutnicka M, et al. Convection-enhanced delivery of AAV vector in parkinsonian monkeys; in vivo detection of gene expression and restoration of dopaminergic function using pro-drug approach. Exp Neurol 2000;164(1):2–14

78. Hurlbert MS, Gianani RI, Hutt C, Freed CR, Kaddis FG. Neural transplantation of hNT neurons for Huntington's disease. Cell Transplant 1999;8(1):143–151

79. Kondziolka D, Wechsler L, Goldstein S, et al. Transplantation of cultured human neuronal cells for patients with stroke. Neurology 2000;55(4):565–569

80. Kaczmarek HJ, Kiefer SW. Microinjections of dopaminergic agents in the nucleus accumbens affect ethanol consumption but not palatability. Pharmacol Biochem Behav 2000;66(2):307–312

81. Fatouros PP, Corwin FD, Chen ZJ, et al. In vitro and in vivo imaging studies of a new endohedral metallofullerene nanoparticle. Radiology 2006;240(3):756–764

82. Bammer R, Augustin M, Strasser-Fuchs S, et al. Magnetic resonance diffusion tensor imaging for characterizing diffuse and focal white matter abnormalities in multiple sclerosis. Magn Reson Med 2000; 44(4):583–591

83. Rose SE, Chen F, Chalk JB, et al. Loss of connectivity in Alzheimer's disease: an evaluation of white matter tract integrity with colour coded MR diffusion tensor imaging. J Neurol Neurosurg Psychiatry 2000; 69(4):528–530

84. Bastin ME, Rana AK, Wardlaw JM, Armitage PA, Keir SL. A study of the apparent diffusion coefficient of grey and white matter in human ischaemic stroke. Neuroreport 2000;11(13):2867–2874

85. Kucharczyk J, Moseley ME. Method and apparatus for use with MR imaging. US Patent No. 6,061,587, May 9, 2000

86. Truwit CL, Liu H. MR-compatible medical devices. US Patent No. 5,964,705, Oct. 12, 1999

87. Truwit CL. Remote actuation of trajectory guide. US Patent No. 5,993,463, Nov. 30, 1999

88. Mendez I, Hong M, Smith S, Dagher A, Desrosiers J. Neural transplantation cannula and microinjector system: experimental and clinical experience. Technical note. J Neurosurg 2000;92(3):493–499

89. Breeze RE, Wells TH Jr, Freed CR. Implantation of fetal tissue for the management of Parkinson's disease: a technical note. Neurosurgery 1995;36(5):1044–1047, discussion 1047–1048

90. Penn RD. The future of drug infusion into the brain. In Gildenberg PL, Tasker RR, eds., Textbook of Stereotactic and Functional Neurosurgery. New York: McGraw Hill; 1997

Index

Note: Page numbers followed by *f* and *t* indicate figures and tables, respectively.

A

Acoustic noise, emitted by MR system, 58
Active tracking, 32–33
Adenoma(s), pituitary
   resection. *See also* Transsphenoidal approach
      iMRI-guided, 122–125, 122*t*–123*t*, 124*f*–128*f*
   skull base surgery for, iMRI and, 180*t*, 182
Advanced multimodality image-guided operating room,
      207–208, 208*f*
AIRIS scanner, 100
   in epilepsy surgery, 157
   and low-field iMRI, 9–10, 10*f*
Airway management, iMRI and, 50–51
American College of Radiology (ACR), safe practice guidelines,
      59–60
American Society for Testing and Materials (ASTM), standards
      for MRI equipment, 63
AMIGO. *See* Advanced multimodality image-guided operating
      room
Aminolevulinic acid fluorescence, 109, 207
Anesthesia, 48–54
   emergence from, 54
   equipment, MRI-compatible, 49–50
   induction, 53
   maintenance, 53
   management, with iMRI, 53
   MRI and, issues in, 48–49, 53
   in MRI environment
      difficulties, 48–49, 53
      emergencies and, 54
   patient preparation for, 62
   provision, with iMRI, problems associated with, 48–49, 53
   quality assurance, 54
Anesthesia machine, MRI-compatible, 50, 51*f*
Aneurysm(s), surgery for, iMRI in, 171–173, 171*t*–172*t*, 172*f*,
      173–174, 173*f*, 174*f*
Arterial spin labeling (ASL), 45
Arteriovenous malformation, surgery for, iMRI in, 171–173,
      171*t*, 174–176, 175*f*
Aspiration, MR-guided
   needle-dependent factors affecting, 33–34
   pulse sequence-dependent factors affecting, 33–34

Astrocytoma
   pilocytic, skull base surgery for, iMRI and, 181*t*, 182
   WHO grade III, resection, iMRI in, 108–117
Awake procedures, 54, 109
   candidates for, 49
   comfort considerations in, 117
   for glioma resection, 162–169
   safety considerations in, 117

B

Biopsy needle, intraoperative visualization, pulse sequences
      for, 33–34
Blood–brain barrier, therapeutic disruption
   MRI-guided, cost-benefit analysis, 244–245
   using MRI-guided focused ultrasound, 236–238
Blood pressure, monitoring
   invasive, 52, 53*f*
   noninvasive, 52, 52*f*
Brain biopsy
   high-field, 73–79
      anesthesia for, 74
      iMRI system for, 73
      instrumentation for, 74, 75*f*
      positioning for, 74
      postoperative care, 79
      preoperative preparation for, 73–74
      procedure, 74–79, 76*f*–78*f*
      prospective stereotaxis for, 76–79, 76*f*–78*f*
      radiofrequency coil placement for, 74, 74*f*
      skull penetration for, 74–75
      trajectory guide for, 74, 75*f*
   low-field, 67–72
      costs, 72
      documentation, 68–69
      instrumentation for, 71, 71*f*
      with intraoperative ultrasound, 70–71, 70*f*
      lessons learned, 71–72
      off-line, 70–71, 70*f*
      on-line, 69–70, 69*f*, 71
      patient education about, 68
      preoperative work-up for, 68, 72
      representative sampling in, 72

Brain biopsy (*Continued*)
  suite for (Oulu, Finland), 67–68, 68*f*
  technique for, 69–71
  MRI-guided
    cost-benefit analysis, 242–244
    historical perspective on, 81
  multimodality imaging in, 70–71, 70*f*, 72
  Oulu (Finland) experience, 67–72
  spectroscopy-guided, 79
Brain mapping
  for epilepsy surgery, 153
  fMRI for, 130, 131, 132*f*, 134–135, 134*f*
  intraoperative, for glioma resection, 165–166, 165*f*
Brain shift, 101, 103*f*, 131, 131*f*, 203–204
  compensation for, in navigation, 217–219, 218*f*
Brainsuite, 187
Brain tumor(s). *See also* Skull base surgery; *specific tumor*
  benign, iMRI-guided surgery for, advances in (future directions for), 202
  primary, iMRI-guided surgery for, advances in (future directions for), 201
  resection
    difficulties, 130–131
    DTI-guided, 139–149. *See also* Diffusion tensor imaging (DTI)
    fMRI-guided, 130–138
    iMRI guidance, 130–131
      advances in (future directions for), 200
      cost-benefit analysis, 242–244
    preoperative imaging for, 130, 130*f*
  robotic laser ablation of, ALA fluorescence and 3D MRI in, 207
  thermal ablation, using MRI-guided focused ultrasound, 236
Burn(s), radiofrequency-related, 58–59
b-value, 41

C
Capnography, 52
Capsulotomy, MR-guided, 23
Carotid endarterectomy, iMRI in, 171–173, 171*t*
Catheter placement, MRI-guided, 80–87
Caverloma(s), susceptibility-weighted imaging, 39
Cavernous angioma, surgery for, iMRI in, 171–173, 171*t*–172*t*
Cavernous malformations
  skull base surgery for, iMRI and, 180*t*, 182
  surgery for, iMRI in, 171–173, 171*t*, 174–176, 175*f*
Cell therapy, MRI-guided, cost-benefit analysis, 244–245
Cerebrovascular surgery, iMRI in, 170–177
  advances in (future directions for), 202
  lesions treated
    locations, 171, 171*t*–172*t*
    numbers, 171, 171*t*–172*t*
    types, 171, 171*t*–172*t*
  procedures, types, 171–173, 171*t*–172*t*
  systems for, 170–171
Cervical discectomy, anterior, iMRI in, 189–190, 190*f*, 191*f*
Cervical trauma, surgery for, iMRI in, 192
Chemical shift imaging (CSI), 42–43
Chiari malformation, suboccipital decompression for, iMRI in, 191–192
Chondrosarcoma, skull base surgery for, iMRI and, 180*t*, 182, 183*f*
Chordoma, skull base surgery for, iMRI and, 180*t*, 182
Choroid plexus papilloma, skull base surgery for, iMRI and, 180*t*, 182
Cingulotomy, MR-guided, 23
Convection-enhanced delivery, 245

Corpus callosum transsection, for epilepsy, 159–160
Craniopharyngioma
  resection, iMRI-guided, pulse sequences for, 36
  skull base surgery for, iMRI and, 180*t*, 182
Craniotomy(ies)
  awake, 109
    comfort considerations in, 117
    for glioma resection, 162–169
    safety considerations in, 117
  at back end of scanner, 20*f*, 26
  iMRI-guided, pulse sequences for, 35–36, 36*f*
Cryogenic system, safety concerns for, 57

D
dB/dt, 58
DBS. *See* Deep brain stimulation
Deep brain stimulation
  electrodes
    MRI and, 59
    MRI-guided implantation, 88–95
      accuracy of placement in, 94
      advances in (future directions for), 94
      brain penetration in, 94
      burr hole location for, 89, 91*f*
      closure, 93–94
      complications of, 94
      equipment for, 88, 89*t*
      final imaging, 94
      guidance sheath and lead, insertion, 91–92, 93*f*
      implantable pulse generator for, placement, 94
      initial exposure, 89–91
      patient positioning for, 88–89, 91*f*
      patient preparation for, 88–89
      pulse sequences for, 88, 90*t*
      technique for, 88
      trajectory guide, mounting, 89–91, 92*f*–93*f*
      trajectory planning, 89, 91*f*
  iMRI-guided stimulator placement for, 23
    cost-benefit analysis, 244
Depth electrode placement, MR-guided, 20, 21*f*, 23, 25*f*
Difficult airway, 50–51
Diffuse axonal injury, susceptibility-weighted imaging in, 39
Diffusion tensor imaging (DTI), 14, 20, 22*f*, 25, 29, 35, 132, 167, 200, 212
  advances in (future directions for), 146–147, 146*f*–147*f*
  challenges, 146–147, 146*f*–147*f*
  clinical applications, 139, 142–144, 143*f*, 144*f*, 145*f*
  fiber tracking, 140–141, 140*f*, 141*f*
    intraoperative, 144–146, 145*f*
  fractional anisotropy maps, 139–140
  glyph representation, 140, 140*f*
  hulls, 141–142
  integration into navigation, 142, 143*f*
  intraoperative, 41–42
    in cerebrovascular surgery, 170
  principles, 139
  pulse sequences for, 41–42, 41*f*
  visualization strategies, 139–142
  volume growing techniques, 140*f*, 141–142
  of white matter tracts, 42
Diffusion-weighted imaging (DWI), 35, 139
  and cerebrovascular surgery, 170, 174, 176
  of high-grade gliomas, 108
dMRI. *See* Magnetic resonance imaging (MRI), diagnostic (dMRI)
Documentation, of brain biopsy, 68–69, 69*f*

Dosimetry, for staff, 60
Double-donut system. *See* Signa SP system
Double inversion-recovery (DIR) pulse sequence, 35
Draeger Fabius MRI-compatible anesthesia machine, 50, 51*f*
Drug therapy, MRI-guided, cost-benefit analysis, 244–245
DSC-MRI. *See* Perfusion MRI, dynamic susceptibility-weighted
    contrast-enhanced
DTI. *See* Diffusion tensor imaging (DTI)
DWI. *See* Diffusion-weighted imaging (DWI)

E

Ear protection, 58
Echo plana imaging
    multi-shot, 30
    single-shot, 30
Echo-time (TE), 30
Electrocardiographic (ECG) monitoring, MRI and, 52
Electrocorticography, intraoperative, 154
Electromagnetic fields, occupational exposure to, safety
    concerns, 60
Eloquent cortex, fMRI of, 130, 131, 132*f*, 134–135, 134*f*
Ependymoma, skull base surgery for, iMRI and, 181*t*, 182
Epidermoid cyst, skull base surgery for, iMRI and, 180*t*, 182
Epilepsy surgery
    advances in (future directions for), 153
    brain mapping for, 153
    corpus callosum transsection in, 159–160
    evolution, 153
    extent of resection, 153
    extratemporal resections for, 157
    iMRI-guided, 153–161
        advances in (future directions for), 160
        clinical experience, 160
        cost-benefit analysis, 244
        development of, 153
        OR set-up for, 154, 155*f*
        pulse sequences for, 37
        systems for, 154
    intraoperative recordings and positioning of electrodes in,
        154–156, 155*f*
    lesionectomies in, 157–159, 159*f*–160*f*
    magnetic resonance spectroscopy for, 43
    temporal lobe resection for, 156–157, 157*f*, 158*f*
Equilibrium magnetization, 29
Espree scanner(s), 25, 26
Evolution 1 robot, 224
Extracranial to intracranial (EC-IC) bypass, iMRI in,
    171–173, 171*t*

F

Fast field echo sequence (FFE) images, 31
Fast imaging with steady precession (FISP), 31, 35, 36*t*
    reverse, 35, 36*t*
    time inversed version, 31
Fast low-angle shot (FLASH) sequence images, 31, 35, 36*t*
Fast-SE, 30
Ferrous objects, internal, 57
Fiber tracking. *See* Tractography
Field strength, and needle visualization, 34, 34*f*
FIESTA, 31
Fluid-attenuated inversion recovery (FLAIR), 30, 35, 36*t*
fMRI. *See* Functional MRI (fMRI)
Foothills Hospital (Calgary), high-field MRI, 20–21, 23*f*
Frequency-encoding direction, and needle visualization, 34, 34*f*
Frequency encoding gradient (Gr), 30

FSE. *See* Fast-SE
Functional imaging
    intraoperative, 39–40, 40*f*
    preoperative, 39–40, 40*f*
Functional MRI (fMRI), 14, 20, 29, 35, 200
    advantages, 131–132, 132*f*
    and extraaxial neoplasms, 15–16
    guidance, of brain tumor resection, 130–138, 167
    of high-grade gliomas, 108
    integration into navigation, 167
    and intraaxial neoplasms, 15
    intraoperative, 130–138, 131*f*
        patient selection for, 132, 133*f*
        procedure for, 135–137, 136*f*
        pulse sequences for, 40–41, 41*f*
        results with, 137–138, 137*f*
        technical aspects, 133–134, 133*f*
    in multimodal navigation, 212, 215–217, 216*f*, 217*f*
    patient selection for, 132, 133*f*
    preoperative, 134–135, 134*f*
        for glioma resection, 167
    pulse sequences for, 40–41, 41*f*
    safety considerations in, 135
    suite for, 135
    and surgical planning, 131–132, 132*f*
    technical aspects, 133–134, 133*f*
Functional neuronavigation
    iMRI-guided, pulse sequences for, 37–38, 38*f*
    pulse sequences for, 39–45
Functional neurosurgery. *See also* Deep brain stimulation;
    Epilepsy surgery
    MRI-guided, cost-benefit analysis, 244

G

Gauss line, 49–50
    and iMRI, 18
GBM. *See* Glioblastoma multiforme
General Electric, Signa. *See* Signa SP system
Georgetown robot, 227
GE Signa. *See* Signa SP system
Glioblastoma(s). *See also* Glioblastoma multiforme
    resection, degree of, 15
Glioblastoma multiforme
    resection
        degree of, 108–109
        iMRI in, 108–117
        survival after, 108–109, 114*f*
    topographical grading, 109
Glioma(s)
    contrast-enhanced imaging, 101
    fMRI of, 131, 132*f*
    high-field MRI, comparison with low-field systems, 106
    high-grade
        aminolevulinic acid fluorescence, 109
        resection
            degree of, 108–109
            iMRI in, 108–117
            intraoperative ultrasound in, 109–110
            low-field iMRI in, 103, 105*t*
            neuronavigation in, 109
            survival after, 108–109, 114*f*
    low-field MRI, 99–107
        advances in (future directions for), 106
        comparison with high-field systems, 106
        pulse sequences for, 101

Glioma(s) (*Continued*)
  low-grade, resection
    field iMRI in, 110
    low-field iMRI in, 103, 104*t*
  magnetic resonance spectroscopy, 43, 43*f*
  preoperative imaging, 130, 130*f*
  resection, 20, 20*f*
    awake craniotomy and iMRI for, 162–169
      anesthesia/analgesia for, 163, 164–165
      imaging, 166
      initial exposure, 164–165
      intraoperative testing, 165–166, 165*f*
      OR set-up for, 162–163
      patient education about, 163
      patient positioning for, 163–164, 164*f*
      patient selection for, 163
      preoperative evaluation/preparation for, 163
      principles, 162
      procedure for, 163
      results, 167–168, 168*f*
      system for, 162
    degree of, 15
    DTI-guided, 142–144, 143*f*, 144*f*, 145*f*
    iMRI-guided
      advances in (future directions for), 106, 117
      effect on course of surgery, 103, 104*t*, 105*f*, 105*t*
      high-field, 106
      indications for, 101–103, 103*f*, 104*f*, 110
      low-field, 99–107
      OR setting for, 110
      outcomes with, 103–106, 110, 111–114
      patient positioning for, 110–111
      pitfalls, 114–117
      pulse sequences for, 36–37, 101
      and repeat contrast clinical application, 115
      and repeat diffusion tensor imaging, 117
      and repeat scanning, 114–115
      and rereferencing, 115, 115*f*–116*f*
      results, 111–114, 113*f*–114*f*
      safety considerations in, 110–111, 117
      scanning procedure for, 111
      surgical procedure for, 111, 112*f*
      technique for, 110–111
    low-field iMRI in, 99–107
Gradient(s), 30
Gradient echo (GRE) pulse sequences, 30
  coherent, 31
  fully refocused, 31
  partially refocused, 31
  spoiled, 31

H

Half Fourier acquisition single-shot turbo spin-echo (HASTE), 30, 31
Health care reform, implications for MRI-guided neurosurgery, 245–246
Hemangioblastoma, skull base surgery for, iMRI and, 180*t*, 182, 183*f*
Hemorrhage, cerebral, susceptibility-weighted imaging in, 39
Hemorrhage scans, 31
High-field MRI
  for brain biopsy, 73–79
  intraoperative (iMRI), in glioma surgery, 106
  market for, 26–27
  pulse sequences for, 37, 37*f*, 37*t*

  suite design, 18–20, 19*f*
    1.5T-systems, 18, 20, 23, 25
    3T-systems, 23, 25
Hitachi Airis low-field iMRI, 9–10, 10*f*

I

Image fusion, 33
Implantable cardiac defibrillator(s), MRI and, 49, 59
Implanted devices, MRI and, 49, 59
iMRI. *See* Low-field MRI, intraoperative (iMRI); Magnetic resonance imaging (MRI), intraoperative (iMRI)
IMRIS. *See* Interventional MR Imaging Systems (IMRIS)
Indocyanine green, 207
Infusion pump(s), 49, 50*f*, 53–54
Interventional device, intraoperative visualization, pulse sequences for, 33–34
Interventional MRI
  equipment for, certification, 63
  patient preparation for, 62
  patient screening for, 62
  staff training for, 61–62
Interventional MR Imaging Systems (IMRIS), 20–26, 23*f*, 187
  in cerebrovascular surgery, 171
  in epilepsy surgery, 154
  in spinal surgery, 187, 187*f*
  surgical suites offered by, types, 26–27
Interventional MRI suite, planning, 61, 62*f*

K

k-space, 30

L

Larmor frequency, 29
Laryngeal mask airway (LMA), 50
Laryngoscope(s), 50
Laser thermal therapy
  iMRI-guided, pulse sequences for, 34–35
  robotic, ALA fluorescence and 3D MRI in, 207
Lesionectomy(ies), for epilepsy, 157–159, 159*f*–160*f*
Low-field MRI, 24. *See also* PoleStar system
  for brain biopsy, 67–72
  intraoperative (iMRI), 13
    advances in (future directions for), 10
    comparison with high-field systems, 106
    experience with
      patient data, 8–9, 9*t*
      technical data, 8–9, 9*t*
    in glioma surgery, 99–107. *See also* Glioma(s)
    image quality in, 100–101, 102*f*
    indications for, 101–103, 103*f*, 104*f*
    Magnetom Open system for, 9, 10, 99, 104*t*, 105*t*
    and MRI-compatible equipment, 8
    pulse sequences for, 35, 36*t*
    safety considerations in, 100
    staff for, 7–8
    suite for (Oulu, Finland), 67–68, 68*f*
    systems for, 99–100, 100*f*
    University of Cincinnati facility for, 9–10, 10*f*

M

Magnetic field(s)
  human exposure to, safety concerns, 57
  static, safety concerns for, 56–57
  time varying, safety concerns for, 58

Magnetic resonance angiography (MRA), 20, 25
  intraoperative, 38
    in cerebrovascular surgery, 170
Magnetic resonance imaging (MRI). *See also* Interventional MRI
  contraindications to, 49, 59
    screening for, 60
  contrast-enhanced, 31
    intraoperative, 38, 38*f*, 39*f*
  diagnostic (dMRI), 3
    in shared-resource facility, 9–10, 10*f*
  functional. *See* Functional MRI (fMRI)
  guidance
    interactive, 32–33, 32*f*
    near-real-time, 32–33, 32*f*
  historical perspective on, 3
  intraoperative (iMRI)
    advances in (future directions for), 86, 106, 199–209
    with awake craniotomy, 162–169
    and cerebrovascular surgery, 170–177
    clinical applications, 200
    contraindications to, 49, 59
    cost-effectiveness analysis, 241–242
    development of, 99, 170, 178
    in epilepsy surgery. *See* Epilepsy surgery
    experience with, 199
    and extraaxial resection, 15–16
    field strengths for, 199
    full access open systems for, 199
    within 5 Gauss line, 18
    high-field, 3, 10, 13
    in high-grade gliomas, 108–117
      advances in (future directions for), 117
      outcomes with, 110, 111–114
      technique for, 110–111
    historical perspective on, 3, 18, 80–81, 99, 178
    indications for, 101–103, 103*f*, 104*f*
    and intraaxial resection, 15
    local RFI shield for, 6–7, 7*f*, 7*t*
    low-field. *See* Low-field MRI, intraoperative (iMRI)
    magnet configurations for, 200
    market for, 26
    mid-field, 12–17. *See also* Signa SP system
    and monitoring complications, 16
    and MRI-compatible equipment, 8, 18
    neurobiopsy using, 14
    neurosurgical applications, 12–14
    OR layout for, 7, 8*f*
    and other electromagnetic devices, 8
    outside 5 Gauss line, 18
    patient mobility for, 26
    in pituitary surgery. *See* Pituitary surgery; Transsphenoidal approach
    pulse sequences for, 31–39. *See also* Pulse sequence(s)
    rear access to scanner for, 20*f*, 23, 25*f*, 26, 26*f*, 27*f*
    resection guidance with, 14–15
    robots compatible with, 224–225
    room shielding for, 6, 7*t*
    scanner mobility for, 20–21, 23*f*, 25–26
    serial imaging and brain shift, 203–204
    in skull base surgery, 178–185
    staff for, 7–8
    and surgical navigation, 4–5, 6*f*
    in surgical oncology, 14
    and surgical planning, 14
    systems for, 170

low-field. *See* Low-field MRI
preoperative, 130, 130*f*
  of high-grade gliomas, 108
principles of, 29–30
safe practice guidelines for, 59–60
Magnetic resonance spectroscopy, 20, 22*f*, 29, 212
  guidance, for brain biopsy, 79
  of high-grade gliomas, 108
  pulse sequences for, 42–43, 43*f*, 44*f*
Magnetization-prepared rapid gradient echo (MP-RAGE) sequence images, 31
Magnetoencephalography, in multimodal navigation, 212, 215–217
Magnetom Open, 9, 10, 99
  in epilepsy surgery, 154
  in glioma surgery, 104*t*, 105*t*
Medulloblastoma, skull base surgery for, iMRI and, 181*t*, 182
Meningioma, skull base surgery for, intraoperative MRI (iMRI) and, 180*t*, 181
Metabolic mapping, magnetic resonance spectroscopy for, 43, 43*f*, 44*f*
Microvascular decompression, iMRI in, 171–173, 171*t*
Mid-field MRI, 24. *See also* Signa SP system
  and degree of resection, 15–16
  intraoperative, development, 12–13
  and monitoring complications, 16
  and resection guidance, 14–15
  in transsphenoidal surgery, 15–16
Minerva robot, 224
Minimally invasive procedures
  at back end of scanner, 23, 25*f*, 26
  iMRI for, pulse sequences for, 31–35
Molecular imaging, 206–208
  and detection of surgical margins, 207
  guidance, and multimodality imaging, 206–207
Monitoring, intraoperative
  American Society of Anesthesiology recommendations for, 54
  MRI and, 48–49, 50, 51–52
MRgFUS. *See* MRI-guided focused ultrasound
MRI-guided focused ultrasound, 233–240
  advances in (future directions for), 238
  advantages, 234
  for blood–brain barrier disruption, 236–238
  for brain tumor ablation, 236
  clinical applications, 236–238
  historical perspective on, 233–234
  intraprocedural monitoring, 236
  intraprocedural targeting, 236
  lesion localization for, 235
  limitations, 234
  mechanism of action, 234–235
  nonthermal (nonablation) procedures using, 236–238
    mechanism of action, 235
  planning for, 235
  preprocedural preparation, 235
  principles, 234
  thermal ablation using, 200, 205–206
    clinical applications, 236, 237*f*, 238*f*
    mechanism of action, 234–235
  validation, 236

N

Navigation. *See also* Neuronavigation
  application accuracy, 213–214
  automatic registration for, 213–215, 214*f*, 215*f*

Navigation (*Continued*)
    brain shift and, 217–219, 218*f*
    diffusion tensor imaging and, 142, 143*f*
    functional MRI (fMRI) and, 167
    image-based, for robotic devices, 205
    implementation in surgical workflow, 212–213
    intraoperative, 204
    intraoperative MRI (iMRI) and, 4–5, 6*f*
    marker fit techniques, 214
    multimodal, 212–221
        techniques, 215–217, 216*f*, 217*f*
    OR set-up for, 213, 213*f*
    with PoleStar system, 4–5, 6*f*
    Slicer system, 12, 13, 13*f*
    updating, 217–219, 218*f*
Navigus system, 23, 25*f*, 33, 71, 71*f*
Navigus trajectory guide, 74, 75*f*
Nerve stimulation, time varying gradient fields and, 58
NeuroArm, 227–231, 228*f*, 229*f*, 230*f*
    clinical trials, 231
    iMRI suite set-up for, 228–229, 228*f*, 229*f*, 231
    in stereotactic procedures, 231, 231*f*
Neurobiopsy, 14, 20, 21*f. See also* Brain biopsy
    iMRI-guided, 14
    MR-guided
        needle-dependent factors affecting, 33–34
        pulse sequence-dependent factors affecting, 33–34
    MR spectroscopic-guided, 20, 22*f*
    sereotactic, 14
    trajectory-guided, combined with magnetic resonance
        spectroscopy, 43
NeuRobot, 226, 226*f*
NeuroCut needle, 71
Neuroendoscopy, MRI-guided, advances in (future directions for),
    202–203
NeuroGate, 71, 71*f*
NeuroMate (robot), 223–224, 223*f*
Neuronavigation. *See also* Navigation
    functional, 212
        iMRI-guided, pulse sequences for, 37–38, 38*f*
        pulse sequences for, 39–45
    intraoperative, 204
    multimodal, 212–221
    in resection of high-grade glioma, 109
Neurostimulation, with depth electrode, 20, 21*f*, 23, 25*f*
Neurosurgery
    functional, MR-guided, 23
    iMRI-guided, 12–16, 18. *See also* Magnetic resonance imaging
        (MRI), intraoperative (iMRI)
        pulse sequences for, 29
    open, MRI-guided, pulse sequences for, 35–39
    perfusion MRI in
        clinical applications, 44
        parameters for, 44
Nuclear imaging, 207
Null point, 30

O

Occupational health and safety, 60, 61*f*
Ommaya reservoir, placement, 20
Onesys Navigator, 68–69, 69*f*
Operating room suite
    electromagnetic devices in, intraoperative MRI and, 8
    for high-field MRI, 18–20, 19*f*
    layout, for intraoperative MRI, 7, 8*f*

    for low-field MRI, 3–11
    for mid-field MRI, 12–17
    MRI in. *See* Magnetic resonance imaging (MRI), intraoperative
        (iMRI)
    shielding, 6, 7*t*
Optical imaging, 207
OR. *See* Operating room
Oximeter(s), MRI-compatible, 51, 52*f*
Oximetry, iMRI and, 51, 52*f*

P

Pacemaker(s), cardiac, MRI and, 49, 59
Percentage of signal-intensity recovery (PSR), 44
Perfusion MRI, 29
    dynamic susceptibility-weighted contrast-enhanced, pulse
        sequences for, 44–45
Phase-encoding gradient (Gp), 30
Philips Intera scanner(s), 18, 19*f*, 20*f*, 23–24
Pial siderosis, susceptibility-weighted imaging in, 39
Picture Archiving and Communication System (PACS), 68
Pituitary surgery, transsphenoidal approach, intraoperative MRI
        (iMRI) and, 15–16, 119–129
    pulse sequences for, 36
Plethysmography, 52
PoleStar N20. *See* PoleStar system
PoleStar system, 18, 19*f*, 24, 26, 100, 101, 101*f*, 187
    control room, 7
    development, 3–4
    in epilepsy surgery, 154
    experience with
        patient data, 8–9, 9*t*
        technical data, 8–9, 9*t*
    future directions for, 10
    in glioma surgery, 104*t*, 105*t*
    images, 4, 4*f*
    intraoperative use, 4, 5*f*
    local RFI shield for, 6–7, 7*f*, 7*t*
    magnet storage cage for, 4, 5*f*
    and MRI-compatible equipment, 8
    OR layout for, 7, 8*f*
    staff for, 7–8
    surgical navigation with, 4–5, 6*f*
    surgical procedure using, 8–9, 9*t*
Politics, and future of MRI-guided neurosurgery, 245–246
Positron emission tomography (PET), 212
Programmable universal machine for assembly (PUMA) robot, 222
Projectile risk, 56–57
Proton density-weighted images, 30
Pseudotumor cerebri, catheter placement for, MRI-guided,
        82*f*–84*f*, 83–84
Pulse oximeter, MRI-compatible, 51, 52*f*
Pulse sequence(s), 29–47
    gradient echo, 30–31
    for intraoperative MRI, 31–39
PUMA. *See* Programmable universal machine for assembly
        (PUMA) robot

Q

Quench, 57

R

Radiofrequency
    burns caused by, 58–59
    specific absorption rates for, 58
    transmission, safety concerns for, 58–59

Radiotracer(s), 207
RAE tube, 50
RAMS. *See* Robot-assisted microsurgery system (RAMS)
Rapid acquisition with relaxation enhancement (RARE), 30, 31
Readout gradient (Gr), 30
Relative cerebral blood volume (rCBV), 44
Relative peak height (rPH), 44
Repetition time (TR), 30
Robot-assisted microsurgery system (RAMS), 225
Robotics, neurosurgical, 222–232
    early systems, 222–224
    for enhanced tool manipulation, 225–226
    historical perspective on, 222, 223*f*
    image-based navigation for, 205
    image-guided, 224–225
        MRI-compatible, 224–225
    for laser ablation of brain tumors, ALA fluorescence and 3D
            MRI in, 207
    for spinal surgery, 227

S

Safety, 56–63
    American College of Radiology (ACR) guidelines for, 59–60
    with MR systems, 56–59
    protocols, for interventional MRI suite, 61–63
SAR. *See* Specific absorption rate(s)
Schwannoma, skull base surgery for, iMRI and, 180*t*,
            181–182, 181*f*
Screening
    device, 60
    equipment, 60
    patient, 59, 62
    personnel, 59–60
SE-echo planar imaging (SE-EPI), 30
SE-inversion recovery (SE-IR), 30
Shared-resource imaging unit, 10, 10*f*
Shunt/shunting, catheter placement for
    MRI-guided, 80–87
        advances in (future directions for), 86–87
        clinical experience, 81–84, 82*f*–84*f*
        development of, 80–81
        methodology, 84–86, 85*f*
        multimodality imaging in, 87
        ultrasound-assisted, 80–81
Signa HDx system, 178–179, 179*f*
Signa SP system, 10, 12, 13*f*, 18, 19*f*, 24, 26, 32, 99, 100*f*, 101
    in cerebrovascular surgery, 170–171
    in glioma surgery, 104*t*, 105*t*
Single voxel spectroscopy (SVS), 42–43
Sinonasal carcinoma, skull base surgery for, iMRI and,
            180*t*, 182
Skull base surgery
    intraoperative MRI (iMRI) and, 15–16, 178–185
        advances in (future directions for), 184
        advantages, 184
        equipment, 179, 179*f*
        imaging technique, 180
        OR set-up for, 179, 179*f*
        outcomes with, 184
        pulse sequences for, 36
        system for, 178–179, 179*f*
    pathology encountered, 180, 180*t*
    technique for, 180
Slicer navigation system, 12, 13, 13*f*
Slice selection gradient (Gs), 30

Specific absorption rate(s), for radiofrequency, 58
Spinal decompression
    posterior, iMRI in, 190–191, 191*f*
    suboccipital, iMRI in, 191–192
Spinal surgery
    intraoperative MRI (iMRI) in, 186–195
        advances in (future directions for), 193–195, 202
        historical perspective on, 186
        Penn State/Wilkes-Barre experience, 187–189, 187*f*,
                188*t*–189*t*
        systems for, 187, 187*f*
    robots for, 227
Spinal tumor(s), surgery for, iMRI in, 192–193, 192*f*, 193*f*
SpineAssist robot, 227, 227*f*
Spin echo (SE) pulse sequences, 30
    T1-weighted, 35, 36*t*
Spin-spin relaxation times, 29
Spoiled gradient echo (SPGR) sequence images, 31
Staff
    occupational exposures, safety concerns, 60
    training, 61–62
Static magnetic field (B$_0$), and safety, 56–57
Steady-Hand robotic system, 225–226, 225*f*
Steady-state free precession (SSFP), 31
Stealth Treon, 171, 179
Stereotactic biopsy, 14
Stereotaxy
    frame-based, 14
    frameless, 14, 21, 32
        in cerebrovascular surgery, 171
        in skull base surgery, 179
    NeuroArm robot and, 231, 231*f*
    optically linked, 32
    prospective, 21–23, 24*f*, 32–33, 33*f*
Subarachnoid hemorrhage, susceptibility-weighted imaging
            in, 39
Superficial temporal artery to middle cerebral artery (STA-MCA)
            bypass, iMRI in, 172
Surgical margin(s), detection, molecular imaging and, 207
Surgical oncology, intraoperative MRI and, 14
Surgical planning
    intraoperative MRI and, 14
    preoperative, *versus* intraoperative decision making, 204
Surgical table(s)
    flexible, 26
    Maquet, 179, 179*f*
Susceptibility-weighted imaging, 14, 29
    clinical applications, 39
    intraoperative, 39
    principles, 38–39
SWI. *See* Susceptibility-weighted imaging
Syrinx, cervicothoracic, catheter placement for, MRI-guided,
            83, 83*f*

T

T$_2$ decay, 29–30
T$_2$· decay, 29–30
Telangiectasia, susceptibility-weighted imaging, 39
Temperature monitoring, intraoperative, 52
Temporal lobe resection, for epilepsy, 156–157, 157*f*, 158*f*
Thermal ablation. *See also* Laser thermal therapy
    MRI-guided, 205–206
        probe-delivered, 205
    MRI-guided focused ultrasound for, 200, 205–206, 234–235,
                236, 237*f*, 238*f*

Thermotherapy, iMRI-guided, pulse sequences for, 34–35
Three-dimensional slicer, 12, 13, 13*f*, 21, 24*f*
Tractography, 14, 20, 41, 41*f*. *See also* Diffusion tensor imaging (DTI)
Transsphenoidal approach, intraoperative MRI (iMRI) and, 15–16, 119–129
   advances in (future directions for), 127–128
   clinical experience, 125–128
   equipment for, 119–120, 121*f*
   historical perspective on, 119
   indications for, 119
   OR set-up for, 119–120, 121*f*
   patient positioning for, 120, 121*f*
   pulse sequences for, 36
   results, 122–125, 122*t*–123*t*, 124*f*–128*f*
   surgical procedure for, 120
   technique for, 120–122
T_1 recovery, 29
TSE. *See* Turbo-SE
Tumor(s). *See also* Brain tumor(s); Spinal tumor(s); *specific tumor*
   grading, 43
   margins, detection, molecular imaging and, 207
   MRI-guided resection
     with high-field strength, pulse sequences for, 37, 37*f*, 37*t*
     pulse sequences for, 35–39
Turbo FLAIR, 15
Turbo-SE, 30
   single-shot, 31
   T2-weighted, 35, 36*t*
Turbo-spectroscopic imaging (TSI), 42–43
T1-weighted images, 30, 35
T2-weighted images, 30, 35

U
Ultrasound. *See also* MRI-guided focused ultrasound guidance, for shunt catheter placement, 80–81
   intraoperative
     in brain biopsy, 70–71, 70*f*
     in glioma resection, 109–110
University of Cincinnati, low-field iMRI facility, 9–10, 10*f*
University of Minnesota
   high-field MRI, 18–20, 19*f*–20*f*, 26
   prospective stereotaxy system, 21–23, 24*f*

V
Vascular malformations
   surgery for, iMRI in, 171–173, 171*t*, 174–176, 175*f*
   susceptibility-weighted imaging in, 39
Venous angioma(s), susceptibility-weighted imaging, 39
Ventriculoperitoneal shunt failure, catheter placement for, MRI-guided, 81–83, 82*f*, 85–86
Verio scanner, 25
Voxel(s), 30

W
White matter tract(s), diffusion tensor imaging, 42, 139. *See also* Diffusion tensor imaging (DTI)

X
xy-plane, 29

Z
z-axis, 29
Zone(s), magnetic resonance risk-related, 59